NUTRITION AND METABOLISM OF THE FETUS AND INFANT

Fifth Nutricia Symposium

NUTRITION AND METABOLISM
OF THE
FETUS AND INFANT

Rotterdam 11–13 October 1978

EDITOR:

H.K.A. VISSER M.D.

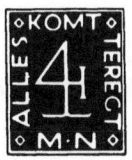

1979

SPRINGER-SCIENCE+BUSINESS MEDIA, B.V.

Library of Congress Cataloging in Publication Data CIP

Nutricia Symposium, 5th, Rotterdam, 1979.
  Nutrition and metabolism of the fetus and infant.

  Includes index.
    1. Fetus – Nutrition – Congresses. 2. Fetus – Growth – Congresses.
  3. Infants (Newborn) – Nutrition – Congresses. 4. Infants (Premature) –
  Nutrition – Congresses. 5. Milk, Human – Congresses. 6. Parenteral feeding
  of children – Congresses. I. Visser, H.K.A. II. Title.
  RG600.N87 1978   612.6'47   79-14263
  ISBN 978-94-009-9320-4   ISBN 978-94-009-9318-1 (eBook)
  DOI 10.1007/978-94-009-9318-1

CONTENTS

SESSION III
NUTRITION OF THE PRETERM INFANT

Chairman: A. Ballabriga

SESSION IV
HUMAN MILK

Chairman: R. Eeckels

* The paper was presented by Dr. Davies.

SESSION V
PARENTERAL NUTRITION OF THE NEWBORN AND INFANT

Chairman: J. H. P. Jonxis

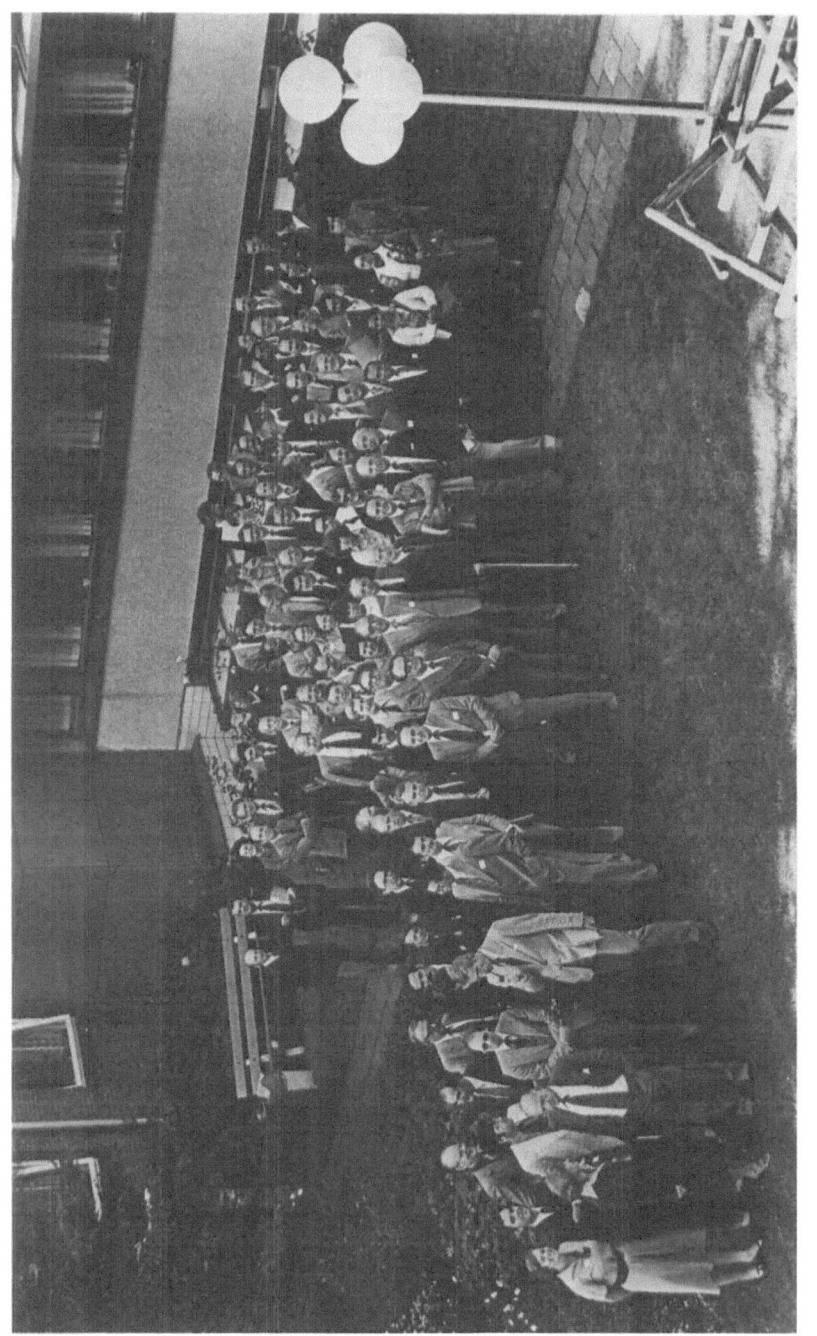

LIST OF PARTICIPANTS

K. VAN ACKER, University of Antwerpen, Department of Pediatrics, Universiteitsplein 1, B-2610 Wilrijk, Belgium.

K. ADRIAENSSENS, University of Antwerpen, Department of Medicine, Universiteitsplein 1, B-2610 Wilrijk, Belgium.

B. I. AGOSTON, Diaconessenhuis Eindhoven, Ds. Th. Fliednerstraat 1, 5600 PD Eindhoven, The Netherlands.

Mrs. A. ALISJAHBANA, Department of Perinatology, R. S. Hasan Sadikin, Jln. Sulanja no. 5A, Bandung, Indonesia.

A. BALLABRIGA, Clinica Infantil de la Seguridad Social, Paseo Valle Hebron S/M, Barcelona, Spain.

Mrs. J. BANDE-KNOPS, Kon. Albertlaan 105, B-3200 Kessel LO, Belgium.

F. C. BATTAGLIA, University of Colorado Medical Center, Department of Pediatrics, 4200 East Ninth Avenue, Denver, Colorado 80262, U.S.A.
Temporary address F. C. Battaglia: Laboratoire de Physiologie du Développement, Place Marcelin-Berthelot, 75231 Paris, Cedex 05, France.

J. D. BAUM, Neonatal Unit, Department of Paediatrics, John Radcliffe Hospital, Headington, Oxford OX3 9DU, Great Britain.

J. BENNEBROEK GRAVENHORST, Department of Obstetrics and Gynaecology, Academic Hospital Leiden, Rijnsburgerweg 10, 2333 AA Leiden, The Netherlands.

H. M. BERGER, Department of Neonatology, Free University of Amsterdam, De Boelelaan 1117, 1081 HV Amsterdam, The Netherlands.

E. R. BOERSMA, Department of Pediatrics, Academic Hospital Rotterdam/Sophia Children's Hospital and Neonatal Unit, Gordelweg 160, 3038 GE Rotterdam, The Netherlands.

J. M. BOON, Department of Pediatrics, St. Radboudziekenhuis, Geert Grooteplein Zuid 20, 6525 GA Nijmegen, The Netherlands.

J. L. VAN DEN BRANDE, Department of Pediatrics, Wilhelmina Children's Hospital, Nieuwe Gracht 137, 3512 LK Utrecht, The Netherlands.

C. A. CANOSA, Hospital Infantil "La Fe", Ciudad Sanitaria de la Seguridad Social, Valencia (9), Spain.

B. CARLSSON, Institute of Medical Microbiology, University of Göteborg, Department of Immunology, Guldhedsgatan 10, 413 46 Göteborg, Sweden.

D. CARTON, University Hospital, Department of Pediatrics, De Pintelaan 115, Gent, Belgium.

E. CASADO DE FRIAS, Universidad Complutense, Facultad de Medicina,

Departamento de Pediatria y Puericultura, Madrid-3, Spain.

CHR. CASSIMOS, University of Thessaloniki, Pediatric Clinic, St. Sophies Hospital, Thessaloniki, Greece.

R. CLARA, Verdussenstraat 8, B-2000 Antwerpen, Belgium.

Mrs. P. A. DAVIES, Hammersmith Hospital, Du Cane Road, London W12 OHS, Great Britain.

Mrs. J. T. DODOIN, University Hospital St. Pierre, Rue Haute 322, 1000 Bruxelles, Belgium.

L. J. DOOREN, Department of Pediatrics, Academic Hospital Leiden, Rijnsburgerweg 10, 2333 AA Leiden, The Netherlands.

R. EECKELS, Academic Hospital Gasthuisberg, Department of Pediatrics, Herestraat 49, 3000 Leuven, Belgium.

E. EGGERMONT, Academic Hospital Gasthuisberg, Department of Pediatrics, Herestraat 49, 3000 Leuven, Belgium.

T. K. A. B. ESKES, Department of Obstetrics and Gynaecology, St. Radboudziekenhuis, Geert Grooteplein Zuid 16, 6525 GA Nijmegen, The Netherlands.

Mrs. N. P. FERNANDO, P.O. Box 465, Safat, Kuwait.

W. P. F. FETTER, Department of Pediatrics, Academic Hospital Rotterdam/ Sophia Children's Hospital and Neonatal Unit, Gordelweg 160, 3038 GE Rotterdam, The Netherlands.

B. FRIIS HANSEN, University of Copenhagen, Department of Pediatrics, Rigshospitalet, Tagensvej 18, 2200 Copenhagen, Denmark.

M. GABR, 163 Tahreer Street, Cairo, Egypt.

G. E. GAULL, Institute for Basic Research in Mental Retardation, 1050 Forest Hill Road, Staten Island, New York, U.S.A.

H. H. VAN GELDEREN, Department of Pediatrics, Academic Hospital Leiden, Rijnsburgerweg 10, 2333 AA Leiden, The Netherlands.

F. GEUBELLE, Université de Liège, Hôpital de Bavière, 4020 Liège, Belgium.

H. L. GREENE, Department of Pediatrics, School of Medicine, Vanderbilt University, Nashville, Tennessee 37232, U.S.A.

L. HAMBRAEUS, Institute of Nutrition, University of Uppsala, Box 551, S-751 22 Uppsala, Sweden.

Mrs. N. HAVERKAMP BEGEMANN, Haarweg 13A, 3959 AM Overberg, The Netherlands.

W. C. HEIRD, Department of Pediatrics, Columbia University, College of Physicians and Surgeons, New York, N.Y., U.S.A.

H. J. HUISJES, Department of Obstetrics, Academic Hospital Groningen, Oostersingel 59, 9713 EZ Groningen, The Netherlands.

D. HULL, University of Nottingham, Medical School, Department of Child Health, Clifton Boulevard, Nottingham NG7 2UH, Great Britain.

F. H. M. JANSEN, Department of Pediatrics, Juliana Children's Hospital, Dr. Van Welylaan 2, 2566 ER The Hague, The Netherlands.

C. T. JONES, University of Oxford, The Nuffield Institute for Medical Research, Headley Way, Headington, Oxford OX3 9DS, Great Britain.

J. H. P. JONXIS, Rijksstraatweg 65, 9752 AC Haren (Gron.), The Netherlands.

G. J. KLOOSTERMAN, Department of Obstetrics, Wilhelmina Gasthuis, 1e Helmersstraat 104, 1054 EG Amsterdam, The Netherlands.

Mrs. J. G. KOPPE, Department of Physiology and Pathology of the Newborn, Wilhelmina Gasthuis, 1e Helmersstraat 104, 1054 EG Amsterdam, The Netherlands.

F. KUIPERS, Emma Children's Hospital, Spinozastraat 51, 1018 HJ Amsterdam, The Netherlands.

H. N. LAFEBER, Department of Pediatrics, Academic Hospital Rotterdam/ Sophia Children's Hospital and Neonatal Unit, Gordelweg 160, 3038 GE Rotterdam, The Netherlands.

B. LAHLOU, 11, rue Allal Ben Abdallah, (ex Rue de l'Horloge), Casablanca, Morocco.

R. DE LEEUW, Department of Physiology and Pathology of the Newborn, Wilhelmina Gasthuis, 1e Helmersstraat 104, 1054 EG Amsterdam, The Netherlands.

B. S. LINDBLAD, Department of Pediatrics, St. Göran's Children's Hospital, Box 12500, S-112 81 Stockholm, Sweden.

H. LOEB, University Hospital St. Pierre, Department of Pediatrics, Rue Haute 322, 1000 Bruxelles, Belgium.

A. H. MARKUM, Jln. Kijai Maja 53 Kebayoran, Jakarta, Indonesia.

N. MATSANIOTIS, University of Athens, St. Sophie's Children's Hospital, Athens 608, Greece.

Z. MAZIEDIE, Ministry of Health, Arabian Gulf Street, Kuwait.

R. A. MCCANCE, 4 Kent House, Sussex Str., Cambridge CB 1 1PH, Great Britain.

J. W. METTAU, Department of Pediatrics, Academic Hospital Rotterdam/ Sophia Children's Hospital and Neonatal Unit, Gordelweg 160, 3038 GE Rotterdam, The Netherlands.

R. DE MEYER, Cliniques Universitaires Saint-Luc, Département de Pédiatrie, Avenue Hippocrate 10, 1200 Bruxelles, Belgium.

R. D. G. MILNER, Department of Child Health, Children's Hospital, Sheffield S10 2TH, Great Britain.

J. C. MOLENAAR, Department of Pediatric Surgery, Academic Hospital Rotterdam/Sophia Children's Hospital and Neonatal Unit, Gordelweg 160, 3038 GE Rotterdam, The Netherlands.

D. NICOLOPOULOS, Alexandra Maternity Hospital, Neonatal Department, Vas. Sophia's Ave., Athens 611, Greece.

A. OKKEN, Department of Pediatrics, Academic Hospital Groningen, Oostersingel 59, 9713 EZ Groningen, The Netherlands.

M. ORZALESI, M.O. Istituto di Puericultura dell' Università, Viale Mancini 3, Sassari, Italy.

Mrs. A. PARDOU, Hôpital Universitaire Brugman, Clinique Obstétricale et Gynécologique, 4, Place Arth. Van Gehuchten, 1020 Bruxelles, Belgium.

R. G. PEARSE, Department of Pediatrics, Academic Hospital Rotterdam/ Sophia Children's Hospital and Neonatal Unit, Gordelweg 160, 3038 GE Rotterdam, The Netherlands.

R. M. PITKIN, Department of Obstetrics and Gynaecology, University of Iowa, Hospitals and Clinics, Iowa City, Iowa 52242, U.S.A.

F. POHLANDT, Universitäts-Kinderklinik, Sektion Neonatologie, Prittwitzstrasse 43, D-7900 Ulm, Germany.

J. QUERO JIMEENEZ, Department of Neonatology, Social Security Hospital "La Paz", Madrid, Spain.

L. H. J. RAMAEKERS, Department of Pediatrics, St. Annadal Hospital, St. Annadal 1, 6214 PA Maastricht, The Netherlands.

M. P. M. RICHARDS, Medical Psychology Unit, Old Cavendish Building, Free School Lane, Cambridge OB 2 3RF, Great Britain.

J. RIGO, Université de Liège, Hôpital de Bavière, Clinique et Policlinique des Maladies de l'Enfance, 4020 Liège, Belgium.

J. H. RUYS, Department of Obstetrics, Academic Hospital Leiden, Rijnsburgerweg 10, 2333 AA Leiden, The Netherlands.

Mrs. L. SACRÉ, Charles Plisnierlaan 23, B-1070 Bruxelles, Belgium.

P. J. J. SAUER, Department of Pediatrics, Academic Hospital Rotterdam/Sophia Children's Hospital and Neonatal Unit, Gordelweg 160, 3038 GE Rotterdam, The Netherlands.

E. D. A. M. SCHRETLEN, Department of Pediatrics, St. Radboudziekenhuis, Geert Grooteplein Zuid 20, 6525 GA Nijmegen, The Netherlands.

R. CH. SENDERS, Wilhemina Children's Hospital, Nieuwe Gracht 137, 3512 LK Utrecht, The Netherlands.

J. SENTERRE, Université de Liège, Hôpital de Bavière, Clinique et Policlinique des Maladies de l'Enfance, 4020 Liège, Belgium.

J. C. L. SHAW, University College Hospital, Medical School, Department of Pediatrics, Huntley Street, London WC1E 6DH, Great Britain.

J. C. SINCLAIR, Department of Pediatrics, McMaster University, Medical School, Hamilton (Ont.) Canada.
    Temporary address J. C. Sinclair: c/o Professor Alex Minkowski, Centre de Recherches Biologiques Néonatales, Université René Descartes, Hôpital Port-Royal, 123, Boulevard Port-Royal, 76574 Paris, Cedex 14, France.

Mrs. S. SKLAVUNU-ZURUKZOGLU, University of Thessaloniki, B Pediatric Clinic, Thessaloniki, Greece.

R. SPRITZER, Department of Pediatrics, Academic Hospital Rotterdam/Sophia Children's Hospital and Neonatal Unit, Gordelweg 160, 3038 GE Rotterdam, The Netherlands.

G. B. A. STOELINGA, Department of Pediatrics, St. Radboudziekenhuis, Geert Grooteplein Zuid 20, 6525 GA Nijmegen, The Netherlands.

J. G. STOLK, Department of Obstetrics and Gynaecology, Free University of Amsterdam, De Boelelaan 1117, 1081 HV Amsterdam, The Netherlands.

SUHARJONO, Department of Child Health, Medical School, University of Indonesia, Jakarta, Indonesia.

R. URRUTIA, P.O. Box 4694, Panama City, Panama.

R. VANHEULE, University of Antwerpen, Universiteitsplein 1, B-2610 Wilrijk, Belgium.

W. VEEGER, Department of Gastroenterology, Academic Hospital Groningen, Oostersingel 59, 9713 EZ Groningen, The Netherlands.

C. VERSLUYS, Department of Neonatology, Free University of Amsterdam, De Boelelaan 1117, 1081 HV Amsterdam, The Netherlands.

J. J. VAN DER VLUGT, Department of Pediatrics, St. Jozefziekenhuis, Van Oldenielstraat 12, 7415 EH Deventer, The Netherlands.

H. C. S. WALLENBURG, Department of Obstetrics, Academic Hospital Rotterdam/Dijkzigt, Dr. Molewaterplein 40, 3015 GD Rotterdam, The Netherlands.

Mrs. E. M. WIDDOWSON, Department of Medicine, Level 5, Addenbrooke's Hospital, Hills Road, Cambridge CB2 2QQ, Great Britain.

A. G. L. WHITELAW, Northwick Park Hospital and Clinical Research Centre, Watford Road, Harrow, Middlesex HA1 3UJ, Great Britain.
Temporary address A. G. L. Whitelaw: Neonatal Unit, The Hospital for Sick Children, 555 University Avenue, Toronto, Ontario, Canada.

Mrs. M. YOUNG, Department of Gynaecology, St. Thomas's Hospital Medical School, London, SE1 7EH, Great Britain.

R. ZETTERSTRÖM, Karolinska Institutet, Department of Pediatrics, St. Göran's Children's Hospital, Box 12500, S-112 81 Stockholm, Sweden.

Participants Nutricia Company

Mrs. I. BECK
Mrs. Y. EXLER-DASBACH
J. M. KOOIJMAN
M. OOSTING
A. W. G. VAN RIEMSDIJK
O. D. SUURENBROEK
C. J. W. WEBER

OPENING

H. K. A. VISSER

It is a great pleasure indeed to welcome all of you at this 5th International Nutricia Symposium, especially our guests from abroad.

Many of you have attended one or more of the earlier symposia. The first one was held in February 1964 at Groningen. The topic was "the adaptation of the newborn infant to extra-uterine life". The second one was in May 1969 at Groningen on "aspects of prematurity and dysmaturity". The third symposium was held in Rotterdam, October 1970 on "metabolic processes in the fetus and newborn infant". The fourth symposium was again organized in Groningen, May 1973. The title was "therapeutic aspects of nutrition".

I have gone through the lists of participants at the earlier symposia. Apart from Professor Jonxis and myself, two of you have attended all symposia: Dr. Widdowson and Dr. Nicolopoulos. A most cordial word of welcome to both of you. We appreciate it that you found it worthwhile to come again. Dr. Widdowson has presented a paper at all symposia and as you have seen in the programme, she will do so this time.

I would like to present special greetings to our guest of honour Professor McCance, who has attended three of the four earlier symposia.

Nutricia Company has been a manufacturer of baby food and dietary products for more than 75 years. The idea to provide funds to organize these symposia originated in the early sixties. Professor Jonxis has been mainly responsible for the organization of the earlier symposia; he is now emeritus-professor, but still very active. We are honoured that he is here and will present a paper.

The papers and discussions of the symposia have been published in books, and it has been rewarding to Nutricia, the editors and the publishers that these books have been received well by the scientific and medical world, and have been quoted many times in the international literature. Part of the success has been due I suppose to the fact that they were published within six months after the time the symposia were held.

We are very grateful to Nutricia Company that it will be possible to continue the organization of these symposia and I hope it will become a tradition in the future.

The topic of this symposium is "nutrition and metabolism of the fetus and infant". There has been great progress in this field of science during the last ten years. This symposium is more or less a continuation of the 3rd symposium we organized here in Rotterdam in 1970. It will be interesting to see how concepts have changed. Five speakers at this symposium also presented papers at the 3rd symposium. This meeting is in some way a reunion of old friends, but at the same time many young clinicians and investigators are now present and it is a great privilege to welcome them. All of us from different disciplines are deeply interested in the problems of nutrition, growth and metabolism of the fetus and infant.

I sincerely hope that this meeting will be as successful as the other symposia.

NUTRITION AND METABOLISM OF THE FETUS

THE ROLE OF INSULIN AND GLUCAGON IN FETAL GROWTH AND METABOLISM

R. D. G. MILNER*

A comprehensive review of hormonal control of fetal development must pay attention to the ontogeny of the endocrine cell, the response of the endocrine cell to stimuli of secretion, hormonal transport in the circulation, the development of hormonal receptors on the effector cell and finally the development of the enzymatic and metabolic response in the effector cell to hormonal receptor activation. Putting to one side the question of whether hormones control or merely modulate fetal growth, the complexity of the subject is so great that any attempt to be comprehensive within the confines of a chapter must necessarily mislead by superficiality. This chapter is therefore an attempt to deal with part of the question in depth in the hope that by dwelling on the pancreatic hormones: insulin and glucagon, some insight will be gained into the general principles that govern hormonal action in the fetus. The development of structure and function in the endocrine pancreas is not considered here because this has been the subject of recent reviews (1, 2, 3). Insulin and glucagon are assumed to be secreted prenatally in the same molecular form as after birth and not to be bound by any "carrier" molecule. The placenta is impermeable to both hormones (4, 5) and insulin or glucagon in the fetal circulation is deemed to be fetal in origin.

Clinical and biological interest in insulin as a fetal growth promoting hormone stems historically from the infant of the diabetic mother (IDM) and subsequently from the realization that insulin, in addition to a glucoregulatory action, has an anabolic role in stimulating amino acid uptake and protein synthesis by cells. But a baby may be heavy in different ways and the action of insulin can only be understood by comparing overall effects on the fetus with the sum of its actions on various organs. It may be that glucagon has little or no direct effect on

* Department of Paediatrics, University of Sheffield, Children's Hospital, Sheffield
S10 2TH, England.

H.K.A. Visser (ed.), Nutrition and Metabolism of the Fetus and Infant, 3–18. All rights reserved.
Copyright © 1979 Martinus Nijhoff Publishers b.v., The Hague/Boston/London.

fetal growth, but glucagon and insulin, besides originating in adjacent cells of the islet of Langerhans, have many opposite endocrine effects and it is difficult to review the action of insulin in fetal life without considering glucagon.

Growth consumes energy and is presumed to proceed optimally in the presence of normal substrate delivery to the fetus. Insulin and glucagon play an important part in the control of storage and mobilization of energy reserves and may thereby have an important if secondary role in regulating fetal growth.

THE WHOLE FETUS

Several groups of workers have injected insulin or glucagon into the fetus in an attempt to study either an acute metabolic effect or a longer action on fetal growth and development. Others have measured fetal plasma concentrations of endogenous hormones and have manipulated these by experimental changes in the mother. Both approaches are interesting since from them a picture, albeit fragmentary, can be got of the action of a hormone on the fetus.

In the last four days of intrauterine life of the rat both plasma insulin and glucagon concentrations were found to rise several fold, but with the preservation of an insulin/glucagon molar ratio of more than 10 (6). Immediately after birth there was a precipitous fall in plasma insulin and a steep rise in plasma glucagon with a consequent drop in the insulin/glucagon ratio to 1 which was maintained during fasting for 16 h (7). If a maternal fast of 96 h was imposed immediately before term, the effect on the fetus was to lower blood glucose and gluconeogenic substrate and to raise blood ketone bodies (8). Plasma insulin fell and glucagon rose, anticipating the changes that occur normally in the immediate postnatal period. There was an increase in activity of key gluconeogenic enzymes in fetal liver of starved pregnancies (*vide infra*) suggesting that maternal starvation might induce precocious fetal gluconeogenesis at the price of impaired fetal growth.

A variety of effects have been described from injecting insulin or anti-insulin serum into rat fetuses. Early reports (9, 10) stated that exogenous insulin injection into the 20 day rat fetus had no effect on the incorporation of ^{14}C from glucose into lipid, glycogen or protein or ^{3}H into fatty acids. Contrary results were obtained subsequently which showed that insulin injection into rat fetuses at term increased the incorporation of

[14]C-glucose into glycogen and that anti-insulin serum produced the opposite effect (11, 12, 13). It is possible that confusion could have arisen because of the high endogenous plasma insulin concentration at the time of exogenous insulin injection. If endogenous insulin were causing a maximum biological action it might not be possible to show a further effect by the injection of exogenous insulin. The action of anti-insulin serum suggests that this might have been the case.

An interesting and technically difficult experiment was performed by PICON (14) who injected rat fetuses with insulin daily for three days. In fetuses collected at 21.5 or 22.5 days, 24 h after the third insulin injection there was a significant increase in fresh weight, dry weight, total body nitrogen, lipid and lipid/nitrogen ratio. These findings suggest that chronic hyperinsulinaemia in the rat fetus at term can result in both an increase in lean body mass and adiposity.

What experiments of nature may be taken as clinical examples of the effects of insulin and glucagon on fetal growth? Much of the interest in the topic stems from the hyperinsulinaemic overweight infant of a diabetic mother (IDM). In the extensive literature on that subject there has been little evidence of scientific rigour in analysing what types of cellular development comprise body weight. The characteristic IDM is overweight mainly due to excess lipid (15) and there is a modest and arguable increase in cell size and number of the lean body mass (16). Subcutaneous fat in normal infants and IDM develops in the last 10–12 weeks of intrauterine life, yet it is inferred that the pancreatic islet hyperplasia, β cell hypertrophy and hyperinsulinaemia antecedes this period of development. If structural and functional β cell pathology does exist in the IDM during the second trimester we may postulate that abnormal adipose development occurs because (? pre-) adipocytes develop insulin receptors at 28-30 weeks gestation. It must not be forgotten however that there is little direct information on pancreatic morphology of IDM or circulating plasma insulin levels before 28 weeks gestation. If, as has been suggested (3), glucose becomes a secretogogue for the human β cell at about 28 weeks gestation, and fetal hyperglycaemia is the key to the pathology of IDM, then hyperinsulinaemia during the last 12 weeks of intrauterine life alone might account for pathological fat accumulation.

The converse has been argued for the infant with transient neonatal diabetes who is hypoinsulinaemic and certainly lacks subcutaneous fat as judged clinically (17). But no clinical or scientific measurement has been made of the lean body mass of these babies. Two siblings with pancreatic agenesis have been reported (18) and in one there was clear, if anecdotal, evidence of a reduction in hepatic cellularity and muscle protein/DNA ratio.

Attempts to mimic diabetic pregnancy or to "insulinectomise" the fetus have had very mixed results (19) largely because of the complexity of the experimental model. It has been difficult to produce a consistently overweight fetus associated with drug-induced maternal diabetes and the techniques employed to deprive the fetus of β cell function have been too imprecise to allow an answer to the question of what action insulin plays in determining fetal growth.

If a chronically catheterized sheep fetus is infused with insulin to produce a rise in plasma concentration within the physiological range there is a fall in blood glucose and increase in glucose utilization (20, 21). Many of the conflicting results in the early sheep experiments arose from a failure to appreciate the need to work with a chronic unstressed preparation. The failure to demonstrate a fall in fetal blood glucose following insulin infusion into the rhesus monkey fetus at 0.9 gestation (22) is open to the same criticism. Alternatively the kinetics of glucose transport across the monkey placenta may be such that it was difficult to influence fetal blood glucose in this way. Plasma free fatty acid levels fell consistently following injection of insulin into the fetus.

The physiological role of glucagon in the human fetus is an enigma. Immunoreactive glucagon is present in human fetal pancreas from week 7 (23) and the a_2 cells are the first in the islet to granulate (24). Fragments of human fetal pancreas of 8 to 20 weeks gestational age incubated or perifused *in vitro* released glucagon consistently in response to arginine or epinephrine, but glucose and acetylcholine were without effect (23, 25). In both normal and streptozotocin diabetic pregnancy, the rhesus monkey fetus at 0.9 term responded to L-dopa infusion with a rise in plasma glucagon concentration, but alanine infusion or insulin-induced hypoglycaemia had no effect (26). When women were given intravenous alanine in labour at term there was a doubling of the mean plasma glucagon in the maternal plasma and umbilical cord blood at delivery 10 to 50 min later (27). The ability of circulating amino acids to influence plasma glucagon concentration in the primate fetus merits further study.

Glucagon infused into newborn infants on the third day of life produced a hypoaminoacidaemia similar to that seen in the adult (28). The gluconeogenic amino acids alanine, glycine, proline and glutamine plus arginine accounted for 60% of the change. On the first day of life an attenuated response to glucagon was seen in normal and small-for-dates infants but IDM were totally insensitive. These results are in keeping with the idea that glucagon is gluconeogenic in the neonate and that glucagon and insulin have opposite actions on gluconeogenesis.

The large changes in plasma glucagon seen in the rat at the time of birth are observed in other species also. Since the autonomic nervous system may be involved the experimental findings are reviewed in some detail. The concentration of glucagon in the cord blood of the newborn infant was low and similar to that in peripheral maternal venous blood (29). At the age of 2 h there was a rise in plasma glucagon concentration which is greater in small-for-dates infants and less in IDM than in normal infants (30). Arginine infusion at the age of 6 h caused a large rise in plasma glucagon (31) but oral alanine evoked a more variable response, causing a rise in the first 24 h but no rise between 25 and 96 h of age (32). Equivocal responses were also obtained from infants aged 12–48 h given nasogastric glucose and casein (33). A clue to the role of glucagon in the human perinatal period comes from a detailed case study of an infant with isolated glucagon deficiency (34). The patient had a birth weight of 3.81 kg at 42 weeks gestation and presented with persistent hypo-glycaemia. Investigations revealed normal insulin secretion, no plasma glucagon response to hypoglycaemia or alanine infusion and severe impairment of gluconeogenesis. The condition appeared to be familial and an autosomal recessive inheritance was suggested. There was no-thing to suggest a role for glucagon in promoting fetal growth.

The futility of seeking a simple metabolic-hormonal interaction for glucagon is best appreciated if the human studies are reviewed in the light of animal experiments. Studies on sheep have suggested that the immediate neonatal surge in plasma glucagon may be causally related to severance of the umbilical cord (35). Lambs were delivered into room air and the umbilical cord left intact and covered with warm saline so that the blood supply to the fetus was undisturbed. The fetal face was covered with a warm saline filled glove. No change in plasma glucagon occurred until the cord was cut 60 min later when a five fold rise occurred in 15 min. This was followed 30 min later by a large rise in plasma FFA. The authors suggested that both events were due to a surge in catechol-amine release triggered by cutting the umbilical cord. In a later study lambs aged 1–3 days were infused with somatostatin which suppressed endogenous insulin and glucagon release (36) and led to a fall in plasma glucose. From the results of infusion with exogenous insulin or glucagon the authors concluded that glucagon is a major hormone for maintaining blood glucose during short term neonatal fasting. A similar conclusion was reached from studies in the rat which indicated that insulin and glucagon affect glucose homeostasis differently, a fall in plasma insulin being the prime factor in triggering glycogen mobilization but a rise in glucagon the prime event initiating gluconeogenesis (37). But there is evidence showing that glucagon is not the only, and possibly not the primary, activator of neonatal gluconeogenesis. Gluconeogenesis in the newborn lamb has been demonstrated within 2 and 4 min of birth at term and to be delayed in two prematurely delivered lambs (139 and 144 days) until breathing was established and the blood fully oxygenated (38). Glucagon infusion at 131 or 144 days into two fetuses caused a rise in blood glucose but no gluconeogenesis. The authors proposed that oxygen availability initiates gluconeogenesis in the newborn lamb. Oxygen or glucagon, or both? The question will not be resolved until simultaneous measurements of the relevant variables are made in one set of experiments. The interaction of blood gases, the autonomic nervous system and the endocrine pancreas is further illustrated by experiments using calves aged 3–6 weeks. Both severe hypoxia or hypercapnia produced large rises in plasma glucagon which were followed by hyperglycaemia and hyperinsulinaemia (39).

LIVER

Rat fetuses injected with insulin at term became hypoglycaemic (40) and formed more hepatic glycogen (11). Conversely fetuses injected with insulin antibody or glucagon became hyperglycaemic and had decreased hepatic glycogen (11, 12, 41). These observations should not tempt the unwary to extrapolate. Although hepatocyte membrane glucagon receptors were demonstrated in 20 day rat fetuses the concentration was less than in neonatal or adult tissues (42, 43). The result was due, not to increased glucagon degradation by fetal tissue or a lack of adenyl cyclase in hepatocyte membranes, but to a paucity of glucagon receptor sites. Binding of ^{125}I glucagon by 15 day fetal hepatic membranes was 1% of the adult level and 23% of that on day 21 (42). In contrast insulin binding on day 15 was 11% of the adult level and 45% of that on day 21. The fetal rat hepatocyte is potentially more sensitive to the action of insulin than glucagon. Both hormones become equipotent, that is achieve their adult membrane binding characteristics by 30 days postnatally.

In a comparative study of the ontogeny of hormone specific binding characteristics, insulin binding by fetal rat liver membranes was 50% that of the adult whereas human growth hormone or ovine prolactin was not bound in appreciable amounts until 40 days postnatally (44). These results are difficult to interpret as growth hormone and prolactin both show greater structural and immunoreactive heterogeneity between species than does insulin. Similar observations were made in the rabbit and, if of physiological significance, suggest that the fetal liver develops receptors to polypeptide hormones at widely differing stages of development.

A comparison of the biochemical ontogeny of the rat and human hepatocyte reveals several similarities especially when enzymic activity is expressed per unit wet liver weight and as a fraction of that found in the adult (45). Of particular interest is the observation that some enzymes which normally appear postnatally in the rat can be evoked by the administration of glucagon to the fetus. For example exogenous glucagon stimulates the activity of tyrosine amino transferase (46, 47), glucose-6-phosphatase (46), phosphoenolpyruvate carboxykinase (PEPCK) (48) and phosphorylase (49). The arginine synthetase system, the rate limiting step in urea biosynthesis increases in the rat from a low level at birth to peak activity on the second postnatal day. Glucagon had no accelerating effect on this system when injected into 19.5–21.5 day fetuses (50), but when added to organ cultures of 18.5 day fetal liver caused a doubling of arginine synthetase activity after 24 h. Insulin had no effect on the liver organ culture system. It is probable that glucagon plays a part in the normal enzymic ontogeny of glycogenolysis and gluconeogenesis and is possible that precocious induction of these pathways may result if hyperglucagonaemia is the consequence of metabolic or drug induced alteration of the fetal environment. GREENGARD (45) suggests that in both rat and man, thyroid hormone, glucocorticoids and glucagon may play a part in controlling patterns of hepatic enzyme development. In this context hormonal interaction must not be forgotten. GIRARD and his co-workers (51) confirmed the induction of glucose-6-phosphatase and PEPCK by exogenous glucagon in 18.5–21.5 day-old rat fetuses. Phosphorylase and glycogen breakdown were not increased by glucagon before day 20.5, but if the fetuses were treated with hydrocortisone on day 18.5, phosphorylase activation by glucagon could be induced prematurely on day 19.5. Insulin administered at birth prevented the normal development of glucose-6-phosphatase or PEPCK but was without effect on hepatic phosphorylase activity and glycogen breakdown.

VILLEE (52) was the first to demonstrate gluconeogenesis by human fetal liver *in vitro* but ethical and technical problems inhibited the further development of this technique until SCHWARTZ and his colleagues performed a series of experiments in which human fetal liver explants were grown in organ culture. The tissue was obtained from fetuses of 5–25 weeks gestational age delivered by hysterotomy for therapeutic abortion. The incorporation of alanine into glucose and glycogen was stimulated by glucagon plus theophylline (53). Unfortunately the two agents were not tested independently and it is not possible to deduce if the effect was mediated by glucagon or theophylline. Insulin abolished the stimulation of gluconeogenesis by glucagon plus theophylline.

Insulin increased tissue glycogen accumulation from fetuses of seven or more weeks gestation and glucagon depleted hepatic glycogen stores from 6 week fetuses (54). When both hormones were present in pharmacological and presumably maximum concentrations, the glucagon effect overrode the insulin effect. Further work (55) led to the conclusion that the two hormones exerted their effect via the D-form of glycogen synthetase and did not influence phosphorylase activity.

When the human fetal liver organ culture was used to study amino acid uptake (56), a-amino isobutyrate accumulation was stimulated by glucagon, dibutyryl cyclic AMP or insulin. The effects of glucagon or dibutyryl cyclic AMP were not additive but the effect of insulin was additive to either, suggesting that insulin worked by a different mechanism to glucagon and that the glucagon effect was transmitted via cyclic AMP. Glucagon sensitivity was demonstrable at 6 weeks gestation (30 mm crown-rump fetus) but insulin responsiveness was not demonstrated below 48 mm crown-rump length. The physiological significance of the same metabolic effect by insulin and glucagon awaits further study.

Isolated, perfused fetal and neonatal canine liver has been employed as a model to investigate the control of glucose production. Fetuses were examined at term and littermates 3 h after delivery were compared with puppies aged 1–5 days. Net glucose production was negligible in the fetus but rose to more than 1 μmol/min · g during the first postnatal day. Gluconeogenesis from lactate rose from negligible rates at birth to account for 21% of glucose production on day 3 (57). Fetal liver did not response to norepinephrine, but postnatal liver did so by increasing glycogenolysis after the capacity for gluconeogenesis had developed. The authors speculated that the two events may be causally related. In a complementary study, pups aged 1–5 days were shown to produce glucose at 55 ± 3 μmol/min · kg body weight (58). If glucagon was infused the rate increased to 81 ± 4 μmol/min · kg. By the use of radio-active gluconeogenic substrates the authors demonstrated that 25% or more of glucose production came from glucose recycled through lactate and pyruvate. The same group (59) using ^{13}C glucose in term normal infants and IDM demonstrated that the mean glucose production rate at 3 h of age in the IDM was 2.5 mg/kg · min compared with 4.2 mg/kg · min in the normal infants. They argued convincingly that the hypoglycaemia characteristic of IDM may be due not so much to accelerated glucose uptake by the lean body mass as inhibition of hepatic glycogenolysis in response to neonatal hyperinsulinism.

HEART

GUIDOTTI and his co-workers (60, 61) pioneered studies of the ontogeny of metabolic responses to insulin using embryonic chick heart as a model. They showed that insulin stimulated glucose uptake at a later stage of development than the incorporation of acetate into lipid, but before the uptake of amino acids and their incorporation into protein. These changes take place early, between the fifth and tenth day *in ovo*.

This methodological approach has been extended more recently using the fetal rat heart. The basal rate of glucose uptake by isolated fetal cardiac muscle fell from day 16 to 22 and remained constant after birth (62). The rate of glucose incorporation into glycogen rose to a maximum on day 18 and cardiac glycogen was at its highest concentration on day 21. Carbon dioxide production from glucose was less than 2% and did not change with age. The addition of a pharmacological concentration of insulin to the incubation increased glucose uptake by a similar fraction (approximately 70%) in 16, 18, 21 day fetuses and 1 day newborn rats. By comparing the digestion of cardiac glycogen with cold or hot potassium hydroxide, the glucose uptake stimulated by insulin was shown to be incorporated into a glycogen moiety that was turning over rapidly (63).

Abnormalities of pregnancy such as maternal alloxan diabetes and fasting have also been studied (64). Fasting for 16 h immediately prior to sacrifice at term caused maternal plasma insulin and glucose concentrations to fall and led to a drop in fetal plasma insulin, hepatic and myocardial glycogen despite a rise in blood glucose concentration. Maternal diabetes induced on day 18 caused maternal and fetal hyperglycaemia, no change in fetal plasma insulin, a fall in fetal hepatic glycogen but a rise in fetal cardiac glycogen concentration. Fetal myocardial glucose uptake *in vitro* was unaffected by maternal diabetes. These results show how a change in circulating substrate concentration can alter tissue carbohydrate in the face of a constant circulating hormone concentration.

In the same model insulin was shown to increase amino acid transport and protein synthesis from the 16th day of gestation onwards (65). The effect was independent of the presence of glucose in the incubation medium, was insulin dose-related and appeared to act by both the alanine and leucine receptor pathways.

Glucagon acted on rat heart at a later stage of development than insulin and by a final common pathway shared with epinephrine which makes easier the analysis of the point at which glucagon failed to act. Fetal rat heart on day 16, 18 and 20 responded to epinephrine with an increase in adenylate cyclase activity and a fall in glycogen concentration but did not respond to glucagon in the same way until 4 weeks postnatally (66, 67). In the 19 day mouse fetus epinephrine and glucagon both caused a depletion of cardiac glycogen and an increase of atrial contraction rate (68). These results illustrate differences between organs, the heart and liver in the development of receptors to glucagon, and differences between related species, the rat and mouse in the time at which glucagon sensitivity appears in the heart. It should be noted however that conflicting results have also been obtained (69). The binding of ^{125}I glucagon and the activation by glucagon of adenylate cyclase was equivalent in 13 and 18 day fetal rat heart homogenates to that in the adult. LEVY et al. (69) suggested that some of the differences might be due to methodology and a further report from CLARK and his colleagues (70) appears to bear this out. In contrast to their earlier findings, they were able to demonstrate activation of adenyl cyclase by glucagon in the presence of 5′ guanylylimidodiphosphate (GMP-PNP, an analogue of guanyl triphosphate (GNP)). They revised their earlier view and concluded that a cardiac receptor for glucagon was present early in the neonatal period of the rat and added that "it remains to be seen if GMP-PNP facilitates the binding of glucagon by receptors or the interaction of glucagon with adenylate cyclase."

Studies have been performed on human fetal heart homogenates of 5–17 weeks gestation (71). Adenylate cyclase could be activated by sodium fluoride at all ages studied, by epinephrine from 6–7 weeks and by glucagon from 8–9 weeks onwards.

MUSCLE AND CONNECTIVE TISSUE

Early experiments indicated that glucose uptake by the fetal rat diaphragm *in vitro* at term was not affected by insulin (10, 72) and that neither insulin nor insulin-antibody influenced the accumulation of radioactive glucose by hind limb muscle. Muscle sensitivity to insulin appeared shortly after birth. More recently contrary results were obtained (73). Insulin at a physiological concentration (5 μU/ml) stimulated the uptake of radioactive 2-deoxyglucose, alpha-amino isobutyric acid or leucine by isolated diaphragm from 20 day fetal to 14 day neonatal rats. Methodological arguments were invoked to explain the differences. The observation has physiological importance: 59% of total body glycogen is in rat fetal muscle on the 21st day compared with 50% on the 20th day (74) and if this can be influenced by circulating insulin there could be important implications for perinatal carbohydrate homeostasis. Ovine growth hormone had no effect on rat diaphragm from term fetuses or 4 day newborns in the stimulation of alpha-amino isobutyric acid uptake (75).

Despite much work on the development of metabolic pathways in fetal rhesus monkey skeletal muscle, little attention has been paid to the hormonal factors involved. Term in the rhesus monkey is 165 days. Fetal thigh muscle at 52 to 61% of term was used to study the effects of insulin (10 μU/ml) or epinephrine (6 $\times$ 10^{-6} M) on carbohydrate metabolism *in vitro* (76). Insulin increased glucose uptake and incorporation into glycogen, lactate and carbon dioxide production. Epinephrine decreased glucose uptake, glycogen content and carbon dioxide production. The two hormones appeared to affect glycogen metabolism as early as 85 days gestation via cyclic AMP and similar enzyme systems to those that operate in the adult.

The availability of human fetal cells that might be representative of the lean body mass is limited but fibroblasts and mononuclear leucocytes have been used to study the biological effects of insulin. Monolayer fibroblast cultures were prepared from fetuses of 78 to 127 days gestational age. Culture in serum-free medium with insulin (0.1 to 100

mU/ml) resulted in the stimulation of glucose uptake, uridine incorporation into RNA and leucine incorporation into protein which persisted
for 60 min after removal of insulin (77). Competitive binding studies
suggested that the prolonged effect was due to persistent interaction of
insulin with its receptor site. Monocytes harvested from the cord blood of
normal newborns bound five times as much insulin as those of healthy
adults (78). The difference was due to increased receptor affinity and in
the number of receptor sites per cell. An inference from both studies is
that insulin may have a biological effect in the lean body mass of the
human fetus from early in prenatal life.

ADIPOSE TISSUE

In comparison to the organs and tissues considered above there is a
surprising paucity of information about the effects of insulin and glucagon on fetal and neonatal adipose tissue. This is partly because adipose
development in the most intensely studied species, the rat, takes place
mainly after birth. In a major review of the development of adipose
tissue (79) emphasis was placed on the physiological and metabolic
differences of brown and white adipose tissue (BAT and WAT) and on
the heterogeneity of WAT between the sexes or from different sites in
the body. The major evidence for a lipogenic effect of insulin remains
the clinical observations on IDM and infants suffering from neonatal
diabetes mellitus.

The actions of glucagon on adipose tissue are complicated. BAT from
newborn rats or rats older than 20 days released glycerol *in vitro* when
exposed to glucagon, but was unresponsive when taken from animals
aged 2–20 days (80). Subcutaneous WAT became responsive to glucagon after day 18 but did not react to the hormone later in life. Ovarian
and epididymal WAT showed an increasing responsiveness to glucagon
with age however. The evidence indicates that glucagon does not have a
primary role in the control of early neonatal lipolysis which is effected by
catecholamine release, but may have an important secondary role by
raising tissue glucose levels via glycogenolysis in WAT and/or hepatic
gluconeogenesis (79).

A naive but important question which still remains to be answered is:
where do adipocytes come from? Fibroblasts grown in tissue culture can
be stimulated to differentiate into adipocytes by prostaglandin F_{2a} or
1-methyl-3-isobutyl xanthine (81). Insulin is necessary for the adipocyte

to fill with lipid but does not seem to play an integral part in the transformation. The relevance of these findings to the ontogeny of adipose tissue remains to be studied.

PLACENTA

The binding of polypeptide hormones by placental tissue has been studied in detail by POSNER (82). Insulin was specifically bound by a human placental membrane fraction, but human growth hormone, human prolactin and glucagon were not. Insulin binding by placental membranes varied between species being highest in monkey and guinea pig and lowest in the rat. Insulin binding was inhibited by somatomedin-like activity (82). The concentration of binding activity was considerably higher at term than early in gestation. Maternal diabetes had no effect on placental insulin binding characteristics. The characteristics of the binding sites were similar to those in other established insulin target tissues. The placental receptor was inferred to be, at least in part, protein since pre-treatment of the membranes destroyed binding activity. The placental membrane fraction possessed insulin degrading activity confirming earlier studies (84).

In a study of placental permeability to insulin at 16 to 20 weeks gestation no evidence was discovered in favour of endogenous radioactive insulin crossing the placenta in either direction or of being sequestered by the placenta (4) in contrast to a previous report of placental sequestration and catabolism of insulin at term (84). Fetal insulin may have a metabolic action on the placenta of physiological importance and/or the placenta may be an important site of insulin catabolism in the feto-placental unit.

SUMMARY

The metabolic effects of insulin and glucagon in prenatal life are reviewed in man and laboratory animals. The two hormones often have opposing actions and their net effect on the fetus is determined not only by the concentration of each hormone in the circulation but also by the development of receptors on target cells. For example in the rat there is an insulin glucagon/molar ratio of 10 late in gestation but insulin receptors have not developed in certain tissues (e.g. skeletal muscle). By contrast in man tissue sensitivity to insulin and glucagon appears early in fetal life but there is not such an extreme molar ratio in favour of either hormone.

Each hormone influences fetal growth indirectly via an effect on the establishment of energy reserves. In normal pregnancy insulin plays the dominant role by stimulating the accumulation of carbohydrate and lipid particularly in the liver and adipose tissue. If substrate delivery is impaired as in maternal starvation, fetal hyperglucagonaemia may occur resulting in fetal glycogenolysis and the premature induction of gluconeogenesis. Glucagon deficiency in the fetus does not appear to impede fetal growth.

Insulin also stimulates amino acid uptake and protein synthesis by fetal cells, but the contribution made in this way to either normal or abnormal fetal growth (infant of a diabetic mother, transient neonatal diabetes mellitus) is unknown.

REFERENCES

1. MILNER, R.D.G. (1974) In: Scientific Foundations of Paediatrics, Davis, J.A. and J. Dobbing eds., W.B. Saunders, Philadelphia, Pa., p. 507.
2. MILNER, R.D.G. (1975) In: Carbohydrate Metabolism in Pregnancy and the Newborn, Sutherland, H.W. and J.M. Stowers eds., Churchill Livingstone, Edinburgh, London and New York, p. 83, first volume.
3. MILNER, R.D.G. (1978) In: Carbohydrate Metabolism in Pregnancy and the Newborn, Sutherland, H.W. and J.M. Stowers eds., Churchill Livingstone, Edinburgh, London and New York, p. 131, second volume, in press.
4. ADAM, P.A.J., K. TERAMO, N. RAIHA, D. GITLIN and R. SCHWARTZ. (1969) Diabetes 18:409.
5. MOORE, W.M.O., B.S. WARD and C. GORDON. (1974) Clin. Sci. Molecular Med. 46:125.
6. GIRARD, J.R., A. KERVRAN, E. SOUFFLET and R. ASSAN. (1974) Diabetes 23:310.
7. GIRARD, J.R., G.S. CUENDET, E.B. MARLISS, A. KERVRAN, M. RIEUTORT and R. ASSAN. (1973) J. Clin. Invest. 52:3190.
8. GIRARD, J.R., P. FERRE, M. GILBERT, A. KERVRAN, R. ASSAN and E.M. MARLISS. (1977) Am. J. Physiol. 232:E456.
9. CLARK JR. C.M., G.F. CAHILL JR. and J.S. SOELDNER. (1968) Diabetes 17:362.
10. BRITTON, H.G. and M. BLADE. (1970) Biol. Neonate 16:370.
11. MANNS, J.G. and R.P. BROCKMAN. (1969) Canad. J. Physiol. Pharmacol. 47:917.
12. PICON, L., F. BAILLY, A. KERVRAN and M. RIEUTORT. (1970) C.R. Acad. Sci. Paris 271:774.
13. RABAIN, F. and L. PICON. (1974) Horm. Metab. Res. 6:376.
14. PICON, L. (1967) Endocrinology 81:1419.
15. OSLER, M. (1960) Acta Endocr. Kbhn. 34:276.
16. NAEYE, R.L. (1965) Pediatrics 35:980.
17. CORNBLATH, M. and R. SCHWARTZ. (1976) Disorders of Carbohydrate Metabolism in Infancy, W.B. Saunders, Philadelphia, Pa., p. 218.

18. SHERWOOD, W.G., G.W. CHANCE and D.E. HILL. (1974) Pediat. Res. 8:360.
19. HILL, D.E. (1976) In: Diabetes and Other Endocrine Disorders during Pregnancy and in the Newborn, Alan, R. ed., Liss Inc. New York, p. 127.
20. SHELLEY, H.J., J.M. BASSETT and R.D.G. MILNER. (1975) Brit. Med. Bull. 31:37.
21. SIMMONS, M.A., M.D. JONES, F.C. BATTAGLIA and G. MESCHIA. (1978) Pediat. Res. 12:90.
22. CHEZ, R.A., D.H. MINTZ, E.O. HORGER III and D.L. HUTCHINSON. (1970) J. Clin. Invest. 49:1517.
23. ASSAN, R. and J.R. GIRARD. (1975) In: Early Diabetes in Early Life, Camerini-Davallos, R.A. and H.S. Cole eds., Academic Press, New York, p. 115.
24. LIKE, A.A. and L. ORCI. (1972) Diabetes 21:511.
25. SCHAEFFER, L.D., M.L. WILDER and R.H. WILLIAMS. (1973) Proc. Soc. Exp. Biol. Med. 143:314.
26. EPSTEIN, M., R.A. CHEZ, G.K. OAKES and D.H. MINTZ. (1977) Am. J. Obstet. Gynecol. 127:268.
27. WISE, J.K., S.S. LYALL, R. HENDLER and P. FELIG. (1973) J. Clin. Endocrinol. Metab. 37:345.
28. REISNER, S.H., J.V. ARANDA, E. COLLE, A. PAPAGEORGIOU, D. SCHIFF, C.R. SCRIVER and L. STERN. (1973) Pediat. Res. 7:184.
29. MILNER, R.D.G., S.K. CHOUKSEY, K.N.P. MICKLESON and R. ASSAN (1973) Arch. Dis. Child. 49:241.
30. BLOOM, S.R. and D.I. JOHNSTON. (1972) Brit. Med. J. 3:453.
31. SPERLING, M.A., P.V. DELAMATER, D. PHELPS, R.H. FISER, W. OH and D.A. FISHER. (1974) J. Clin. Invest. 53:1159.
32. WILLIAMS, P.R., R.H. FISER JR., M.A. SPERLING and W. OH. (1975) New Engl. J. Med. 292:612.
33. SALLE, B.L. and A. RUITON-UGLIENGO (1977) Pediat. Res. 11:108.
34. VIDNES, J. and S. ØYASAETER. (1977) Pediat. Res. 11:943.
35. GRAJWER, L.A., M.A. SPERLING, J. SACK and D.A. FISHER. (1977) Pediat. Res. 11:833.
36. SPERLING, M.A., L.A. GRAJWER, R.D. LEAKE and D.A. FISHER. (1977) Pediat. Res. 11:962.
37. SNELL, K. and D.G. WALKER. (1978) Diabetologia 14:59.
38. WARNES, D.M., R.F. SEAMARK and F.J. BALLARD. (1977) Biochem. J. 162:627.
39. BLOOM, S.R., A.V. EDWARDS and R.N. HARDY. (1977) J. Physiol. 269:131.
40. PICON, L. and A.B. MONTANE. (1968) C.R. Acad. Sci. Paris 271:774.
41. HUNTER, D.J.S. (1969) J. Endocrinol. 45:367.
42. BLAZQUEZ, E., B. RUBALCAVA, R. MONTESANO, L. ORCI and R.H. UNGER. (1976) Endocrinology 98:1014.
43. VINICOR, F., G. HIGDON, J.F. CLARK and C.M. CLARK JR. (1976) J. Clin. Invest. 58:571.
44. KELLY, P.A., B.I. POSNER, T. TSUSHIMA and H.G. FRIESEN. (1974) Endocrinology 95:532.
45. GREENGARD, O. (1977) Pediat. Res. 11:669.
46. GREENGARD, O. and H.K. DEWEY (1967) J. Biol. Chem. 242:2986.
47. WICKS, W.D. (1968) J. Biol. Chem. 243:900.
48. YEUNG, D. and I.T. OLIVER. (1968) Biochem. J. 108:325.
49. PHILLIPIDIS, H. and F.J. BALLARD. (1970) Biochem. J. 120:385.
50. SCHWARTZ, A.L. (1972) Biochem. J. 126:89.
51. GIRARD, J.R., D. CAQUET, D. BAL and I. GUILLET. (1973) Enzyme 15:272.
52. VILLEE, C.A. (1953) J. Appl. Physiol. 5:437.
53. SCHWARTZ, A.L. and T.W. RALL. (1975) Diabetes 24:650.

54. SCHWARTZ, A.L., N.C.R. RAIHA and T.W. RALL. (1975) Diabetes 24:1101.
55. SCHWARTZ, A.L. and T.W. RALL. (1975) Diabetes 24:1113.
56. SCHWARTZ, A.L. (1974) Biochem. Biophys. Acta 362:276.
57. CHLEBOWSKI, R.T. and P.A.J. ADAM. (1975) Pediat. Res. 9:821.
58. ADAM, P.A.J., G. GLAZER and F. ROGOFF. (1975) Pediat. Res. 9:816.
59. KALHAN, S.C., S.M. SAVIN and P.A.J. ADAM. (1977) New Engl. J. Med. 296:375.
60. GUIDOTTI, G.G., G. GAJA, L. LORETI and P.P. FOA. (1963) Fedn. Proc. 23:410.
61. GUIDOTTI, G.G., L. LORETI, G. GAJA, G. RANGOTTI and P.P. FOA. (1965) Fedn. Proc. 24:511.
62. CLARK JR. C.M. (1971) Am. J. Physiol. 220:583.
63. CLARK JR. C.M. (1973) Diabetes 22:41.
64. VINICOR, F., D. KOHALMI and C.M. CLARK, JR. (1974) Diabetes 23:662.
65. CLARK JR. C.M. (1972) Biol. Neonate 19:379.
66. CLARK JR. C.M., B. BEATTY and D.O. ALLEN. (1973) J. Clin. Invest. 52:1018.
67. CLARK JR. C.M., D.O. ALLEN and J.F. CLARK. (1977) Endocrinology 100:989.
68. WILDENTHAL, K., D.O. ALLEN, J. KARLSSON, J.R. WAKELAND and C.M. CLARK JR. (1976) J. Clin. Invest. 57:551.
69. LEVEY, G.S., S. MARTIN, B.A. LEVEY, W. COPENHAVER and E. RUIZ. (1974) Proc. Soc. Exp. Biol. Med. 146:425.
70. YOUNT, E.A., C.F. CLARK and C.M. CLARK JR. (1976) Pediat. Res. 10:851.
71. PALMER, G.C. and W.G. DAIL JR. (1975) Pediat. Res. 9:98.
72. FELIX, J.M., M.T. SUTTER, B.J. SUTTER and R. JACQUOT. (1971) Horm. Metab. Res. 3:71.
73. FRICKE, R. and C.M. CLARK JR. (1973) Am. J. Physiol. 224:117.
74. DE MEYER, R., P. GERARD and G. VERELLEN. (1970) In: Metabolic Processes on the Foetus and Newborn Infant, Jonxis, J.H.P., H.K.A. Visser and J.A. Troelstra eds., H.E. Stenfert Kroese N.V., Leiden, Holland, p. 281.
75. NUTTING, D.F. (1976) Endocrinology 98:1273.
76. BOCEK, R.M., M.K. YOUNG and C.H. BEATTY (1973) Pediat. Res. 7:787.
77. FUJIMOTO, W.Y. and R.H. WILLIAMS (1977) In Vitro 13:268.
78. THORSSON, A.V. and R.L. HINTZ. (1977) New Engl. J. Med. 297:908.
79. HAHN, P. and M. NOVAK. (1975) J. Lipid Res. 16:79.
80. HAHN, P. (1971) Pediat. Res. 5:126.
81. RUSSELL, T.R. and R. HO. (1976) Proc. Natal. Acad. Sci. U.S.A. 73:4516.
82. POSNER, B.I. (1974) Diabetes 23:209.
83. MARSHALL, R.N., L.E. UNDERWOOD, S.J. VOINA, D.B. FONSHEE and J.J. VAN WYK. (1974) J. Clin. Endocrinol. Metab. 39:283.
84. BUSE, M.G., W.J. ROBERTS and J. BUSE. (1962) J. Clin. Invest. 41:29.

PROTEIN TURNOVER RATE IN FETAL ORGANS:
THE INFLUENCE OF INSULIN

MAUREEN YOUNG*, JANE HORN* and DAVID L. NOAKES**

The Fetus

"Open for business during alterations"

A. G. STREETER

Streeter was an embryologist, but such a description must be equally applicable to every aspect of the biochemistry of development which forms the basis of all the structural rearrangements accompanying growth in the fetus and after birth.

In fetal tissues, as in regenerating liver and malignant growths (1, 2, 3), both the extracellular and intracellular concentrations of free amino acids are higher than in the adult, and indicate that a faster turnover rate of the tissue proteins accompanies their deposition. Measurement of protein synthetic rate confirms this; the half life for mixed protein was found to be about 2 days in newborn rat and mouse brain in comparison with 8 days in the adult (4, 5). SCHOENHEIMER's (6) concept of the dynamic state of the body protein may be exhibited to its full extent in the fetus and newborn, where the endocrine systems are relatively immature and the genetically determined regulation of biochemical processes is not yet fully expressed. A fast turnover rate of body constituents may also influence the total nitrogen requirements of growing animals. In the lamb "in utero", the placental transfer rate of amino acids, measured from the umbilical veno-arterial difference and blood flow, has been found to be considerably greater than the quantity of amino acids laid down as protein in a given time (7). Further, infants require an intake of over 1.5 g N/kg body weight per day in comparison with 0.7 N/kg per day in the adult, and a greater proportion of essential amino acids, 43% and 19% of the total nitrogen respectively (8).

* Department of Gynaecology, St. Thomas's Hospital Medical School, London, SE1 7EH.
** Department of Surgery and Obstetrics, Royal Veterinary College Field Station, North Mimms, Herts.

H.K.A. Visser (ed.), Nutrition and Metabolism of the Fetus and Infant, 19–27. All rights reserved.
Copyright © 1979 Martinus Nijhoff Publishers b.v., The Hague/Boston/London.

Our own interests in protein synthesis rate in the tissues of fetal organs arose primarily out of the current view that increased insulin production by the fetal pancreatic islets might be one of the causes of the macrosomia of the large infant of a diabetic mother, whose blood glucose is not well controlled (9), and the further possibility that insulin might be a growth hormone in the normal infant. Growth rate in the human infant can only be measured by the weight increment in a known time, but in the experimental animal, the qualitative nature of the protein accumulation accompanying growth, may be investigated by the nitrogen (10) and amino acid (11) composition of the organs and carcass, and by the relationship of these to the DNA and RNA content of the tissues (12). All these observations are made over relatively long time periods, but a variety of short term methods are also in use for measuring protein synthetic rate utilizing the rate of uptake by the protein of a labelled amino acid "*in vivo*" (13, 14). These techniques require the maintenance of steady state specific activity in the free amino acid precursor pools which are, unfortunately, not easy to identify precisely; the specific activity of the intracellular or plasma pools is usually used in the calculations.

Protein Synthetic Rate in the Lamb "in utero"

Fetal lambs were chosen for the investigation of protein synthetic rate because they are large enough for repeated blood sampling to check on steady state conditions, and prolonged glucose infusions are known to release insulin from their pancreatic islets towards the end of gestation (15). The studies were made at 135 days' gestation on lambs weighing 2.41 kg ($\pm$ 0.17); indwelling catheters had been inserted into one carotid artery and jugular vein one or two days previously, with the ewe under ketalar anaesthetia (16, 17). The method of continuous infusion of a labelled amino acid, modified from that of WATERLOW and STEPHEN, was used to measure protein synthetic rate (18). L-^{14}C lysine was given intravenously for 6 hr, and its rate of uptake by the protein in the steady state, estimated by determining the specific activity of the labelled lysine bound in this pool, and relating it to that in the intracellular free amino acid pool. These values were obtained by sacrificing the fetus, removing the organs quickly and homogenising aliquots in cold 10% trichloracetic (TCA) solution. The amino acid content of the precipitated proteins and supernatant were determining using a Technicon amino acid analyser, TSM 1; the radioactivity associated with the lysine was also measured.

Fractional protein synthesis rates were calculated from the ratio of the specific activities in the protein bound (S_B) and the intracellular pools (S_i), using the equations for rapidly turning over tissue described by PAIN and GARLICK (19). A curve was plotted for different S_B/S_i ratios against a rate constant k, the % synthesis per day and, using the measured values for specific activities, k was read from this curve. the results were expressed as protein half life, $t_{\frac{1}{2}}$ in days.

The half life of the mixed proteins of fetal organs in six fetuses is compared with those in the newborn and adult sheep in table 1. The mean values of about one day in brain, liver and heart are very short in

Table 1. *Changes with age in mixed protein half life in sheep (days, mean ±S.E.)*

	Fetus 135 days	Lamb* 3 days	Adult** 1 year
Brain	1.62 ± 0.41	–	–
Liver	0.67 ± 0.15	0.7 ± 0.05	6.9
Skeletal muscle	7.81 ± 2.96	3.1 ± 0.19	40.7
Cardiac muscle	1.00 ± 0.24	2.3 ± 0.42	21.6
"n"	6	6	4

* SOLTESZ et al. (21)
** BUTTERY et al. (20)

comparison with the adult (20), but are comparable with those in the newborn lamb (21), with the exception of skeletal muscle; the half life of placental proteins is similar to that in the fetal liver. This lack of differentiation between the tissues might have been anticipated in the rapidly developing young animal. The fetal and newborn protein half lives are half those found in the brains of 2 to 3 day old rats using a similar technique (4, 5, 22). The marked differentiation in the mixed protein half life seen between the tissues of the adult ewe has also been observed in the adult mouse (23).

GARLICK et al. (18) have shown that there is a direct relationship between protein synthetic rate and growth rate in the young rat, and LAJTHA and DUNLOP (22) have compared isotope incorporation rates with protein deposition rate in the cerebral hemispheres and cerebellum in the growing rat. As seen in table 2, deposition was about 20–25% of

Table 2. *Changes with age in protein metabolism in the rat brain*
      (mg protein per 100 g tissue protein per hour)

	Cerebrum			Days	Cerebellum		
	8	18	37		8	18	37
Protein deposition	0.46	0.18	0.01		0.80	0.28	0.01
Incorporation of label	1.71	0.88	0.58		2.06	1.06	0.78
Breakdown	1.25	0.70	0.57		1.26	0.78	0.58

from LAJTHA and DUNLOP (22)

the rate of incorporation of labelled amino acid at the end of the first week of life, decreasing to about 1% by 27 days of age. Incorporation rate decreased by 60% during this time and breakdown, the difference between incorporation and deposition, rather less. Therefore, both incorporation and breakdown rates are high when deposition rates are fastest during growth. The incorporation rate which we have measured in the lamb is faster than in the young rat, but the deposition or accumulation rate of protein is slower in the lamb than in the growing rat (10).

Protein consists of a heterogeneous mixture of nitrogenous compounds with various half lives and, during 6 hr of L-^{14}C lysine infusion in the lamb, the protein with a faster synthetic rate will be preferentially labelled. In the adult mouse, LAJTHA et al. (23) found that brain protein consisted mostly of elements having a half life of about 10 days, whilst nearly all the liver proteins had an average half life of 26 hours; in the kidney there were 2 components, about equally represented, which had half lives of 18 hours and 2.6 days respectively. The short half of the proteins in fetal organs which we, and others, have observed may be due either to the presence of a greater proportion of the rapidly turning over proteins, or to some difference in fetal physiology which allows the whole spectrum of tissue proteins to be turning over more rapidly. The latter may be due to a greater rate of supply of substrates in the fetus than in the adult for organ blood flow is high (24) and the blood tissue barriers more permeable (22). Moreover, the basic turnover characteristics of proteins may be less restrained in the fetus due to the immaturity of the endocrine systems "in utero". Alternatively, the proteins themselves may be different during growth (22).

The Influence of Insulin on Protein Synthetic Rate "in utero"

The evidence that insulin might directly influence fetal protein synthetic rate is conflicting. PICON (25) observed that fetal rats given intramuscular insulin "in utero" were heavier than control litter mates, and contained a greater amount of nitrogen and a larger lipid/N ratio. Insulin has also been shown to enhance the rate of incorporation of labelled amino acids into the proteins of a variety of adult and fetal isolated tissues "in vitro" (26, 27, 28, 29); JEFFERSON et al.(30) consider that this may be due to the reinforcement of an imperfect medium lacking the necessary hormones to maintain a normal synthesis rate "in vitro". MORTIMORE and MONDON (31) found that insulin reduced the tissue free amino acid pool in the perfused rat liver, but did not enhance amino acid uptake by the protein. PAIN and GARLICK (19) observed no influence of insulin on protein turnover rate in normal rat skeletal muscle using the continuous infusion method "in vivo"; however, insulin partially reversed the depressed protein synthetic rate observed in streptozotocin diabetic animals, and this may be analogous to the influence of insulin "in vitro".

The effect of insulin on protein turnover rates in the tissues of the fetal lamb were studied by infusing the hormone at rates of less than 0.5 U/kg/hr, and from 0.5 to 1.7 U/kg/hr, simultaneously with the ^{14}C lysine during the 6 hr infusion period. The average steady state plasma insulin levels were 111 and 161 μU/ml in comparison with the resting levels of 15 and 18 μU/ml respectively.

The most striking effect of the hormone was the reduction in the plasma and tissue free amino acid pools. The fall in plasma concentration was 30% and 60% with the low and high rates of insulin infusion in comparison with 10% during the experimental period in the control group just described (table 3). Tissue free lysine concentrations were always greater than in the plasma, ranging from one and a half times greater in the brain to five times the concentration in liver. These free pools were reduced threefold in liver and cardiac muscle, and fivefold in skeletal muscle during the low rates of infusion; similar changes were observed at the high rates of infusion, except that the fall in muscle was more profound. Such a fall in tissue free amino acid concentration strongly suggests a marked reduction in protein catabolism in each organ, with the exception of the brain where the changes may have been secondary to the fall in the circulating plasma levels. An increased

Table 3. *Effect of insulin on free lysine pools in fetal lambs (lysine, mean $\pm$ S.E.)*

		Free in body fluids	
	Control	Insulin U/kg/h	
		< 0.5	≥ 0.5
Preinfusion Plasma	99.8 ± 3.5	53.0 ± 6.1**	95.7 ± 13.8
End infusion	92.9 ± 6.4	×36.5 ± 4.4**	37.8 ± 5.9**
Brain	162.6 ± 20.6+	94.8 ± 15.6*	123.0 ± 26.4
Liver	522.0 ± 100.0	210.1 ± 54.8**	237.6 ± 75.1
Skeletal muscle	505.6 ± 121.5	108.3 ± 45.1**	20.6 ± 1.20*
Cardiac muscle	360.8 ± 751.	129.6 ± 20.8**	105.0 ± 11.6
n	6	6	3

1. Free lysine is expressed as μM for plasma and $\mu mole. kg^{-1}$ wet weight in tissues.
2. Significantly different from control ($p < 0.02$)**
   ($p < 0.05$)*
3. End infusion value slightly significantly lower than preinfusion value ($p < 0.10$)×.
4. Significantly lower than liver within group ($p < 0.05$)+.

metabolism of the lysine may also have contributed to the reduction in tissue concentrations, for the counts associated with lysine were a smaller proportion of the total counts following insulin infusion, particularly in muscle.

The fractional protein synthesis rates calculated from the ratios of the specific activities of lysine in the protein and intracellular pools are shown in figure 1. Insulin, at the lower infusion rates, apparently reduced the protein synthetic rate in each organ; in skeletal and cardiac muscle, the half life was trebled, and in brain it was doubled but, due to the large variation in the results, only that for cardiac muscle was significant. The half life of liver protein was only slightly lengthened. Since catabolism is also decreased, such a reduction in synthetic rate would not be incompatible with protein accumulation provided the final balance of anabolism and catabolism is changed in favour of the former. It is, however, not known what influence the low levels of tissue free amino acids have on protein synthesis "in vivo", so the observations have been repeated during constant infusions of either amino acids or glucose,

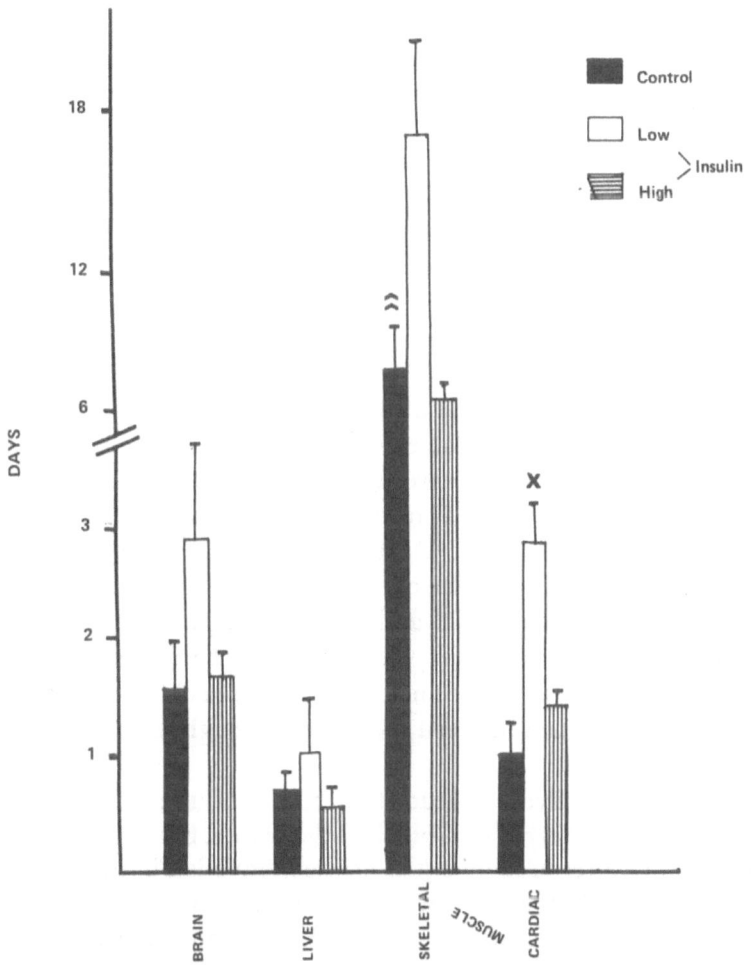

Fig. 1. Effect of insulin on mixed protein half life in fetal lambs (days, mean ± S.E.).
p = < 0.05^x from control fetus
p = < 0.02^â within group

to maintain their normal plasma and tissue levels; the results, so far, suggest that low substrate levels do not influence protein synthetic rate, as measured over a 6 hr period, either in the presence or absence of insulin.

Theoretically, whole body protein synthesis rate could have been measured following the infusion of labelled lysine from its total flux or metabolic clearance rate. Our calculations for the whole body provided very large values in comparison with the measured retention rate of protein in the lamb (10). This may be explained by the loss of labelled amino acid available for uptake by the protein, due to its rapid metabolism which was also found for other amino acids in the newborn lamb (21) and rat (22), and to transplacental flux of the label into the mother.

CONCLUSIONS

Fetal protein and amino acid metabolism is in a more dynamic state than in the adult. The faster deposition rate of protein in the growing animal is accompanied by both a quicker incorporation of labelled precursors and a faster breakdown rate, and an elevation of the tissue free amino acids. The free amino acids are also more quickly metabolised than in the adult.

Fractional organ synthesis or turnover rates, in the fetal lamb, calculated from the uptake of L-^{14}C lysine in the steady state "in utero" provided values for the half life of mixed protein of about a day in the brain, liver and cardiac muscle, and seven days in skeletal muscle; these are comparable with turnover rates found in the newborn brain of smaller species. The values are much shorter than in the adult ewe or rat, with less differentiation between the organs, as might be anticipated in the growing animal.

A six to tenfold increase in steady state plasma insulin level apparently reduced the fractional organ protein synthetic rate, but such a change is difficult to interpret because of the marked reduction in the free tissue amino acids which may influence synthetic rate by reducing the substrate supply. However, a reduction in this pool does indicate a fall in protein catabolic rate. The macrosomia and increased nitrogen content of the large infant of diabetic mothers may occur because the increased insulin secretion alters the balance between anabolism and catabolism of protein in favour of the former, whilst the congenital disturbances, which also occur in these infants, may be caused by the changes in metabolism in the major target organs of insulin, skeletal muscle and heart, and the alterations in the inter-organ traffic of amino acids, and other metabolites which ensues.

ACKNOWLEDGEMENTS

The work would have been impossible without good colleagues, Mrs. Sylvia Chrystie, Mark Stern, Ian Sloan.

REFERENCES

1. YOUNG, M. (1976) In: Fetal Physiology and Medicine, Beard, R.W. and P.W. Nathanielsz eds., W.B. Saunders, London, p. 59.
2. RYAN, W.L. and M.J. CARVER. (1966) Nature (Lond.) 212:292.
3. CHRISTENSEN, H.N., J.T. ROTHWELL, R.A. SEARS and J.A. STREICHER. (1948) J. biol. Chem. 175:101.
4. DUNLOP, D.S., W. VAN ELDEN and A. LAJTHA. (1975) J. Neurochem. 24:337.
5. OJA, S.S. (1967) Ann. Acad. Sci. Fenn. (Med.) 131:7.
6. SCHOENHEIMER, R. (1942) The Dynamic State of Body Constitutents. Harvard Univ. Press, Cambridge, Mass.
7. LEMONS, J.A., E.W. ADCOCK, D.M. JONES, M.A. NAUGHTON, G. MESCHIA and F.C. BATTAGLIA. (1976) J. clin. Invest. 58:1428.
8. MUNRO, H.N. (1974) Acta Anaesth. Scand. Suppl. 55:66.
9. HOET, J.J. (1969) In: Foetal Autonomy, Wolstenholme, G.E.W. and M. O'Connor eds., Ciba Foundation Symposium. J. & A. Churchill, London, p. 186.
10. BLAXTER, K.L. (1964) In: Mammalian Protein Metabolism, Munro, H.N. and J.B. Allison eds., Academic Press, New York, London, vol. II, p. 173.
11. SOUTHGATE, D.A.T. (1971) Biol. Neonate 19:272.
12. WINICK, M., J.A. BRASEL and P. ROSSO. (1972) In: Nutrition and Development, Winick, M. ed., vol. 1, p. 49. J. Wiley, New York.
13. WATERLOW, J.C., P.J. GARLICK and D.J. MILLWARD. (1978) Protein turnover in Mammalian Tissues and in the Whole Body. Elsevier, North-Holland, Amsterdam.
14. LAJTHA, A. and D. DUNLOP. (1976) In: Subcellular Mechanisms in Reproductive Neuroendocrinology, Naftolin, F., K.J. Ryan and I.J. Davies eds., Elsevier Scientific Publishing Co., Amsterdam, p. 63.
15. BASSETT, J.M. and D. MADILL. (1974) J. Endocr. 62:299.
16. CHRYSTIE, S., J. HORN, I. SLOAN, M. STERN, D. NOAKES and M. YOUNG. (1977) Proc. Nutr. Soc. 36:118A.
17. YOUNG, M., D. NOAKES, J. HORN, I. SLOAN and S. CHRYSTIE. (1977) Ann. Rech. Vet. 8:499.
18. GARLICK, P.J., D.J. MILLWARD and W.P.T. JAMES. (1973) Biochem. J. 136:935.
19. PAIN, V.M. and P.J. GARLICK. (1974) J. biol. Chem. 249:4510.
20. BUTTERY, P.J., A. BECKERTON and R.M. MITCHELL. (1975) Proc. Nutr. Soc. 34:91A.
21. SOLTESZ, GY., J. JOYCE and M. YOUNG. (1973) Biol. Neonate 23:139.
22. LAJTHA, A. and D. DUNLOP. (1974) Adv. in Behav. Biol. 8:215.
23. LAJTHA, A., L. LATZKOVITS and J. TOTH. (1976) Biochim. Biophys. Acta 425:511.
24. RUDOLPH, A.M. and H.A. HEYMANN. (1974) Ann. Rev. Physiol. 36:187.
25. PICON, L. (1967) Endocr. 81:1419.
26. ASPLUND, K. (1975) Hormone Res. 6:12.
27. CLARK, C.M. (1971) Biol. Neonate 19:379.
28. GUIDOTTI, G.G., A.F. BORGHETTI, B. LUNEBURG and G.C. GAZZOLA. (1971) Biochem. J. 122:409.
29. VILLEE, D. (1975) In: Early Diabetes in Early Life, Camerini-Davalos, R.A. and H.S. Cole eds., Academic Press, London, p. 78.
30. JEFFERSON, L.S., D.E. RANNELS, B.L. MUNGER and H.E. MORGAN. (1974) Fed. Proc. 33:1098.
31. MORTIMORE, G.E. and C.E. MONDON. (1970) J. biol. Chem. 5:375.

FETAL INGESTION AND METABOLISM
OF AMNIOTIC FLUID PROTEIN

ROY M. PITKIN, M.D.*

INTRODUCTION

It is well known that the fetus, at least from mid-gestation onwards, regularly swallows amniotic fluid. The most direct evidence supporting this phenomenon comes from amniographic studies in which radiopaque material injected into the amniotic sac can be demonstrated radiographically in the fetal alimentary tract some hours later (1). An example of such a study is illustrated in figure 1.

Fetal swallowing of amniotic fluid plays an essential role in regulating amniotic fluid volume; in fact, it is generally acknowledged that this mechanism represents the principal route of amniotic fluid removal during the last half of pregnancy. In certain abnormal states such as fetal malformations which interfere with deglutition by the fetus, polyhydramnios or accumulation of excessive amounts of amniotic fluid is a consistent finding.

Whether amniotic fluid ingestion plays a physiologic role in addition to volume regulation is uncertain. An immunologic function, in which antibodies might be acquired passively by the fetus, has been suggested by several observations. Particularly intriguing is the question of whether or not fetal swallowing fulfills a role in fetal nutrition. On the one hand, there does not appear to be any theoretical need for enteral nutrition in the fetus, in view of the normally abundant transplacental mechanism of providing the nutrients necessary for growth and development. On the other hand, however, certain findings suggest that fetal swallowing may play some function in nutrition during intrauterine life. The concentration of protein in amniotic fluid decreases progressively throughout the last half of gestation (2, 3), suggesting the possibility of a nutritive function of ingested amniotic fluid (4). Moreover, conditions in which

* Department of Obstetrics and Gynecology, University of Iowa, Iowa City, Ia., U.S.A.

H.K.A. Visser (ed.), Nutrition and Metabolism of the Fetus and Infant, 29–41. All rights reserved.
Copyright © 1979 Martinus Nijhoff Publishers b.v., The Hague/Boston/London.

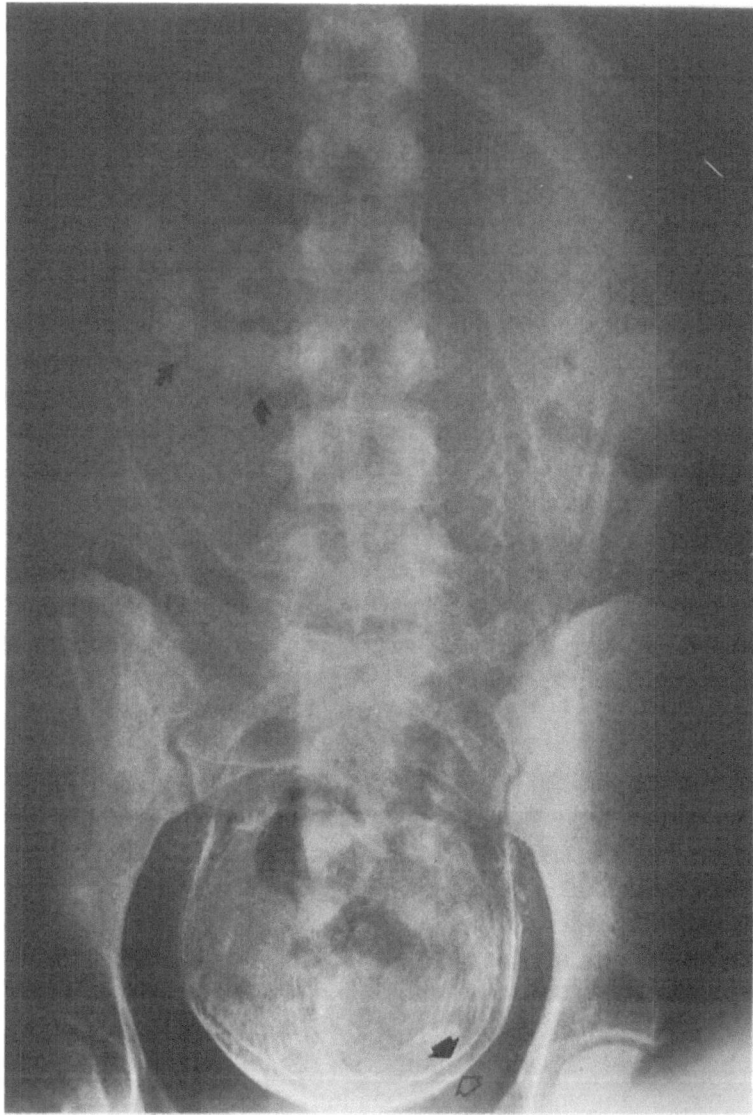

Fig. 1. Amniogram and fetogram of term fetus taken 18 hr after intra-amniotic injection of 30 ml diatrizoate meglumine. Arrows indicate concentration of contrast material in the fetal colon, confirming previous fetal ingestion of amniotic fluid.

fetal swallowing cannot occur, such as congenital esophageal atresia, have been noted to be associated with retarded fetal growth (5).

If ingested amniotic fluid is to represent a potential source of protein nutrition for the fetus, the protein must be either absorbed intact in the alimentary tract or hydrolyzed into its constituent amino acids which are then available for protein synthesis in fetal tissues. It is the purpose of this paper to review the evidence relating to these questions and, in particular, to examine the phenomenon of fetal digestion of amniotic fluid protein and its utilization by the fetus.

FETAL GASTROINTESTINAL DEVELOPMENT

The gastrointestinal tract originates from both entoderm and a mesoblastic mesenchymal layer, the former giving rise to the epithelial lining (including glandular tissues) and the latter to the muscular, vascular, and serosal layers. Differentiation and maturation of the digestive system generally proceed from proximal to distal portions (i.e., from cephalad to caudad). Rotation of the gastrointestinal tract in a counterclockwise direction is a characteristic feature of the fifth and sixth week of intrauterine life. By the end of the first trimester, the gross anatomic aspects of the fetal stomach and small and large intestines resemble those of postnatal life. The principal morphologic change of the last two-thirds of fetal life is that of growth, the small intestine elongating 500 to 1000-fold during this time. The length of the small bowel at term is 3 or 4 times the crown-heel length (i.e., 150 to 200 cm).

Functional development of the gastrointestinal tract, reviewed in detail recently by GRAND and associates (6), follows a series of intricate and interrelated steps. The ability of the small intestine to transport amino acids actively across its mucosa can be demonstrated in vitro by 12 weeks' gestational age, corresponding with the appearance of dipeptidases in the intestinal brush border at this time, and does not change during the last two-thirds of intrauterine life. Thus, the functional sequence of fetal gastrointestinal development depends largely on acquisition of the ability to digest nutrients into absorbable components. In the adult, some digestion of protein into peptides occurs in the stomach and this probably occurs in the fetus as well since peptic activity can be demonstrated as early as 16 weeks' gestational age. Stomach digestion is probably not fully operative until relatively late, however, in view of the finding that hydrochloric acid secretion does not appear until about

32 weeks. The pancreatic enzyme trypsin, one of the principal proteolytic enzymes, is detectable at approximately 16 weeks but tryptic
activity remains low until 28 weeks or so, when it increases markedly.
Enterokinase, which first appears at 26 weeks, seems to represent the
regulatory mechanism for trypsin secretion. Enterokinase activity during
the interval of 26 to 30 weeks is approximately 6% that of older children
and by term reaches 20% that of childhood.

Thus, the ability of the fetal gastrointestinal tract to digest nutrients is
reasonably well-developed by the last few weeks of intrauterine life.
Protein can be broken down into peptides and amino acids and then
absorbed. The question of whether or not the fetus and newborn can
absorb whole protein molecules, considered in greater detail below, is
a controversial issue with considerable significance in relation to the
transfer of passive immunity.

PREVIOUS REPORTS

In 1965 PRITCHARD (7) reported the first quantitative study of deglutition by the human fetus. Using an approach in which ^{51}Cr-labeled
erythrocytes were injected into the amniotic sac and then the meconium
passed by the neonate was collected and analyzed, he demonstrated
that the volume of fetal swallowing at term averaged approximately 450
ml per 24 hr. By means of radioiodinated serum albumin (RISA) also
administered intra-amniotically, the half-life of the injected protein in
amniotic fluid was determined to be $24\frac{1}{2}$ hr. Moreover, nearly all of the
radioactivity which disappeared from the amniotic sac ultimately appeared in the maternal urine, indicating that the injected RISA had
been de-iodinated in the fetus and the free radioiodine transferred to the
maternal circulation to be excreted by the maternal kidney. Thus, these
observations provided indirect evidence of the ability of the fetal gut to
metabolize ingested amniotic fluid protein, at least to the extent of de-
iodination.

In a comprehensive report published in 1972, GITLIN and colleagues
(8) examined the turnover of several types of amniotic fluid proteins
labeled with radioiodine. It was found that the rate of protein clearance,
at least 80% of which occurred by fetal swallowing, was virtually identical for the proteins of various molecular weights studied, with a half-life
averaging 29 ($\pm$ 3) hr in women at term but not in labor. The mean
volume of amniotic fluid cleared of protein under these conditions was

342 ml per 24 hr. However, the amount ingested by individual fetuses varied in direct relation to the amniotic volume present. GITLIN and associates noted, as had PRITCHARD, that a large portion of the protein-bound radioactivity disappearing from the amniotic sac was ultimately excreted in the maternal urine as protein-free radioactivity, implying fetal digestion and absorption.

While it is generally thought that, at least in the adult, protein must be hydrolyzed into amino acids and small peptides to be absorbed, there exists some indirect evidence that the developing gastrointestinal tract may be able to absorb protein molecules intact. This question has been examined by LEV and ORLIC in two animal species (9, 10). Horseradish peroxidase, a protein with a molecular weight of approximately 40000 daltons, was injected into the amniotic sacs of pregnant rats at term and electron microscopic examination of the fetal intestine 6 to 18 hr later documented the presence of the macromolecular protein in the absorptive cells and underlying vascular endothelium (9). These same investigators carried out similar studies in pregnant rhesus monkeys with results identical in some respects but different in others (10). Light and electron microscopic examination of the fetal intestine 7 hr after intra-amniotic administration of horseradish peroxidase documented the presence of absorbed peroxidase granules in intestinal epithelial cells of 2 of 3 term fetuses and of one immature fetus. However, one term fetus exhibited no evidence of absorption of intact protein. Moreover and more significantly, no animals demonstrated peroxidase granules beyond absorptive cells (i.e., in extracellular or vascular spaces), suggesting that the primate fetus may be able to take up whole protein molecules into its intestinal cells but not release them intact. Thus, species differences appear to exist with respect to protein-absorptive ability and it seems likely that the capacity to absorb macromolecular protein is minimal in primates compared with lower mammals (11).

PRESENT STUDY

Methods

The present study, described in detail elsewhere (12), utilized a biologically-synthesized protein prepared as follows: A growing pig was rendered protein-deficient by placing it on a protein-free diet for 5 days and by removing approximately 30 ml of plasma on days 1, 3 and 5 of the diet. The pig was then fed a high protein diet and given 1 mCi ^{35}S-L-methonine by intraperitoneal injection. Four days later the animal was exsanguinated and the plasma thus harvested was of high specific activity (282×10^3 dpm/ml) with virtually all of the radioactivity precipitable in trichloracetic acid. This plasma, containing protein synthesized biologically from ^{35}S-L-methionine with specific activity of 5700 dpm/mg protein, was then utilized to investigate the fate of amniotic fluid protein in the pregnant rhesus monkeys (*Macaca mulatta*).

Eleven pregnant monkeys, all in the gestational interval of 130 to 160 days (corresponding to the last 20% of gestation in this species), underwent transabdominal amniocentesis with removal of 5 ml of amniotic fluid and replacement with an equivalent volume of ^{35}S-labeled protein. Delivery was accomplished by cesarean section at daily intervals from 1 to 7 days later. At delivery, samples of amniotic fluid, maternal blood, and fetal blood were obtained for analysis. The fetus was then killed by injection of an overdose of pentobarbital and dissected. Samples of lung, liver, skeletal muscle, and cerebral cortex were taken. The fetal alimentary tract was removed intact after clamping the cardiac end of the stomach and the rectosigmoid junction and carefully opened to permit collection of the contents of the stomach, duodenum, jejunum, ileum, and transverse colon. Samples of the alimentary tract wall at each of these levels were obtained. All specimens were sampled in triplicate.

Each sample was treated with trichloracetic acid (TCA) in order to differentiate between TCA-soluble and TCA-insoluble fractions. In the case of fluid samples, a measured volume was mixed with an equivalent amount of 10% TCA and then washed twice with 5% TCA. In the case of tissue samples, a weighed portion was homogenized with 5% TCA and rewashed twice. The combined supernatents from each sample were prepared for liquid scintillation counting by addition of Instagel (Packard Instrument Co., Downers Grove, Illinois, U.S.A.). The combined precipitates were first dissolved in Nuclear Chicago Solubilizer (Amersham Searle Corp., Chicago, Illinois, U.S.A.) and then prepared for liquid scintillation counting by addition of Instagel.

The specimens were analyzed for ^{35}S-activity in a Packard 3380 liquid scintillation counter with absolute activity analyzer. The resulting disintegrations per minute (dpm) were corrected for radioactive decay by expressing the values as equivalent to the day the radioactive plasma was harvested. The TCA-precipitable fraction of each fluid and tissue sample was considered to represent protein and is hereafter referred to as such. The TCA-soluble fraction represented principally the sulfur-containing amino acids, methionine, cystine, and cysteine. For convenience, the TCA-soluble material is hereafter designated "amino acids" although it should be acknowledged that it probably also contained small amounts of peptides and inorganic sulfates as well.

The protein content of each sample was estimated by measuring the nitrogen level with a Coleman nitrogen analyzer and multiplying this value by 6.25.

Results

The disappearance of ³⁵S-protein following its injection into amniotic fluid, as illustrated in figure 2, was logarithmic and the half-time was 1.1

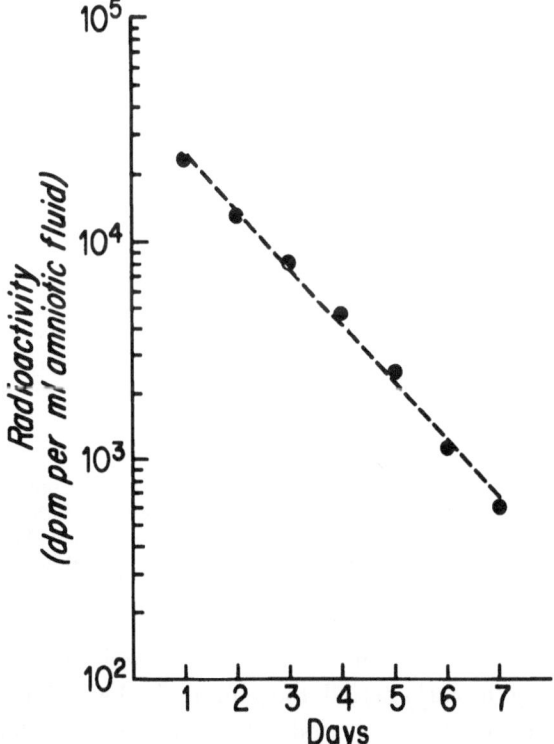

Fig. 2. Amniotic fluid protein radioactivity after injection of ³⁵S-protein into amniotic sac. Note logarithmic ordinate. Half-time of amniotic fluid protein = 1.1 days. (Reproduced with permission from Amer. J. Obstet. Gynecol. 123:356, 1975).

days. This finding implies that slightly less than half of amniotic fluid protein is cleared per 24 hr, a value entirely consistent with earlier studies (7, 8) indicating that the term fetus swallows amniotic fluid in daily amounts equivalent to approximately half the volume of fluid present.

Figure 3 illustrates the radioactivity profiles in the fetal alimentary tract contents as a function of time since injection into the amniotic fluid.

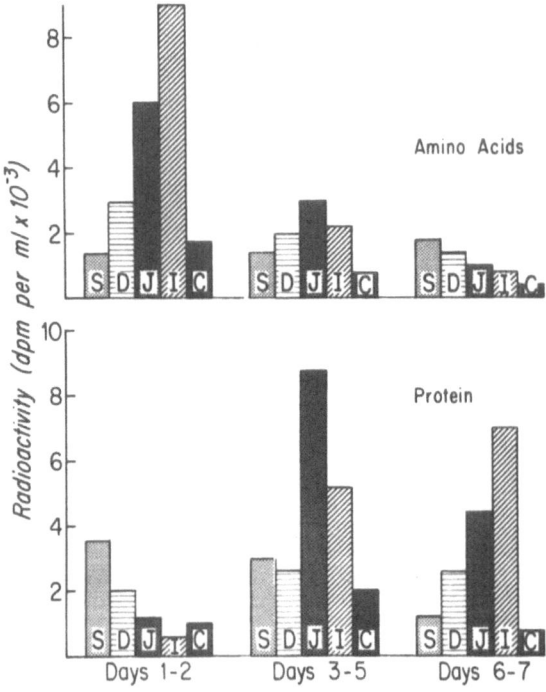

Fig. 3. Radioactivity in fetal alimentary tract contents after intra-amniotic injection of 35S-protein. Upper panel ("amino acids") refers to TCA-soluble radioactivity. Lower panel ("protein") refers to TCA-insoluble radioactivity. S = stomach, D = duodenum, J. = jejunum, I = ileum, C = colon. (Reproduced with permission from Amer. J. Obstet. Gynecol. 123:356, 1975).

In relative terms, the levels of amino acid radioactivity were highest in the ileum during the early period, the jejunum in the middle period, and the stomach during the late period. The early finding of high levels of amino acids in the distal small intestine likely reflects the progressive proteolysis along the course of the bowel whereas the late finding of high levels in the stomach probably reflects swallowing of amniotic fluid which by that time had accumulated substantial quantities of radioactive amino acids from fetal urinary excretion. An exactly opposite pattern was exhibited by radioactive protein levels in the gut with highest levels in the stomach early and in the ileum late. The high stomach levels early undoubtedly reflected fetal swallowing of amniotic fluid containing a relatively high concentration of radioactive protein. The finding that protein levels late were highest in the distal small bowel contents is more difficult to explain. It probably reflects protein synthesis within the intestinal epithelium, utilizing amino acids from the gut contents, with these epithelial cells then desquamated and propelled along the course of the alimentary tract.

Protein synthesis within the alimentary tract wall was demonstrated by the finding of high levels of ^{35}S-labeled protein in these tissues. In fact, the highest concentration of ^{35}S-labeled protein occurred in the wall of the small intestine, especially the ileum where levels 8 or 10 times that in liver were encountered.

Radioactive amino acids were found in fetal serum and their levels as a function of time were strikingly similar to those of maternal serum and amniotic fluid (fig. 4) with peak values on the third day after injection.

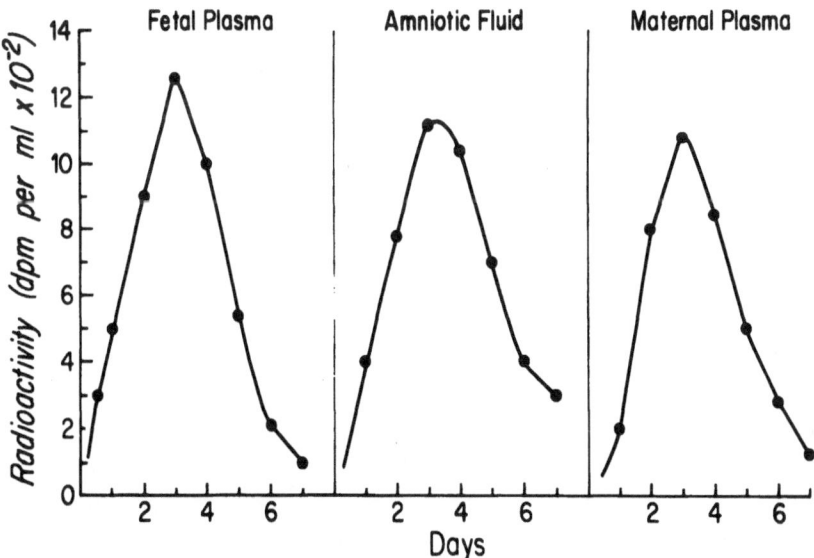

Fig. 4. Radioactivity in amino acids in fetal plasma, amniotic fluid, and maternal plasma after intra-amniotic injection of ^{35}S-protein. (Reproduced with permission from Amer. J. Obstet. Gynecol. 123:356, 1975).

This basic similarity likely reflects the relatively free exchange of amino acids between these three compartments. Careful examination, however, reveals the fetal plasma values to be slightly but consistently greater than those in either maternal serum or amniotic fluid during the first three days when levels were rising, suggesting that the primary source is the fetus.

Specific activity of plasma proteins, illustrated in figure 5, was consistently greater in fetus than in mother. Moreover, the peak specific activity in fetal plasma protein occurred on day 4, one day after the maximum level of radioactivity in amino acids in fetal plasma. This interval is consistent with the known synthesis time of 12 to 48 hr for albumin (13), the principal plasma protein.

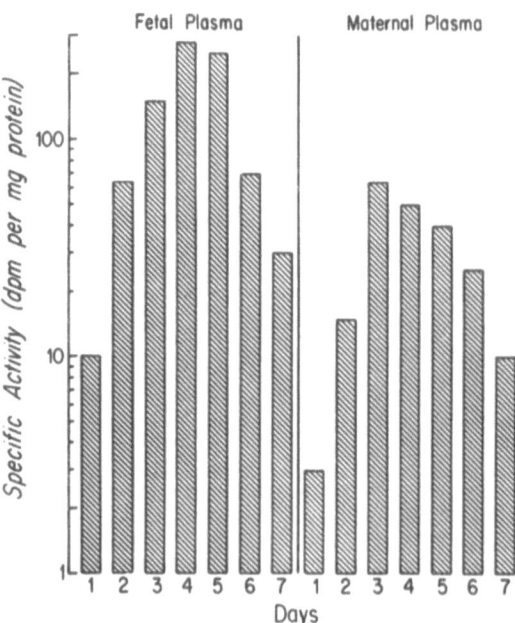

Fig. 5. Specific activity of plasma protein in mother and fetus after intra-amniotic injection of ^{35}S-protein. (Reproduced with permission from Amer. J. Obstet. Gynecol. 123:356, 1975).

SUMMARY AND SPECULATIONS

The observations of the present investigation, as well as those of several previously reported studies, indicate clearly that the fetus swallows amniotic fluid and, moreover, that the protein thus ingested is hydrolyzed in the fetal alimentary tract into its constituent amino acids. As illustrated diagramatically in figure 6, the amino acids liberated by proteolysis are absorbed and may have any of several fates. They may be

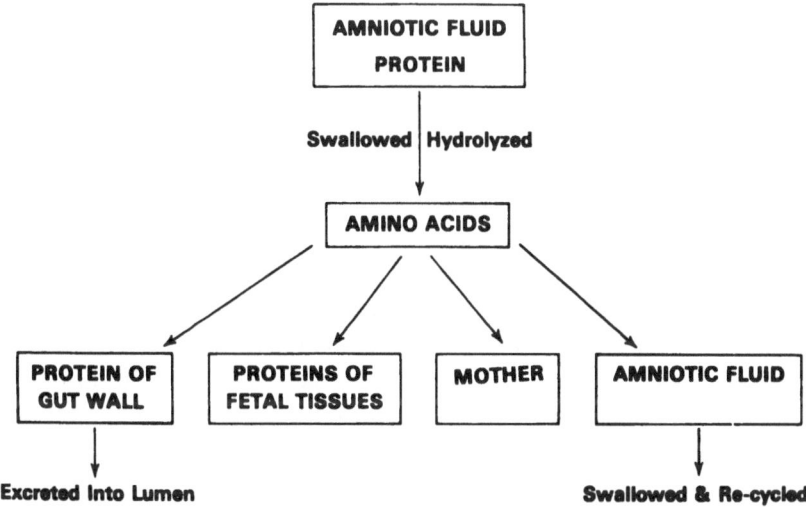

Fig. 6. Diagrammatic representation of the fate of amniotic fluid protein. See text for explanation.

(a) utilized in protein synthesis in the intestinal epithelium (part of which is later excreted into the gut lumen, (b) transported by blood to be incorporated in protein synthesis in any fetal tissue, (c) transferred across the placenta to enter the maternal pool, or (d) excreted into amniotic fluid to be swallowed again and recycled.

Fetal swallowing is of obvious importance in maintaining amniotic fluid volume (i.e., in preventing excessive amniotic fluid accumulation) during late intrauterine life. Why the fetus needs the capacity, as it has been here demonstrated to possess, to digest and absorb protein is considerably more obscure. The placenta serves its role in fetal nutrition quite adequately, at least under normal circumstances, and any nutritive function of amniotic fluid must be small indeed. For example, assuming average daily swallowing by the term human fetus of 300 ml of amniotic fluid containing protein in the amount of 300 mg/dl, approximately 1 g of protein per day would be provided, which probably represents no more than 10 or 15% of the protein requirements of the term fetus. Yet it must be acknowledged that the fact the fetus *does* ingest and metabolize amniotic fluid protein represents some sort of teleologic argument of purpose. Indeed, the clinical observation that congenital malformations interfering with swallowing, especially esophageal atresia (5), seem to be associated with intrauterine growth retardation further suggests a function of fetal deglutition in nutrition of the fetus. Thus, in spite of what appears to be at most a minor role in a quantitative sense, ingestion and digestion of amniotic fluid protein may serve some important function in preparing the fetal gastrointestinal tract for the proteolytic activity essential after birth.

Finally, demonstration that the fetus ingests, absorbs, and utilizes nutrients from the amniotic fluid raises the possibility of taking therapeutic advantage of this mechanism. A preliminary report (14) describing the intra-amniotic injection of amino acid mixtures in cases of suspected fetal growth retardation has provided some basis for cautious optimism regarding such an approach. The concept of "feeding the fetus" via the amniotic route is nothing more than an intriguing speculation at present. Yet it rests on a reasonable physiologic basis and, if both efficacy and safety can be demonstrated, might someday have clinical application.

REFERENCES

1. McLain, C.R., Jr. and P.T. Russell. (1970) Am. J. Obstet. Gynecol. 107:673.
2. Bishop, E.H. (1974) Int. J. Gynaec. Obstet. 12:117.
3. Prevedourakis, C., G. Papaevangelou, M. Garidi and D. Kaskarelis. (1975) Int. J. Gynaec. Obstet. 13:87.
4. Mandelbaum, B. and T.N. Evans. (1969) Am. J. Obstet. Gynecol. 104:365.
5. Cozzi, F. and A.W. Wilkinson. (1969) Arch. Dis. Childh. 44:59.
6. Grand, R.J., J.B. Watkins and F.M. Torti. (1976) Gastroenterology 70:790.
7. Pritchard, J.A. (1965) Obstet. Gynecol. 25:289.
8. Gitlin, D., J. Kumate, C. Morales, L. Noriega and N. Arevalo. (1972) Am. J. Obstet. Gynecol. 113:632.
9. Lev, R. and D. Orlic. (1972) Science 177:522.
10. Lev, R. and D. Orlic. (1973) Gastroenterology 65:60.
11. Baintner, K. Jr., (1973) Gastroenterology 65:695.
12. Pitkin, R.M. and W.A. Reynolds. (1975) Am. J. Obstet. Gynecol. 123:356.

13. JEEJEEBHOY, K.N., J. HO, G.R. GREENBERG, M.J. PHILLIPS, A. BRUCE-ROBERTSON and U. SODTKE. (1975) Biochem. J. 146:141.
14. HELLER, L. (1974) In: Parenteral Nutrition in Infancy and Childhood, Bode, H.H., and J.B. Warshaw eds., Plenum Press, New York and London, p. 206.

SOME OF THE CONSEQUENCES OF INTRA-UTERINE GROWTH RETARDATION

H. N. LAFEBER*, C. T. JONES** and T. P. ROLPH**

INTRODUCTION

About 5–14% of all live born children in Western Europe and the United States weigh 2500 g or less at birth (1–4). In other parts of the world this figure can be much higher, in India for instance it is about 27% (5). Approximately one third of these children are born small for gestational age (2). There are a number of clinical conditions commonly associated with these small newborn babies that are thought to have experienced intra-uterine growth retardation. These are summarized in table 1. The causes of the growth retardation are various. It occurs after infections such as rubella (32), or in association with drugtaking such as narcotics and alcohol (33–36) or as a result of genetic factors such as in Down's syndrome (37). However in most cases the causes are either unexplained

Table 1. *Clinical manifestations of intrauterine growth retardation.*

Clinical condition	Incidence	References
Asymmetric organ growth	+++	(6, 7, 8)
Hypoglycaemia	++	(9, 10, 11, 12, 13)
Polycythaemia	++	(14, 15, 16)
Haemoglobin rise	++	(14, 15)
Erythropoietin rise	++	(17)
Impaired gluconeogenesis	+	(18, 19, 20)
Depleted energy stores:		
glycogen	+	(21, 22)
fat	++	(23, 24, 25, 26)
Delay of skeletal growth	++	(27, 28)
Higher incidence of asphyxia	+	(14, 29)
Relatively few neurological disorders		
on examination	++	(30, 31)

* Erasmus University Rotterdam, Department of Pediatrics, Academic Hospital Rotterdam/Sophia Children's Hospital and Neonatal Unit, Rotterdam, the Netherlands.
** University of Oxford, Nuffield Institute for Medical Research, Oxford, England.

H.K.A. Visser (ed.), Nutrition and Metabolism of the Fetus and Infant, 43–62. All rights reserved.
Copyright © 1979 Martinus Nijhoff Publishers b.v., The Hague/Boston/London.

or there are indications of poor uterine or placental circulation (38). These latter conditions are frequently associated with toxaemia of pregnancy, hypertension, smoking, and multiple pregnancy (4, 39–43) or with direct evidence of vascular disorders such as abruption and premature separation of the placenta (6, 7, 44, 45). It is generally thought that reduced nutrient supply to the fetus is the consequence of these (46). By comparison malnutrition has a small but significant effect on fetal body weight (47). In animals severe protein and calorie malnutrition can cause large reductions in fetal weight with proportional effects on organ weight (48–50). A detailed description of the events occurring in intrauterine growth retardation is unlikely to come directly from human studies.

While it is clear that there can be some postnatal compensation for intrauterine growth retardation such as in "catch-up growth" in body weight (51–55) or in the postnatal growth of the brain (56–58), the long-term physiological consequences of this condition are not clear. It is known that the catch-up growth is not complete in many cases (51–58). Also the impairment of hepatic gluconeogenesis that has been suggested for the small-for-dates infant (18, 19, 20) may explain the higher incidence of ketotic hypoglycaemia that occurs in such infants later in childhood (19, 59).

ANIMAL STUDIES

To understand the causes and consequences of intrauterine growth retardation and to investigate the factors regulating fetal growth several approaches to causing intrauterine growth retardation in experimental animals have been used. It has been induced by reducing placental blood flow with uterine artery ligation (60–68) or microsphere injection into the placenta (69) and by reducing placental mass through surgical reduction of endometrial caruncles prior to conception (70–73) or ligation of interplacental vessels in the primate (74–76). In this review the data from such studies will be compared with that from man and that from our own investigation with the growth retarded fetal guinea pig. In our experiments one uterine artery of the pregnant guinea pig at 30 days of gestation was ligated essentially as described for the rat by WIGGLES-WORTH (60). The growth retarded fetal guinea pigs were compared with their littermate controls from the unoperated uterine horn 20 or 30 days later (fig. 1).

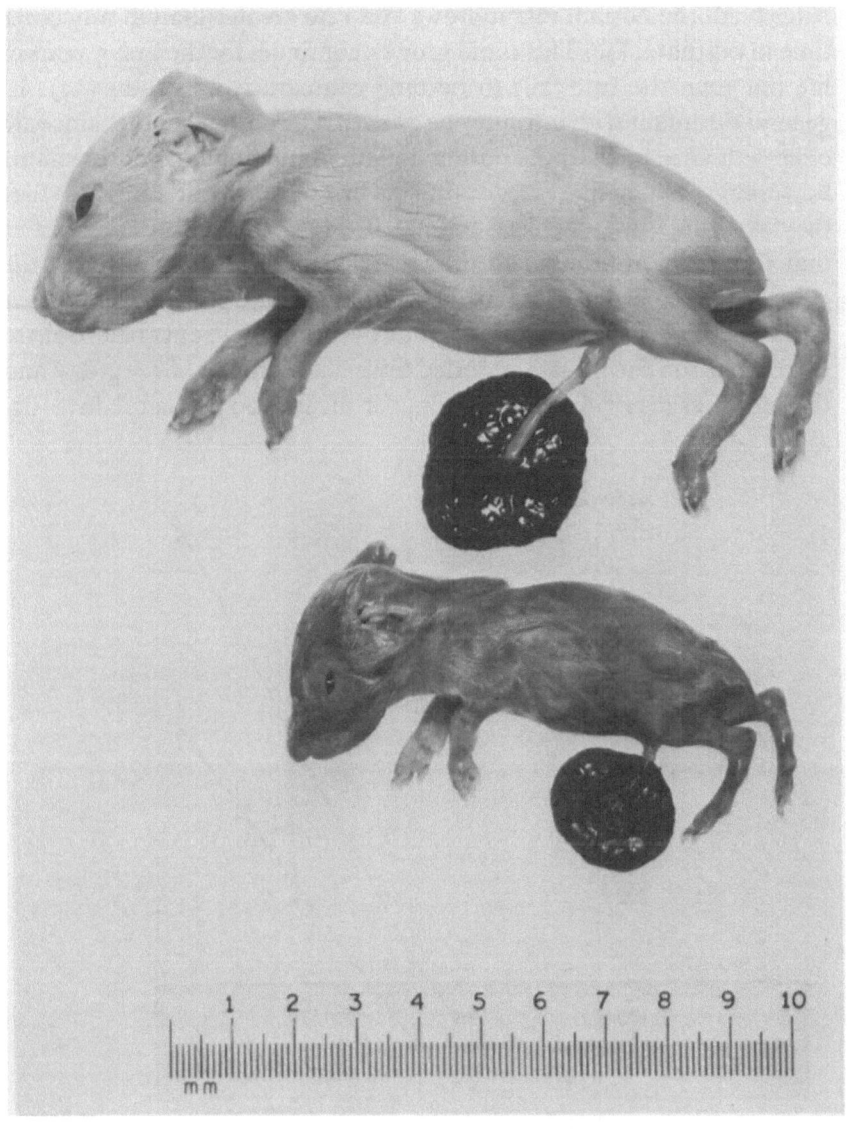

Fig. 1. Normal and intrauterine growth retarded 61 day fetal guinea pigs after 30 days of uterine artery ligation. The weight of the growth retarded fetus (lower) was 18 g and that of its normal littermate from the unoperated horn was 61 g (upper). Both were born alive.

PRE- AND POSTNATAL GROWTH

After birth the normal infant grows at a rate greater than at any other time in postnatal life. This rapid growth continues for the first 3 years of life but then the rate falls to become comparatively steady (77). In general the infant with intrauterine growth retardation has the same rate of growth after birth as the normal infant. Some small-for-dates infants however grow at higher rates during the first 6 months after birth, so that they eventually may achieve normal size (54, 58). This demonstrates that the major restriction to growth is intrauterine. Similarly in the guinea pig the normal postnatal growth rate at 10.6 g/day (over the first 20 days) is higher than that of 4.2 g/day over the last 20 days before birth. By comparison the growth retarded fetus has a growth of 1.7 g/day and this increases over 5 fold to 9.1 g/day for the first 20 postnatal days (fig. 2).

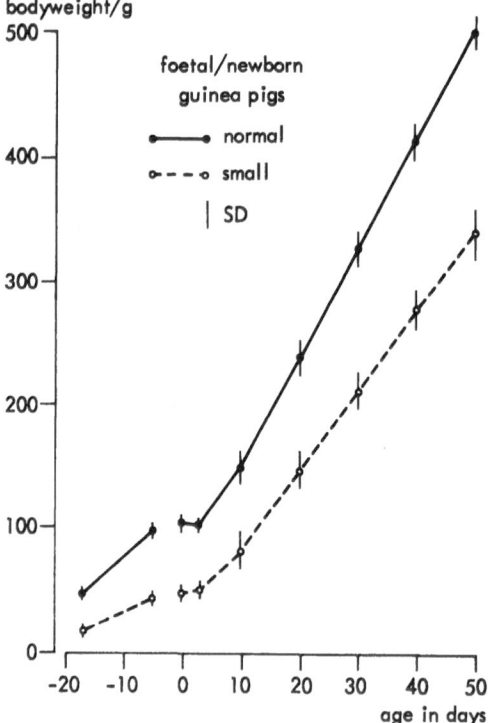

Fig. 2. Pre- and postnatal growth of normal (●) (n = 102) and intrauterine growth retarded guinea pigs (○) (n ·· 102).

ASYMMETRIC ORGAN GROWTH

A consistent feature of intrauterine growth retardation both in the animal experiments and in man is an asymmetric effect on organ growth (fig. 3). The reduction in the length of the fetus is much less than the fall in body weight. While there is a significant fall in brain weight in all

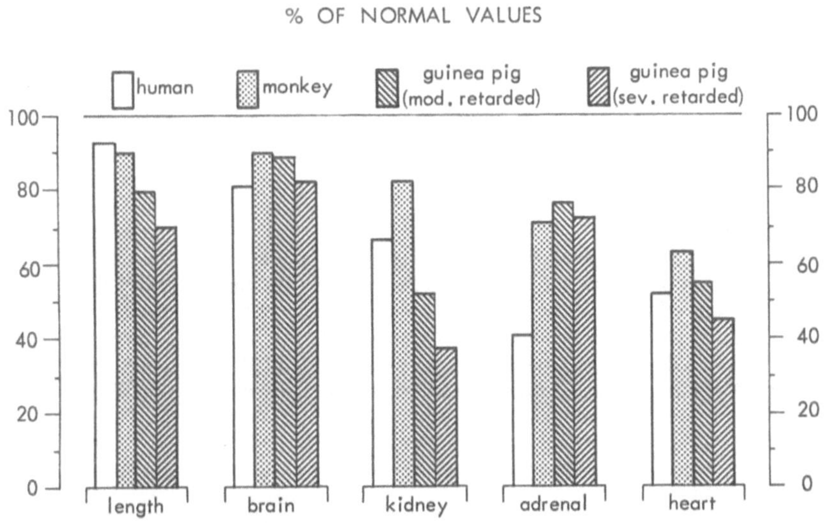

Fig. 3A. See caption to figure 3B.

studies this is much less than the change in body weight. The fall in the weight of the lung, kidney and heart is more or less in proportion to body weight. In contrast the weight of the liver and the spleen is much more reduced than body weight (fig. 3). The effects on the endocrine glands are variable particularly for the adrenal (fig. 3).

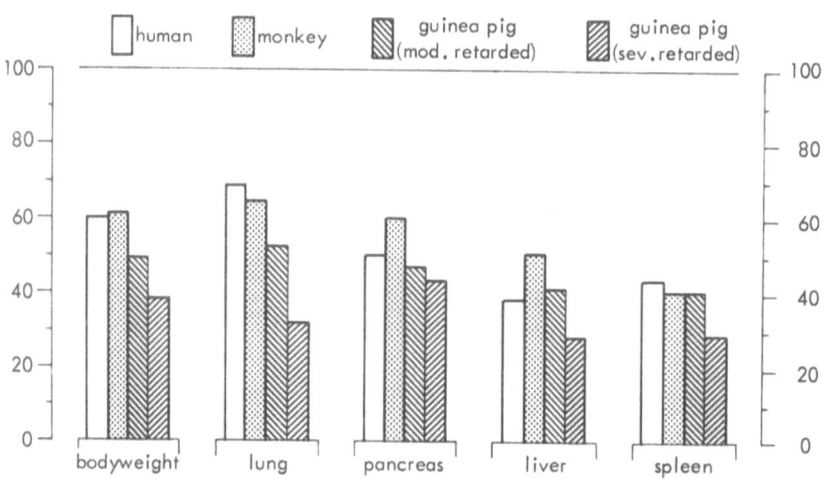

Fig. 3B.

Comparative organ size in growth retarded fetuses of man, monkey and guinea pig. The human data (□) is taken from (6, 8) and that of the monkey (▧) from (74, 75). The data for the guinea pig refers to 60–63 day fetuses studied after 30 days of uterine artery ligation. These fetuses are divided into those moderately retarded (▨) (mean body weight ± SD = 42.8 ± 4.9 g(40)) and those severely retarded (▨) (mean body weight ± SD = 30.2 ± 4.8 g (20)). Normal body weight at this age is 85.0 ± 11.0 (60).

THE PLACENTA

An important question of the growth retarded condition is the extent to which placental function is affected. Is the transport potential of the placenta reduced? Does it make compensatory adjustments in the way it handles nutrients or in its secretion of hormones to the mother and the fetus? At present the data are largely anatomical. There are numerous reports indicating changes in gross placental anatomy in association with growth retardation that have been used to suggest a fall in the effective exchange area of the placenta (6, 45, 46, 79–81). There are also reports of an increase in the fetal/placental weight ratio which has led to the suggestion that the fetus compensates for the reduction in placental weight (70, 80). However infarctions are frequently seen in the placenta of the growth retarded fetus (6, 45, 46, 78, 79) and in the guinea pig, for instance, these can cover a large part of the placenta (fig. 4). The effect of this for the 60–63 day fetal guinea pig is to decrease the fetal/placental weight ratio from 16.7 ± 2.2 (52) to 13.2 ± 2.1 (18) (P < 0.001). Moreover placental weight correlates well with fetal weight over the latter third of gestation in the normal but not in the growth retarded fetal guinea pig (fig. 5).

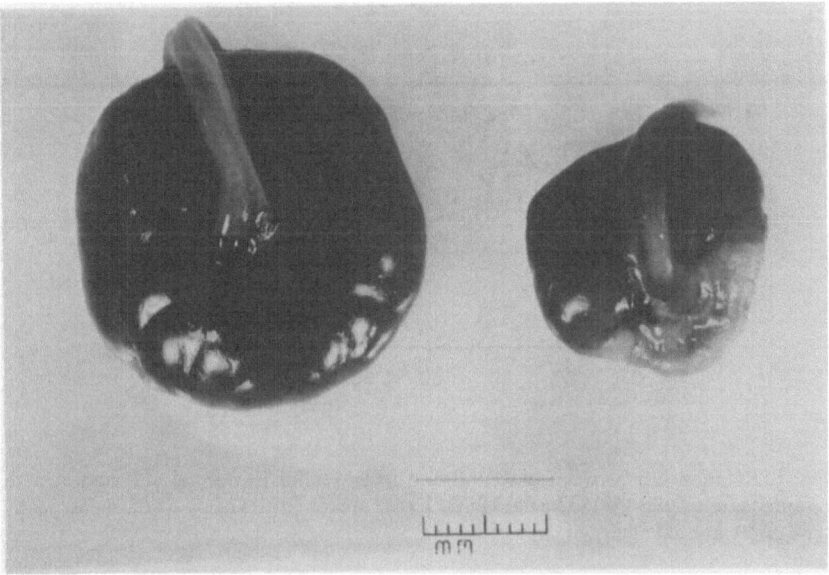

Fig. 4. The placentae of a normal (left) and intrauterine growth retarded (right) fetal guinea pig (percentage of normal body weight = 42%). Note the infarction in the placenta of the small fetus.

There is some preliminary evidence from studies with radio-active analogues that nutrient transport from the mother to the growth retarded fetal rat is less than that to the normal weight littermate (82).

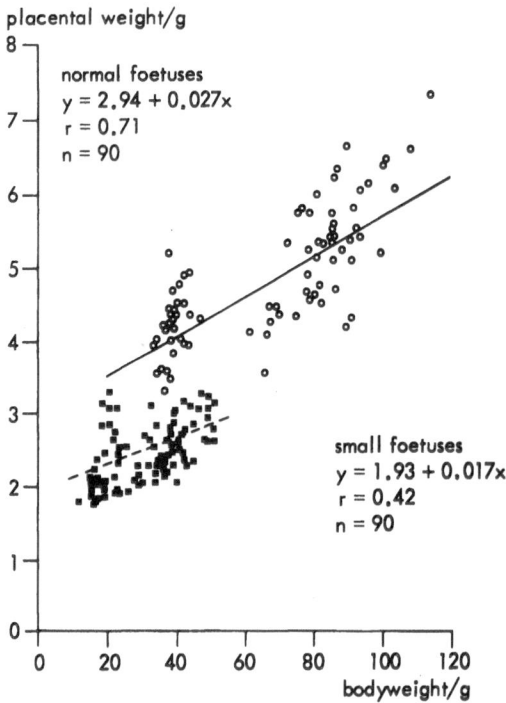

Fig. 5. Relationship between placental and fetal weights in normal (O) and growth retarded guinea pigs (■). The data in each case are for fetuses of 49–51 days and 60–63 days of gestational age.

FETAL METABOLISM

An impairment of placental transport is suggested by the frequent occurrence of low blood glucose concentration in growth retarded fetuses (table 2). Plasma free fatty acid concentrations are similarly low, which may also relate to a modification of placental transport as in a number of species some of the free fatty acids in the fetal circulation are of maternal origin (83). The existence of fetal hypoxaemia also supports this view (71). The elevated alanine concentration in the plasma of growth retarded fetuses and human newborns (table 2) is probably a consequence of reduced metabolism by the peripheral tissues, while the high ammonia concentration probably reflects a poorly developed urea cycle (see below).

Immediately after birth hepatic glycogen and triglyceride deposits are

Table 2. *Plasma metabolite and hormone concentration of growth retarded fetuses and human newborns.*

	Percentage of normal values			
Species	Man	Sheep	Rat	Guinea Pig
Foetal body weight	65***	75**	66***	38***
Glucose	80*	55**	70***	61***
Alanine	184*	70**	151**	234**
Ammonia	137*	-	--	925***
Free Fatty Acids	100–125[a]	84*	77**	56***
Insulin	100–140[a]	47**	46*	39***
Glucagon	153	..	129	480
References	(18, 86, 88)	(71, 72, 73)	(84, 62, 85)	[b]
	(11[a], 87[a])			

[a] data refers to plasma samples taken 2–24 hr after birth, all other data in this table refers to venous cord blood.
[b] data of growth retarded fetal guinea pigs at 60–63 days of gestation after 30 days of uterine artery ligation.
* $P < 0.05$ ** $P < 0.01$ *** $P < 0.001$.

important energy stores that are rapidly mobilized. In the small-for-dates newborn infant it has been suggested that the hepatic glycogen stores are less than normal (table 3) and that this may therefore contribute to the neonatal hypoglycaemia. Unfortunately in these studies it is not possible te exclude the effects of the poor neonatal condition prior to death. Animal studies show no consistent picture. The hepatic glycogen concentration of the growth retarded fetus is less than normal in the rat (61–65, 90–91), unaffected in the monkey (74, 75) and higher than normal in the guinea pig (table 3). In addition to the chemical measurements, hepatocytes of growth retarded fetal guinea pigs show much more glycogen in their cytoplasm than do controls (fig. 6). In general triglyceride stores in adipose tissue and particularly in the liver are reduced by intrauterine growth retardation (table 3). Thus although reduction of glycogen stores, whether they are hepatic, in the heart or in skeletal muscle (table 4), is not a common feature of intrauterine growth retardation, a reduction in mobilizable triglyceride stores probably is.

Because of the large changes in liver and skeletal muscle mass associated with growth retardation gross changes in organ composition might be expected. In addition to the changes in glycogen and triglycerides the activities of a variety of enzymes are much affected (table

Table 3. *Energy stores in growth retarded fetuses and human newborns*[b].

	Percentage of normal values			
Species	Man	Monkey	Rat	Guinea Pig
Foetal body weight	30–60[***]	65[***]	66[***]	38[***]
Liver				
glycogen wt/g liver	35	100	43–81[***]	164[**]
wt liver/g bwt.		98	45[***]	125
triglycerides				
wt/g liver		19[*]	–	56[*]
wt liver/g bwt.		21[*]	–	53[*]
Adipose tissue				
perirenal fat				
wt/g bwt.		..	–	90[***]
interscapular fat				
wt/g bwt.		..	62[**]	–
Total fat wt/g bwt.	reduced	--	73[**]	–
References	(21–26)	(74–76)	(61–64) (89–91)	[a]

[a] data of growth retarded fetal guinea pigs at 60–63 days of gestation after 30 days of uterine artery ligation.
[b] data refers to growth retarded fetuses near term and where appropriate to human growth retarded newborns shortly after birth.
[*] $P < 0.05$ [**] $P < 0.01$ [***] $P < 0.001$.

4). Hexokinase activity is increased in liver and skeletal muscle, while that of phosphofructokinase, phosphoenolpyruvate carboxykinase and some enzymes associated with the metabolism of amino acids and with the urea cycle is reduced (table 4). The relative changes in the hexokinase/phosphofructokinase ratio may explain the maintenance of glycogen synthesis despite the hypoglycaemia and low plasma insulin concentration. The low activity of phosphoenolpyruvate carboxykinase is consistent with the suggested impairment of the hepatic gluconeogenesis in this condition (18–20). The low activities of some of the aminotransferases indicate reduced rates of peripheral amino acid metabolism and are consistent with the elevated plasma amino acid concentration. The low activity of carbamyl phosphate synthetase is consistent with the poor rate of urea synthesis in the liver of the growth retarded fetus (unpublished observations).

Livers from growth retarded fetuses have proportionately less cytosol,

Table 4. *Changes in tissue composition and enzyme activities of liver, heart and skeletal muscle of the growth retarded fetal guinea pig*[a].

| | Percentage of normal values | | | | | |
| Foetal organ | Liver | | Heart | | Skeletal muscle | |
Percentage of gestation	75	90	75	90	75	90
Glycogen	314**	164**	104	164*	91	127
Triglycerides	177*	56*	224*	225*	–	–
Hexokinase	160**	188***	106	108	100	136
Phosphofructokinase	40**	38***	62*	71	73*	50**
Phosphoenolpyruvate carboxykinase	31***	17***	–	–	–	–
Aspartate aminotransferase	63*	77**	105	96	82	72*
Alanine aminotransferase	<10	12***	<10	56*	58	38*
Glutamate dehydrogenase	23***	27***	101	97	104	100
Carbamyl phosphate synthetase	27*	19**	–	–	–	–
$(Na^+ + K^+)$-ATPase	–		107	93	–	–
Ca^{++}-ATPase	–		69*	81	90	52***

[a] data of growth retarded fetal guinea pigs at 49–51 and 60–63 days of gestation after 20 and 30 days of uterine artery ligation.
* $P < 0.05$ ** $P < 0.01$ *** $P < 0.001$.

fewer mitochondria and less endoplasmic reticulum (fig. 6). These also have more haematopoietic cells than controls, although this in no way accounts for the enzyme changes. A low Ca^{2+}-ATPase activity in skeletal muscle in the growth retarded fetal guinea pig (table 4) suggests an effect on the functional development of this organ. The effects of growth retardation on the heart are less pronounced than for the liver or skeletal muscle, although there is also a much lower activity of alanine amino-transferase and phosphofructokinase in these hearts, the latter probably contributing to the maintenance of the cardiac glycogen concentration.

Many of the effects of growth retardation on the fetal guinea pig are consistent with delays in the processes of normal development. An important question to be answered is by which mechanism restriction of intrauterine growth rate brings about selective changes in organ growth and composition. It is likely that a reduced supply of nutrients via the placenta is a primary cause. Of the secondary causes, one of the major

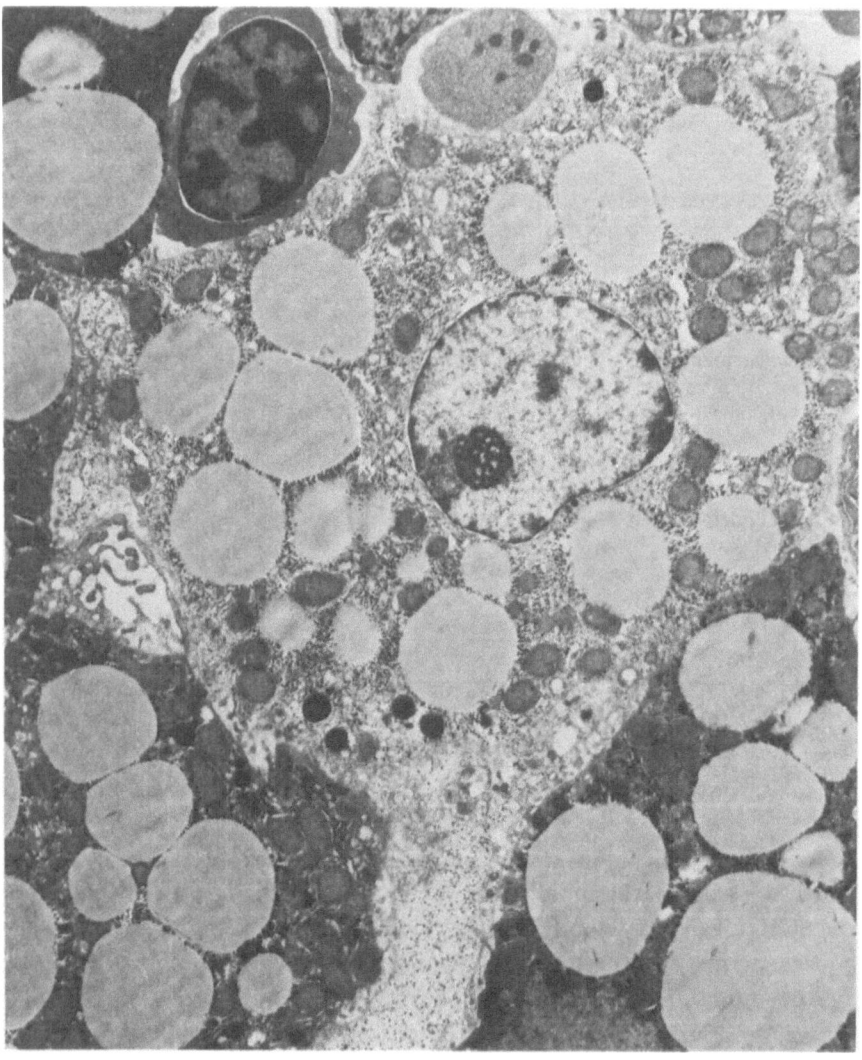

Fig. 6A. See caption to figure 6B.

hormonal consequences of this condition is a lower plasma insulin concentration and elevated glucagon/insulin ratio (table 2). Insulin is probably an important growth-promoting hormone for the fetus (92). Moreover, it is essential for the normal proliferation of many cells and particulary of hepatocytes (93, 94).

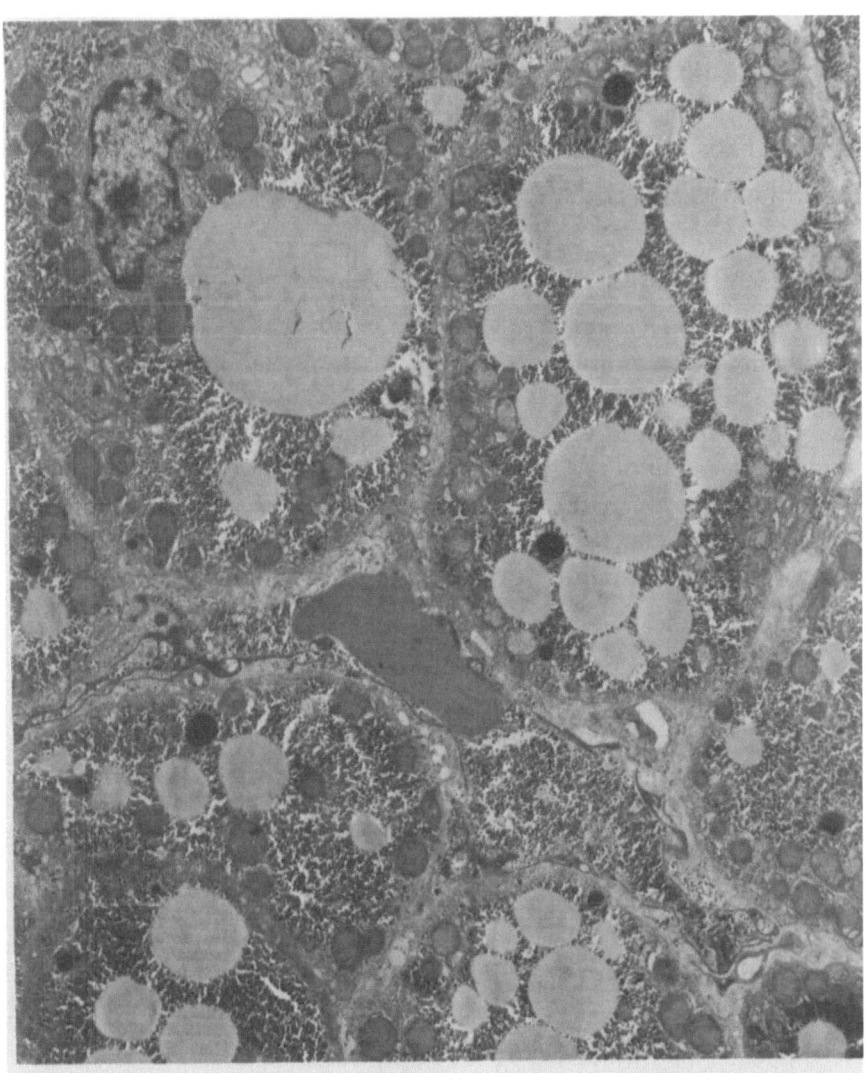

Fig. 6B.

Hepatocyte structure in the liver of normal (A) and growth retarded (B) fetal guinea pigs. The normal fetus was 62 days and the growth retarded was 61 days of gestational age. Linear magnification is × 1000. Note that the hepatocyte of the growth retarded fetus has more glycogen and less fat, mitochondria and cytosol.

A persistent low plasma insulin concentration may promote the growth of those tissues that are relatively insulin insensitive like the brain against those like liver and skeletal muscle that are sensitive to the hormone. In the growth retarded fetus the relationship between glucose and insulin is still maintained and thus changes in nutrient supply are probably the primary determinant of the fetal responses.

BRAIN GROWTH

Even though in growth retarded fetuses the growth of the brain is maintained relative to that of the other organs (fig. 7), it is clear that there is a significant reduction in its mass. Moreover, it is striking that in the various species in which intrauterine growth retardation has been studied the extent of the reduction in brain mass (i.e. 15–20%) is very similar (fig. 7). The reduction in brain mass is associated with a similar fall in DNA, RNA and protein content (table 5). Whether this in all cases is associated with a fall in neuronal and glial cell content is not clear.

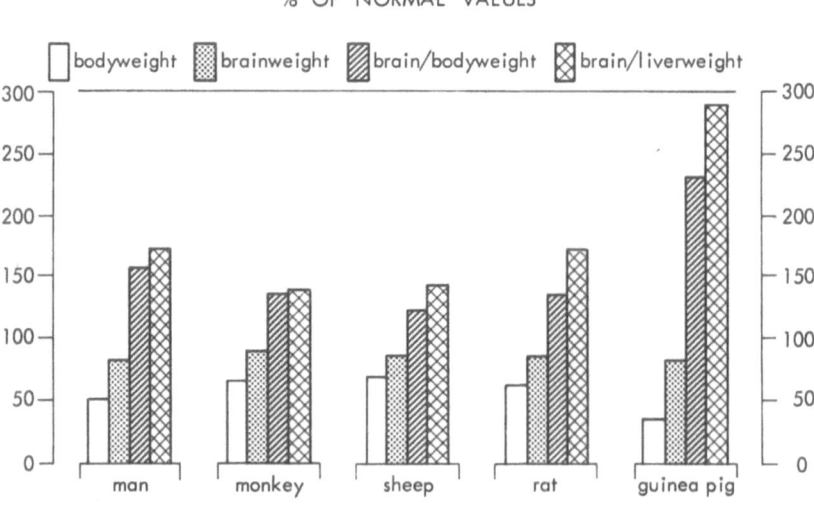

Fig. 7. The relative size of the brain in growth retarded fetuses of a number of species. The data for man is from (8), that for the monkey from (74–76), that for the sheep from (69) and that for the rat from (62). Data of the guinea pig refers to 60–63 day fetal guinea pigs after 30 days of uterine artery ligation.

Table 5. *Changes in brain composition of growth retarded fetuses*[b].

Species	Percentage of normal values					
	Man	Monkey	Rat	Rabbit	Guinea pig	
Foetal body weight	61**	65***	67	85***	48**	38***
Cerebral weight	79*	90*	91	87***	86**	79***
Total cerebral DNA	81	87	99	88***	93*	72**
Total cerebral RNA	-	91*	104	–	71**	69**
Total cerebral protein	89	74	95	85***	81	74
References	(98)	(74)	(99, 100)	(67)	[a]	

[a] data of growth retarded fetal guinea pigs at 60–63 days of gestation after 30 days of uterine artery ligation.
[b] data refers to growth retarded fetuses near term; the human data refers to growth retarded fetuses from 34 weeks to term.
* $P < 0.05$ ** $P < 0.01$ *** $P < 0.001$.

There are examples of restricted brain growth causing a deficit in neuronal and in glial cell numbers and in the extent of myelination (95–97). In addition in growth retarded fetal guinea pigs the rate of prenatal myelination is slower than normal (unpublished observations). The extent to which any prenatal deficit can be made up postnatally is unclear and is likely to vary with the species. Brain development is largely postnatal in the rat, is pre- and postnatal in man and is prenatal in the guinea pig (101) although even here some postnatal neurogenesis occurs (102). In man available clinical data suggests that if the growth restriction occurs after 26 weeks, at which time much neurogenesis and some myelination has occurred (103), the brain mass is reduced but there is postnatal compensation probably to produce a normal sized brain. Growth restriction before 26 weeks causes permanently stunted brain growth and neurological damage (56).

SKELETAL GROWTH

Another organ system that is affected by intrauterine growth retardation is the skeletal system. There are reports of poor skeletal development in small-for-dates newborn infants (27, 28). Similarly growth retarded fetal guinea pigs have poor skeletal development (fig. 8). This is associated with low activity in fetal plasma of factors promoting sulphate incorporation into cartilage (unpublished observations).

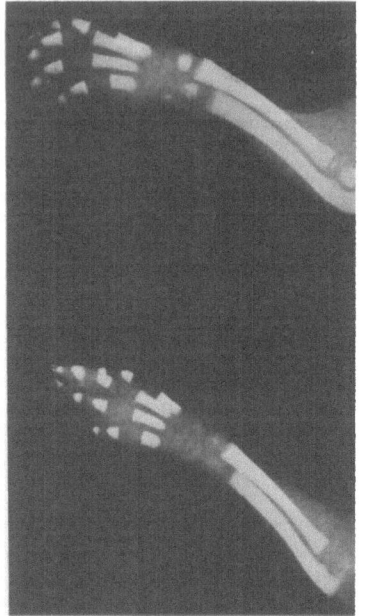
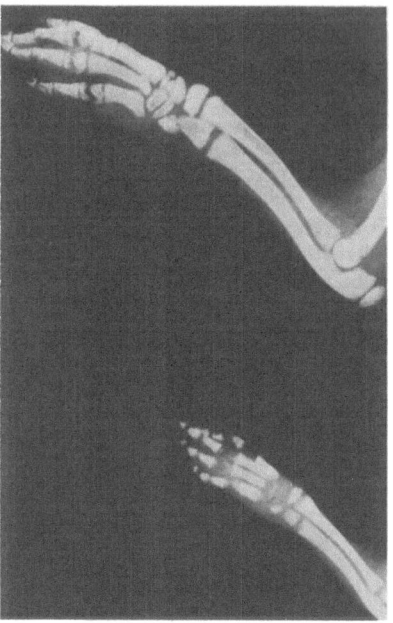

A   B

Figs. 8A + B. X-ray pictures of the forelimbs of normal (upper) and growth retarded (lower) fetal guinea pigs of 50 (A) and 61 (B) days of gestational age. The body weight and body length were respectively 33.0 g and 19.3 g (10.1 cm and 8.4 cm) in the 50 day fetuses (A) and 82.2 g and 23.6 g (14.5 cm and 9.7 cm) in the 61 day fetuses (B). Note the delayed ossification in phalanges, carpals, metacarpals, radius and ulna of the growth retarded fetuses.

SUMMARY

Intrauterine growth retardation affects the normal development of at least the liver, spleen, bone, pancreas, adrenal and to a lesser extent that of the heart and the brain. Many of the effects are indicative of delays in development. These may be caused by a reduced nutrient supply and secondarily by changes in circulating insulin and glucagon. The post-natal consequences of this condition have not been extensively investigated although there is ample evidence from man of hypoglycaemia, polycythaemia and neurological disorder.

ACKNOWLEDGEMENTS

This work was completed during the tenure of a Sophia Foundation Research Fellowship (H.N.L.) and a Medical Research Council Scholarship (T.P.R.) with the help of grants from the Royal Society, the Medical Research Council and the Sophia Foundation for Medical Research. We wish to thank Professor G.S. Dawes and Professor H.K.A. Visser for their interest and encouragement.

REFERENCES

1. GEYERSTAM, G. (1969) Public Health Reports 84:939.
2. GRUENWALD, P. (1964) Pediatrics 34:157.
3. LUBCHENCO. L.O.. D.T. SEARLS and J.V. BRAZIE. (1972) J. of Pediatrics 81:814.
4. SCOTT, K.E. and R. USHER. (1966) Amer. J. Obstet. Gynecol. 94:951.
5. SHARMA, U. (1968) Indian J. Pediat. 35:454.
6. GRUENWALD, P. (1963) Biol. Neonate 5:215.
7. GRUENWALD, P. (1968) In: Aspects of Praematurity and Dysmaturity. Jonxis, J.H.P., H.K.A. Visser and J.A. Troelstra eds., Stenfert Kroese, Leiden, Holland, p. 37.
8. NAEYE, R.L. (1965) Arch. Pathol. 79:284.
9. NELIGAN, G.A., E. ROBSON and J. WATSON. (1963) Lancet 1:1282.
10. LUBCHENCO, L.O. and H. BARD. (1971) Pediatrics 47:831.
11. BLUM, D., J. DODION, H. LOEB, P. WILKIN and P.O. HUBINOT. (1969) Arch. Dis. Childh. 44:304.
12. CORNBLATH, M., G.B. ODELL and E.Y. LEVIN. (1959) J. of Pediatrics 55:545.
13. CORNBLATH, M., S.H. WYBREGT, G.S. BAENS and R.I. KLEIN. (1964) Pediatrics 33:388.
14. LUGO, G. and G. CASSADY. (1971) Amer. J. Obstet. Gynecol. 109:615.
15. HAWORTH, J.C., L. DILLING and M.K. YOUNOSZAI. (1967) Lancet 2:901.
16. HUMBERT, J.R., H. ABELSON. W.E. HATHAWAY and F.C. BATTAGLIA. (1969) J. of Pediatrics 75:812.
17. FINNE, P.H. (1966) Acta Paed. Scand. 55:478.
18. HAYMOND, M.H.. I.E. KARL and A.S. PAGLIARA. (1974) New Engl. J. Med. 291:322.
19. CORNBLATH, M. and R. SCHWARTZ. (1976) In: Disorders of Carbohydrate Metabolism in Infancy. W.B. Saunders Company, Philadelphia, Pa., p. 167.
20. MESTYAN, J., G. SOLTESZ, K. SCHULTZ and M. HORVATH. (1975) J. of Pediatrics 87:409.
21. SHELLEY, H.J. and G.A. NELIGAN. (1966) Brit. Med. Bull. 22:34.
22. DAWKINS, M.J.R. (1964) Proc Roy. Soc. Med. 57:1063.
23. BRANS, Y.W., J.W. SUMNERS, H.S. DWECK and G. CASSADY. (1974) Ped. Res. 8:215..
24. DAUNCEY, M.J., G. GANDY and D. GAIRDNER. (1977) Arch. Dis. Childh. 52:223.
25. METTAU, J.W., H.J. DEGENHART, H.K.A. VISSER and W.P.S. HOLLAND. (1977) Ped. Res. 11:1097.
26. METTAU, J.W. 1978. Measurement of Total Body Fat in Low Birth Weight Infants. Thesis, Rotterdam.

27. SCOTT, K.E. and R. USHER. (1964) New Eng. J. Med. 27:822.
28. WILSON, M.G., H.I. MEYERS and A.H. PETERS (1967) Pediatrics 40:213.
29. LOW, J.A., R.W. BOSTON and S.R. PANCHAM. (1972) Am. J. Obstet. Gynecol. 113:351.
30. FITZHARDINGE, P.M. and E.M. STEVEN. (1972) Pediatrics 50:50.
31. DRILLIEN, C.M. (1972) Develop. Med. Child. Neurol. 14:575.
32. COOPER, L., R. GREEN, S. KRUGMAN et al. (1965) Amer. J. Dis. Childh. 110:416.
33. RAYE, J.R., J.W. DUBIN and J.N. BLECHNER. (1977) Biol. Neonate 32:222.
34. NAYE, R.L., W. BLANC, W. LE BLANC and H.A. KHATAMEE. (1973) J. Pediat. 83:1055.
35. ZELSON, C., E. RUBIO and E. WASSERMAN. (1971) Pediatrics 48:178.
36. JONES, K.L., D.W. SMITH, A.P. STREISSGUTH and N.C. MYRIANTHAPOULOS. (1974) Lancet 1:1076.
37. POLANI, P.E. (1974) In: Size at Birth, CIBA Foundation Symposium 27, Associated Scientific Publishers, Amsterdam, p. 127.
38. DAWES, G.S. (1974) In: Size at Birth, CIBA Foundation Symposium 27, Associated Scientific Publishers, Amsterdam, p. 383.
39. BUTLER, N. (1974) In: Size at Birth, CIBA Foundation Symposium 27, Associated Scientific Publishers, Amsterdam, p. 379.
40. DE SOUZA, S.W., R.W. JOHN and B. RICHARDS. (1976) Brit. J. Obst. Gynaec. 83:292.
41. LOW, J.A. and R.S. GALBRAITH. (1974) Obst. and Gynec. 44:122.
42. GRUENWALD, P. (1970) Biol. Neonate 15:79.
43. MILLER, H.C., K. HASSANEIN and P.A. HENSLEIGH. (1976) Amer. J. Obstet. Gynecol. 125:55.
44. GRUENWALD, P., H. LEVIN and H. YOUSEM. (1968) Amer. J. Obstet. Gynecol. 102:604.
45. FOX, H. (1975) In: The Placenta and Its Maternal Supply Line, Gruenwald, P. ed., MTP Co. Ltd., Lancaster, p. 197.
46. GRUENWALD, P. (1974) In: Size at Brith, CIBA Foundation Symposium 27, Associated Scientific Publishers, Amsterdam, p. 3.
47. SMITH, C. (1947) J. of Pediat. 30:229.
48. LEE, C.J. and B.F. CHOW. (1965) J. Nutrition 87:439.
49. CHOW, B.F. and C.J. LEE. (1964) J. Nutrition 82:10.
50. WIDDOWSON, E.M. and R.A. McCANCE. (1963) Proc. Roy. Soc. B. 158:329.
51. BECK, G.J. and B.J. VAN DEN BERG. (1975) J. of Pediatr. 86:504.
52. McCANCE, R.A. and E.M. WIDDOWSON. (1974) Proc. Roy. Soc. B. 185:1.
53. CRUISE, M.O. (1973) Pediatrics 51:620.
54. FITZHARDINGE, P.M. and E.M. STEVEN. (1972) Pediatrics 49:671.
55. OUNSTED, M. and T.E. TAYLOR. (1971) Dev. Med. Child. Neurol. 13:421.
56. FANCOURT, R., D.R. HARVEY, A.P. NORMAN and S. CAMPBELL. (1976) Brit. Med. J. 1:1435.
57. WALLIS, S., D. SHAMSI and D. HARVEY. (1977) In: Poor Intrauterine Fetal Growth, Salvadori, B. and A. Bacchi Modena eds., Centro Minerva Medica, Rome, p. 567.
58. BABSON, S.G. (1970) J. of Pediatrics 77:11.
59. GRUNT, J.A., M.C. McCARRY, A. McCOLLUM and J.D. GOULD. (1970) Yale J. Biol. Med. 42:420.
60. WIGGLESWORTH, J.S. (1964) J. Pathol. Bacteriol. 88:1.
61. HOHENAUER, L. and W. OH. (1969) J. Nutr. 99:23.
62. ROUX, J.M., C. TORDET CARIDROIT and C. CHANEZ. (1970) Biol. Neonate 15:342.

63. NITZAN, M. and H. GROFFMAN. (1971) Biol. Neonate 17:420.
64. OH, W., M.D. D'AMODIO, L.L. YAP, L. HOHENAUER and J.A. GUY. (1970) Amer. J. Obstet. Gynec. 108:415.
65. HOHENAUER, L. (1971) Pädiatr. u. Pädol. 6:1.
66. LUGO, G., L. O'NEIL and G. CASSADY. (1971) Amer. J. Obstet. Gynec. 110:358.
67. VAN MARTENS, E., S. HAREL and S. ZAMENHOF. (1975) Biol. Neonate 26:221.
68. DIETZMANN, K. and W. LESSEL. (1976) Exp. Path. Bd. 12:309.
69. CREASY, R.K., C.T. BARRETT, M. DE SWIET, K.V. KAHANPAÄ and A.M. RUDOLPH. (1972) Amer. J. Obstet. Gynec. 112:566.
70. ALEXANDER, G. (1964) J. Repr. Fert. 7:307.
71. ROBINSON, J.S., C.T. JONES, J.R.G. CHALLIS and G.D. THORBURN. (1976) Ped. Res. 10:891.
72. ROBINSON, J.S., I HART, C.T. JONES and G.D. THORBURN. (1977) Brit. J. Obst. Gynec 84:535.
73. JONES, C.T. and J.S. ROBINSON. (1979) In: Maternal Affects on Fetal Growth and Development, 4th International Symposium of the British Society of Developmental Biology, Balls. M. and D. Newth eds., Cambridge University Press.
74. HILL, D.E. (1974) In: Size at Birth, CIBA Foundation Symposium 27, Associated Scientific Publishers, Amsterdam, p. 99,.
75. MYERS, R.E., D.E. HILL, A.B. HOLT, R.E. SCOTT, E.D. MELLITS and D.B. CHEEK. (1971) Biol. Neonate 18:379.
76. HILL, D.E., R.E. MYERS, A.B. HOLT, R.E. SCOTT and D.B. CHEEK. (1971) Biol. Neonate 19:68.
77. TANNER, J.M. (1962) In: Growth at Adolescence, Blackwell Scientific Publications, Oxford.
78. ROBERTSON, W.B., J. BROSENS and G. DIXON. (1975) In: Human Placentation, Brosens, J., G. Dixon and W.B. Robertson eds., Excerpta Medica, Amsterdam.
79. GRUENWALD, P. (1975) In: The Placenta and Its Maternal Supply Line, Gruenwald, P. ed., MTP Co. Ltd., Lancaster, p. 336.
80. THOMSON, A.M., W.Z. BILLEWICZ and F.E. HYTTEN. (1969) Brit. J. Obstet. Gynaec. 76:865.
81. MYERS, R.E. and T. FUJIKURA. (1968) Amer. J. Obstet. Gynec. 100:846.
82. NITZAN, M., S. ORLOFF and J.D. SCHULMAN. (1977) Ped. Res. 11:410.
83. JONES, C.T. (1976) Biochem. J. 156:357.
84. MANNIELLO, R.L., A.J. ADAMS and P.M. FARRELL. (1977) Ped. Res. 11:840.
85. GIRARD, J.R., C. CHANEZ, A. KERVAN, C. TORDET CARIDROIT and R. ASSAN. (1976) Biol. Neonate 29:262.
86. RUBALTELLI, F.F., P.A. FORMENTIN and L. TATO. (1970) Biol. Neonate 15:129.
87. WILLIAMS, P.R., R.H. FISER, M.A. SPERLING and W. OH. (1975) New Engl. J. Med. 292:612.
88. MELICHAR, V., M. NOVAK, V. SABATA, P. HAHN and O. KOLDOVSKY. (1965) Phys. Bohem. 14:553.
89. COGNEVILLE, A.M., N. CIVIDINO and C. TORDET CARIDROIT. (1975) J. Nutr. 105:982.
90. CHANEZ, C., C. TORDET CARIDROIT and J.M. ROUX. (1971) Biol. Neonate 18:58.
91. NITZAN, M. and M. GROFFMAN. (1970) Isr. J. Med. Sci. 6:697.
92. BASSETT, J.M. and C.T. JONES. (1976) In: Fetal Physiology and Medicine, Beard, R.W. and P.W. Nathanielsz eds., W.B. Saunders Co. Ltd. London, p. 158.
93. LEFFERT, H.L. and K.S. KOCH. (1977) In: Growth, Nutrition and Metabolism of Cells in Culture, Rothblad, G.H. and V.J. Cristofals eds., Academic Press Inc. New York, Vol. 3, p. 225.

94. STARZL. T.E., A. FRANCAVILLA, C.G. HALGRINSON, F.R. FRANCAVILLA, K.A. PORTER, T. BROWN and C.W. PUTMAN. (1973) Surg. Gynec. and Obst. 137:179.
95. DOBBING, J. and J. SANDS. (1977) Arch. Dis. Childh. 48:757.
96. DOBBING, J., J.W. HOPEWELL and A. LYNCH. (1971) Exp. Neurol. 32:439.
97. CULLEY, W.J. and R.D. LINEBERGER. (1968) J. of Nutr. 96:375.
98. CHASE, H.P., N.N. WELCH, C.S. DABIERE, N.S. VASAN and L.J. BUTTERFIELD. (1972) Pediatrics 50:403.
99. WINICK, M., J.A. BRASEL and P. ROSSO. (1972) In: Current Concepts in Nutrition Vol. 1 Nutrition and Development, Winick, M. ed., John Wiley and Sons, p. 49.
100. WINICK, M. (1976) Malnutrition and Brain Development, Oxford University Press, New York, p. 106.
101. DOBBING, J. and J. SANDS. (1970) Brain Res. 17:115.
102. ALTMAN, J. and G.D. DAS. (1967) Nature 214:1098.
103. DOBBING, J. (1973) In: Applied Neurochemistry, Davison, A.N. and J. Dobbing eds., Blackwell Scientific Publications, Oxford.

DISCUSSION

PAPER BY R.D.G. MILNER

M. Young: What age were the human fetuses whose livers Schwartz studied? Christensen's early work showed that fetal guinea pig liver did not accumulate AIB very actively until after birth. (CHRISTENSEN, H.N. and J.B. CLIFFORD. (1963) J. Biol. Chem. 238:1743.)

R.D.G. Milner: Schwartz studied human fetal livers from 6 to 20 weeks gestational age. The metabolic actions that I described were demonstrable in all cases by 8–9 weeks and suggest that the human fetal hepatocyte becomes sensitive to glucagon before insulin.

I think there may be important species differences in the balance of the metabolic action of the hormones, which await further study, especially between primates and other commonly studied experimental animals.

C.T. Jones: Just a note of caution on receptors. Usually if you take adult tissues there is only a small proportion, a few percent, of the total receptors required for the metabolic action of the hormone. This is illustrated well in the rabbit fetus, for instance at about 29 days there is very little binding, if any binding, of glucagon to the hepatocyte and between then and 5 days postnatal there is a very large increase in binding. However, in the perfused liver both at 29 days of fetal life and at 5 days postnatal the same rise in cyclic AMP and substantial glycogenolysis occur at physiological glucagon concentrations.

R.D.G. Milner: Yes I take that point. I think it is going to be important to continue to perform experiments in parallel, those which are essentially a bioassay of receptors and those which are direct radio-immunological studies of receptor populations upon the cells.

A. Ballabriga: Do you have some experience with insulin receptors in placenta membranes at different gestational age of the animals?

We have recently studied this in 26 human placentas, devided in 3 groups – full-term, small-for-dates and preterm but normal for gestational age – and we found maximal values for insulin receptors between 20 and 28 weeks gestational age. The amount of insulin receptors is very much reduced in the small-for-dates group as compared with the other two groups.

R.D.G. Milner: No, I did not deal with other tissues, because of time, in this presentation.

M. Young: May I ask Professor Ballabriga whether he looked at mixed membranes in the placenta or whether he separated the surface microvillous membranes from the intracellular membranes?

A. Ballabriga: This is a very interesting question. We speak only about affinity for insulin receptors in placenta membranes, and we cannot specify if they are from the maternal or the fetal side of the placenta. We obtained highly purified membranes from placentas immediately after birth, using ultracentrifugation. Purity of the membrane fraction was controlled by measuring 5-nucleotidase activity and with electron microscopy.

PAPER BY M. YOUNG

C.T. Jones: This is always technically a very difficult experiment to do. I wondered, specifically looking at some of your free amino acids and the specific activity of the amino acids, about the effects of the method of collecting your samples. Presumably the fetal samples were collected quite a long time after death. We know that this may have an important effect on the turnover of amino acids and possibly on amino acid uptake. To what extent, you think, the values that you actually finally measure represent the concentrations that exist in vivo?

M. Young: I think that the concentrations of free amino acids that we measure are perfectly all right. There is data showing that changes in free amino acids do not occur rapidly after tissues are excised. (HOLLENBERG,

M., N. Hombo and A.J. Samorodin. (1976) Am. J. Physiol. 231:1445.)
We were very aware of the problems because it takes about five minutes
to get all the tissues out of a fetal lamb. I am not so worried about the free
amino acid levels as the amount of radio activity which we find in them,
and I think that the specific activity in our intracellular fluid is possibly a
little on the low side. But we have courage in that our values for protein
synthetic rate are very similar to those which other people have found in
smaller animals, in which you are able to get at your tissues more quickly.

C.T. Jones: It seems very difficult to do the control experiments, so that
you can actually establish whether or not in the fetal sheep there were
changes occurring between the time you put the animal down and the
time you collected your samples.

M. Young: Well it is very easy to show that if you leave them a quarter or
half an hour, there might be an increase in free amino acids levels, not a
decrease.

R.M. Pitkin: You did not report any values in erythrocytes and I wonder
if you examined those, specifically free amino acid levels and protein
synthesis, under the conditions of your experiment.

M. Young: No. Just the organs which I showed you.

B.S. Lindblad: Dr. Young, I wonder whether the effect of insulin on
protein synthesis in the placenta can be compared with other maternal
tissues?

M. Young: All the measurements that I showed you were made in the
fetus in utero with indwelling catheters in the fetal jugular vein and
carotid artery. These fetal values were compared with those found in the
adult ewe by Buttery et al. (Buttery, P.J., A. Beckerton and R.M.
Mitchell. (1975) Proc. Nutr. Soc. 34:91A.)

B.S. Lindblad: Has anyone studied the uptake in heart, or muscle, or
other organs of the mother during pregnancy? We have been studying
(Fredholm, B., B.S. Lindblad, B. Persson, M. Stangenberg and
L. Stange. The acute effects of insulin-induced hypoglycaemia in pregnant diabetic women. In manuscript.) the diurnal variation of different

parameters in the blood of pregnant diabetics and also the variation of
the plasma levels of free amino acids during 24 hours. There is quite a
variation normally, but in the pregnant diabetic there was very little
variation. The pregnant diabetic women also had higher than normal
fasting levels of free amino acids in plasma. We then studied the effect of
insulin when given to the diabetic pregnant mother. The plasma concentrations of amino acids normally fall very rapidly after insulin injection.
But they did not in the pregnant diabetic women. We might call this
"insulin insensitivity". We repeated these studies after delivery and then
these mothers responded normally to insulin. So, I wonder if there is
something in the pregnant state that makes you "insensitive" to insulin
and that is why I was asking if anyone ever measured the effect of insulin
on the protein synthesis in other tissues of the pregnant mother.

M. Young: To my knowledge, no. The only experiments which have been
done in the intact animal on the effect of insulin on protein synthetic rate
are those of Pain and Garlick; they studied muscle specifically, because
that was their interest. (PAIN, V.M. and P.J. GARLICK. (1974) J. Biol.
Chem. 249:4510.) I has no effect on protein synthetic rate in the normal
rat, and I cannot tell you whether they were male or female; but insulin
did partially restore the protein synthetic rate in the muscle of rats that
were made diabetic by streptocytocin.

S. Sklavunu: In your experiments you used adult insulin; we know that
there is also a fetal insulin. Do you know if experiments have been done
with fetal insulin, and with the antagonists of adult insulin?

M. Young: Not that I know of. We used bovine insulin in fetal lambs.

E. Eggermont: In regard to the lower protein half life you found in fetal
tissues, do you think this is due to the lower concentration in fetal tissues
or to the increase of lysosomal activity?

M. Young: I don't know. I only know there is a very heterogeneous
mixture of proteins in all tissues. It looks as though the proteins with short
half life may be present in a higher concentration in fetal tissues or else
there may be a greater turnover of every single protein in the fetal tissue,
which seems more likely, because you have to have this continuous
rearrangement of structures in the fetus.

G.J. Kloosterman: We studied 120 cases of maternal diabetes and we could conclude that if we start treatment early in pregnancy, there is almost no overweight of the baby afterwards. (KLOOSTERMAN, G.J. (1977) Diabetes en zwangerschap. Verh. Koninkl. Acad. Geneesk. België, 39, nr. 4:181.) The difference in birth weight between these babies and normal controls was only 100 g. If we started treatment after 20 weeks and specially after 30 weeks of pregnancy we were not able to bring down the birth weight of the baby. Could it be that insulin receptors develop in the first 20–30 weeks of pregnancy, that could perhaps explain our findings? It seems that starvation is very important in the last 10 weeks of pregnancy, but in maternal diabetes it seems that the first 20 of 30 weeks of pregnancy are the most important. I am wondering what the explanation could be.

M. Young: I think that I should pass that on to Professor Milner.

R.D.G. Milner: The only comment I would make is that we have to think not only about quantity of control, the number of weeks, but also about the intensity of control and I would be interested to know whether you controlled the diabetic women to normal euglycaemia.

G.J. Kloosterman: We kept the blood glucose values very strictly between 4 and 8 mmole. The perinatal mortality in these 120 cases of insulin treated women was 3.0. All women were treated with insulin before pregnancy and 30% of them had juvenile diabetes. I think these results are an indication of very thorough treatment. And nevertheless if women came in the last weeks of pregnancy with not a very severe degree of diabetes, we were not able to bring down the weight of the baby. In this group the babies had an overweight on the average of more than 800 g, where as it was 100 g in the babies of the mothers who came before 20 weeks of pregnancy.

I think the explanation could be that insulin receptors develop in the first 20–30 weeks of pregnancy.

R.D.G. Milner: Not an explanation but a speculation.

J.C.L. Shaw: There is one point that has always interested me about insulin in pregnancy. Though we may treat a diabetic early in pregnancy and reduce the weight of the fetus, the incidence of congenital malfor-

mations does not seem to alter much. (GABBE, S.G. et al. (1977) Amer. J.
Obstet. Gynec. 129:723.) This suggests that insulin may be necessary
very early on in pregnancy. Perhaps, therefore, to minimise all the effects
of diabetes on the fetus it will be necessary to establish good control before
conception takes place.

PAPER BY R.M. PITKIN

R.A. McCance: I was extremely interested in this paper, because I have
long known that the swallowing of amniotic fluid is very important for
the fluid metabolism of the fetus. There is one historical point that should
interest this gathering. I believe the man that made the first observation
on swallowing of amniotic fluid was a Dutchman, De Snoo. He used
methylene blue. (DE SNOO, K. (1937) Monatsschr. Geburtsh. u. Gynäk.
105:88.)

R.M. Pitkin: I have elsewhere acknowledged the original work of De
Snoo. He also reported that the injection of saccharine seems to alleviate
the problem of polyhydramnios, the implication being if you make the
amniotic fluid taste good the fetus will swallow more of it. That paper has
been widely quoted as a reference. (DE SNOO, K. (1937) Monatsschr.
Geburtsh. u. Gynäk. 105:88.) We have tried to investigate this in a
somewhat different way using iodinated albumin in primates and measuring the excretion of radioacitivity in the maternal urine, our thesis
being that if the fetus drinks more amniotic fluid, the pregnant animal
will excrete more radioactivity earlier. While this seemed to us somewhat
simplistic but rather a good idea to try, it did not work out well, and we
were unable to find out the difference between saccharine and other
sugars in effect on taste.

F.C. Battaglia: In your calculation of the 300 ml of amniotic fluid that
might be swallowed a day, you are making the assumption that that fluid
with any of its nutrients – protein, carbohydrates, what ever – is completely cleared. Why don't you subtract from that the solutes added to
amniotic fluid, since the total amount is not changing each day appreciably. In other words, most of us refer to nutrients as a *net* addition of
carbon and nitrogen to the organism.

R.M. Pitkin: That would be another way of calculating it. I had not thought of it that way but, in order to do this, one would than have to know what is added. You are quite right that amniotic fluid does stay in balance in terms of its osmolality, what is added ought to be what is provided to the fetus on a given day. This would need to be estimated under experimental conditions of a chronic sort of preparation where you could obtain some reliable data regarding contributions to amniotic fluid, where it comes from and on a time basis. If that could be done I think it would be an alternative way of calculating it.

B.S. Lindblad: I would like to say to Professor McCance that in England, in 1651, Harvey suggested (cited by: NEEDHAM (1931) Chemical embryology, Cambridge Univ. Press, Cambridge) that the fetus was nourished also by mouth, by ingestion of the amniotic fluid. We are increasingly aware of the non-function of the pancreas during total intravenous alimentation. May we look at the ingestion of the amniotic fluid as important for the development of the endocrine function of the gastrointestinal canal?

R.M. Pitkin: I think that is a very important point; you are thinking in terms of enzyme induction or something similar. The fact that swallowing of amniotic fluid exists almost implies that it has a purpose.

B.S. Lindblad: It could be an important problem to the pediatric surgeon. I would like to know how the pancreas functions in newborns with atresias of the gastrointestinal canal.

R.M. Pitkin: I don't know. The question you are asking is what happens in a newborn with, for instance, duodenal atresia where swallowing has not occurred. I cannot comment on that, particularly about the ability to digest proteins.

B. Friis Hansen: Professor McCance brought up the question of fluid metabolism. I have always been surprised and intrigued by the fact that up to delivery the fetus can swallow some 400–500 ml of water per kg per day. Yet after delivery and particulary in small premature infants we are very happy if they can take 5 ml glucosewater or milk. Therefore, life would be so much easier if we knew how we could do the trick of making the newborn infant swallow fluids in these quantities, even if it was not milk, during the first days after birth.

J.C.L. Shaw: Alcorn et al. (J. Anat. 123:649–660, 1977) have made some observations on the fetal lung which might have a bearing on the function of fetal swallowing. They cannulated the fetal trachea in chronic sheep preparations. If lung liquid was allowed to drain freely there was a substantial reduction in both lung tissue weight, and differentiated type II alveolar cells. In contrast, if the trachea was ligated and lung liquid allowed to accumulate, the lung tissue weight was increased and the number of differentiated type II alveolar cells increased. It therefore seems possible that fetal swallowing might have an effect on morphological development of the intestine. It would be interesting to devise an experiment to study this point.

R.M. Pitkin: That would have to be done early in gestation. It has been done in the monkey in late gestation but only to demonstrate its role in producing polyhydramnios, not its morphological role as you suggested.

J.C. Sinclair: In regard to Dr. Battaglia's previous comment, I believe that we would keep the terminology clear if we referred to the energy intake via fetal swallowing of amniotic fluid as the gross energy intake of the fetus by this route. Because the fetus is excreting energy into the amniotic fluid in his urine, and perhaps occasionally from the gastrointestinal tract, we could make a second calculation of the energy excretion into amniotic fluid. Have you in fact calculated the gross energy content of amniotic fluid in human pregnancy at or near term, resulting not only from protein but from other nutrients in the amniotic fluid, and made a calculation, given the volume of fetal swallowing, of the approximate gross energy intake via fetal swallowing at term?

R.M. Pitkin: No, we have not. It would be easy to do by determining the energy content with a calorimeter, but we have not done it.

M. Gabr: If I understood correctly you explained the high level of protein in the ileum by synthesis in situ of new enterocytes from the broken down ingested protein. Would exudation be another possibility to explain this high protein content in the ileum?

R.M. Pitkin: It has been demonstrated that the capacity for the small bowel in the dog to lose protein is quite substantial. Whether this occurred as a result of desquamation of cells or exudation of protein I think is not quite clear. We determined protein, and do not know if this is intracellular protein or free protein. You are right, exudation is quite possible.

PAPER BY H.N. LAFEBER

E.M. Widdowson: I hope Dr. Jones will forgive me if I once again bring up the question of fat. We produced retarded growth in the fetal guinea pig by a different method, by severely undernourishing the mother. We produced similar effects to yours, but it was surprising that these growth retarded fetuses had as high a percentage of fat in their bodies as the normally grown ones. Of course the total amount was less, but the percentage was just the same. (WIDDOWSON, E.M. (1974). In: Size at birth. Ciba Foundation Symposium 27 (new series). K. Elliott and J. Knight eds., Elsevier North-Holland, p. 65.) In the figure you showed about perirenal fat, I saw that it was almost as much retarded as the total weight. You did not give any figures for the interscapular fat; we found that the retarded animals had interscapular fat that weighed as much as that in the normal animals, so as a percentage of the total weight it was much higher. I would like to ask once again why do these undernourished fetuses continue to deposit fat?

H.N. Lafeber: We did not measure interscapular fat in the guinea pig. We only measured perirenal fat. But I don't know any explanation why in this type of growth retardation there is a reduction in body fat and why there is not in malnutrition. May be Dr. Jones may have an answer to that question.

C.T. Jones: I think we are dealing with two entirely different situations. If I can mention the malnutrition situation first. In that case, as for instance Professor Hull has shown with the rabbit, you get a mobilization of maternal adipose tissue and elevation of free fatty acids in maternal circulation with an increased transfer to the fetus. In the uterine growth retardation produced by uterine artery ligation you have no increase in mobilization of fat from maternal adipose tissue. There is one striking thing that Dr. Lafeber did not mention. In those fetuses that are moderately retarded, what I mean by that is that those are 40–50% of normal weight, the free fatty acid concentration of the blood is not depressed and, if anything, the hepatic tryglyceride concentration in those fetuses is increased. This is consistent with what you see in fetuses of malnourished guinea pig mothers, as Dr. Widdowson has shown. In the severely retarded fetuses, by that I mean those which are 25–30% of normal weight, the circulating free fatty acid concentration in the fetus is no more than half of normal and the hepatic tryglyceride stores are much less than normal. So in answer to Dr. Widdowson, the two situations are different but the situation in intrauterine growth retardation produced by uterine artery ligation is also complicated and the effect that you observe depends upon the degree of the growth retardation.

T.K.A.B. Eskes: Does it make any difference at what stage of pregnancy you ligate the artery?

H.N. Lafeber: We did not investigate this in the guinea pig, because for practical reasons we choose only midgestation. There are other studies which indicate that the later the ligation the less some of the changes in various organs. (HILL, D.E. (1974) In: Size at birth. Ciba Foundation Symposium 27 (new series). K. Elliott and J. Knight, eds., Elsevier North-Holland, p. 116.)

T.K.A.B. Eskes: My second question if I may. Do all placentas have infarcts?

H.N. Lafeber: No. All of them are small as you could see in the relation between fetal and placental weight.

T.K.A.B. Eskes: You were very critical in weighing placentas. I know that the chairman of this session spent almost his whole life in weighing placentas. What do you suggest, should we stop weighing placentas and instead calculate surface areas?

H.N. Lafeber: No, certainly not, but you will agree that just simple weight is not a criterium for function. May be with new techniques we might have new opportunities to assess placental function better than just by weight. That is all I can say.

G.J. Kloosterman: Weight is a primitive and poor criterium for function and endeavours to weigh the brain of individuals as a criterium for intelligence belong to the past. Partly this is also true for the placenta. If the mother smokes heavily during pregnancy, then the weight of the placenta stays almost the same and the weight of the fetus goes down with 10%. The same phenomenon exists if there are many infarcts in the placenta. Then its function (fetal weight) goes down and its weight stays the same. Nevertheless, as a tool to examine large groups and to make comparisons between groups, the weight still is and will stay to be a very important criterium, if used with intelligence, like Dr. Lafeber did.

R. Eeckels: In a study in African newborns we have some data which indicate that the weight of the infant is more related to the surface of the placenta than its weight. Would that agree with your figures or did not you measure surfaces?

H.N. Lafeber: We did not measure surfaces of the placentas.

G.J. Kloosterman: I always wondered how it is possible to get an accurate measure of the surface of the placenta, but if it is possible than I agree that it is more important than placental weight.

R. Eeckels: I agree that it is more difficult to have good data for surfaces than for weight. But still if you accept that the data were not exact, the differences were quite striking.

M. Young: In animal studies, Dr. Widdowson and I made some estimations of the functional capacity of placentas of fetuses of mothers who were on a low calorie diet or a diet low in protein but with adequate calories. (YOUNG, M. and E.M. WIDDOWSON. (1975) Biol. Neonate 27: 184.) There were retardations in growth on both diets. At the end of gestation, we injected a single dose of AIB, which is a non-metabolisable amino acid, and we related the transfer of that amino acid to the placental weight and to the fetal weight. We found a reduction in transfer per gram of placenta in calorie malnutrition, but a smaller reduction in transfer rate in the low protein group. Such a functional test can only be done in animals.

C.A. Canosa: About ten years ago we studied twenty placentas from severely malnourished mothers from poor and isolated rural Guatemalan villages, and compared them with placentas from twenty well-nourished mothers from Iowa City. Some of the relevant results were as follows: weight and total water were similar; the total amount of DNA in the Guatemalan placentas was half that in those from Iowa; the cell concentration of zinc and chromium was different in the Guatemalan placentas: zinc was markedly increased and chromium very much decreased. (DAYTON, D.H., L.J. FILER and C.A. CANOSA. (1969) Fed. Proc. 28:488; CANOSA, C.A., D.H. DAYTON, L.J. FILER and S.J. FOMON. (1968) XII Intern. Congr. Ped., Mexico, Dec. 1.) This work was later continued by the MIT group in Boston. Perhaps we could link these findings to some of the remarks made by Professors Ballabriga and Milner about the sensitivity of the target cells of placentas in well and poorly nourished mothers. Professor Milner was referring to normal full-term infants and Professor Ballabriga to "small for dates". The speculation is that when there is a decreased number of, as well as altered, placental cells, the sensitivity of the target cells – whether to glucagon or to insulin – could be markedly increased.

The second comment I would like to make is about intrauterine linear growth of long bones as an index of fetal maturation. We determined intrauterine bone growth in two groups of newborns from 26 to 37 weeks of gestation, of which one group was AGA and the other was SGA. The study shows that the length of long bones at the same gestational ages was similar in the two groups. (CANOSA, C.A., F. PEREZ CANDELA, F. FOLCH, L. SAN ROMAN and J. MARTINS FILHO. (1976) Rev. Esp. Red. 32:537; CANOSA, C.A. (1976) (Abstract) Eur. Soc. Ped. Res., Rotterdam.) Thus, it is possible to speculate that intrauterine linear bone growth could be used as an accurate and precise index to determine fetal age and maturation. Further studies are in progress.

G.B.A. Stoelinga: I was very impressed by your findings about the delay in skeletal development. I wonder if you have data bout catch-up growth in skeletal development after birth, and if this was related with catch-up growth in height.

H.N. Lafeber: We don't have many data on the follow-up of growth retarded newborn guinea-pigs. Simply because it is practically very difficult to do this type of study. I mentioned briefly that we have some evidence in the growth retarded fetuses just before birth, that there is a lower activity of factors that stimulate incorporation of sulfate into cartilage. These studies are only preliminary; and I don't know if this might have some effects on skeletal development after birth.

A. Ballabriga: I should like to emphasize how difficult it is to make a correlation between biochemical findings in the brain and function later on. We have measured in brain homogenates N-acetylneuraminic acid as a chemical marker for gangliosides and the total plasmalogen as chemical marker for synaptogenesis. Total levels were lower in brains of small-for-dates as compared with normal full-term infants or preterm infants with normal birth weight for gestational age. All infants died during the first days of life. How to relate these findings with the functional development? This will depend on the eventual catch-up growth later on and on many environmental factors. Final mental ability does not depend only on nutrition, it plays an important role, but not a unique role. Other factors, as environmental, play an important role. It is for this reason that extrapolation of data concerning animal species to the human is so very difficult.

H.N. Lafeber: I totally agree with that. We only used simple measurements of DNA, RNA and protein for basic information but have made no attempt to relate the results to a delay of functional brain development or neurological damage.

GENERAL DISCUSSION

B.S. Lindblad: I would like to comment on Dr. Lafeber's paper. I was interested to see that in your guinea pigs there was a correlation between the biochemical findings and the degree of growth retardation. We are all aware of the heterogeneous nature of the small-for-dates syndrome in the human. It is therefore important to characterise our materials carefully. For instance, when we studied newborn babies of severely malnourished mothers in Addis-Abeba (GEBRE-MEDHIN, M.U. LARSSON, B.S. LINDBLAD and R. ZETTERSTRÖM. (1978) Acta Paediatr. Scand. 61:213.), we thought that the main cause of growth retardation would be the maternal malnutrition. However, the findings suggested that placental insufficiency was an important factor. So, although this is a difficult problem, we should try to subdivide our human material into possible aetiological groups.

H.N. Lafeber: Within our model of placental insufficiency, we subdivided our guinea pigs into two groups: moderately and severely retarded.

Moderately means about 50% of normal and severely is about 30% of normal. And in general we find that many of the changes in the moderate groups are more pronounced in the severe group. For instance a change of brain weight which is relatively small in the moderate group, is really severe in the severely retarded group. Also many of the changes in organ maturation, for instance in the liver and skeletal muscle, are also much more pronounced in this severe group.

C.T. Jones: Certainly in animal studies it is clearly possible to divide groups, that is to compare maternal malnutrition against placental insufficiency. In the clinical situation I think that our clinical colleagues are trying to interpret from a heterogeneous group what has been the cause of the growth retardation.

There are some indications from animal studies that there are some major differences between the two groups, that is the placental insufficiency is usually associated with asymmetrical effects on organ growth, while severe maternal malnutrition is usually associated with a proportional reduction in the mass of the organs. Another intriguing difference which clearly should be investigated is that in for instance the growth retarded sheep which is produced by the placental insufficiency model, the circulating prolactin concentrations in the fetus are only about 3% of normal, whereas if you produce growth retardation in the rat by maternal malnutrition than the circulating prolactin concentration is higher than normal. So there is a subtle difference between the two different conditions, that may on the one hand explain why organ growth is different in the two conditions, and perhaps may be responsible for other rather subtle changes in organ composition.

F.C. Battaglia: Just two comments. I think when you were presenting tables that compared species, perhaps some of the confusion would disappear if you had tested the significance of some of the differences. You were talking about a 98% of normal for cerebral DNA in one species for example, we may be making too much of the fact that it is not 100%, so I think we need to know the significance of the differences that are on the tables to be able to make some decisions about what are real species differences and what are not.

The other is, I think it is risky to measure arterial concentrations of solutes in fetal blood, and drift into the pattern of interpreting this as a reflection of umbilical substrate flow. We have good data in the sheep to show that this could be quite misleading. You can have an increase of umbilical uptake of glucose in the face of hypoglycaemia, or a decrease of umbilical uptake in the face of hypoglycaemia. I think all it is telling you is the arterial concentrations in the fetus. The question I have to Dr. Jones is to hear how he interprets the increase of fetal liver glycogen concentration in the face of a decrease in plasma insulin and an increase in plasma glucagon.

C.T. Jones: I think that that was certainly a very surprising observation and it indicates a way in which the fetus is attempting to compensate this hypoglycaemia and hypoinsulinaemia. The only evidence that we have that would suggest a mechanism, is this quite large reduction in the phosphofructokinase/hexokinase ratio and that these livers are capable, at physiological glucose concentrations, of taking up glucose adequately and incorporating it into glycogen. It is surprising that this occurs together with hypoglycaemia and it certainly makes us to ask some questions about the mechanisms controlling glycogen deposition.

I think that it is likely that what is happening is that the lower phosphofructokinase activity is ensuring that more of the glucose, that is taken up, is incorporated into glycogen and is then diverting it from glycolysis.

G.E. Gaull: There has been some concern expressed for sorting out the aetiology of what is going on in man. I would like to return to the animal models for a moment and ask Dr. Lafeber and Dr. Jones whether they have made any measurements of oxygen and the removal of acidic compounds in the model they are looking at. This is a propos of Dr. Widdowson's question about the difference between maternal malnutrition and this model in which you have ligated the uterine artery. I wonder whether some of the questions that have been asked about malnutrition and your model might be sorted out by this consideration.

C.T. Jones: Did you say oxygen?

G.E. Gaull: I said oxygen, among other things. I mean there is a difference in ligating a artery and between having a pure reduction in the delivery of substrates. You are also limiting other things.

C.T. Jones: Well, by nutrient substrates of the fetus, I would include oxygen, I would not consider it as separately from general nutrient supply to the fetus. It is difficult to study this in the guinea pig, there certainly is an increase in packed cell volume in the growth retarded guinea pig. The best model to investigate this is in the chronically-catheterized sheep, where the PO_2 falls from about 23 to about 15 in association with the intra-uterine growth retardation, and there is an increase in packed cell volume. This is the model in which the placental mass is grossly reduced. The picture that one has from the guinea pig and the sheep is that probably there is a lower PaO_2, which may indicate a reduction in oxygen transport to the fetus and there is a compensatory increase in packed cell volume.

R.A. McCance: I would like to get back to Dr. Pitkins paper again. I don't think any work has been done on the swallowing of amniotic fluid in species other than man. I may be wrong about this but it is important with regard to the fluid metabolism of the fetus. Animals' fetuses behave differently. One can remove the kidneys from some and they survive, but others do not, and for different reasons. If you ligate the vitelline vessels in rodents you can get the most alarming effects on fluid metabolism in the fetus, and the fetus always dies. (LE GOASCAGNE, C. (1964) Bull, de L'Assoc. Anatomistes 49:1065; MOTT, J.C. (1973) In: Barcroft Symposium on "Foetal and neonatal physiology", Comline, K.S., K.W. Cross, G.S. Dawes and P.W. Nathanielsz, eds., Cambridge University Press, p. 166.)

R.M. Pitkin: In smaller mammals, rats and guinea pigs, I don't know that it has been done.

E. Eggermont: I have also a question for Dr. Pitkin. When you looked for the intraluminal protein in your fetuses, did you estimate the concentration of the proteins and did you try to characterize the nature of the proteins?

R.M. Pitkin: No, we did not. We simply measured radioactivity in either TCA soluble or insoluble fractions, so we did not characterize the protein. As far as the plasma protein is concerned we assumed, but this is only an assumption, that this is primarily albumin, just because that is the major plasma protein. It does of course contain methionine and the other sulfur containing amino acids.

M. Orzalesi: I would like to come back to the question of Dr. Gaull concerning the role of oxygen deprivation in the two experimental models of intrauterine growth retardation. Obviously, when you ligate the uterine artery, you impair not only the flow of nutrients and oxygen, but also the transfer of it. There is a different situation when you have malnutrition of the mother. Then not enough fuel is available, but whatever is available the fetus can burn much better than when it is oxygen deprived. There is also clinical evidence for at least two types of intrauterine growth retardation, one which is associated with oxygen deprivation and one which is not. I am thinking of the ultrasound measurements of biparietal diameter, which indicate the two different patterns of growth retardation. All other things being equal, the type that is associated with oxygen deprivation, probably is more dangerous and produces more damage, particularly to the brain.

I think that in animal experiments one has to estimate the amount of oxygen available to the fetus.

I like to ask a question to Dr. Pitkin, which goes back to the question of Professor Friis Hansen, concerning the mechanism of swallowing in the fetus, which seems to disappear after the fetus is born prematurely. What do we know about the physiological mechanism of swallowing in utero, in relation to breathing, taste, osmolality, temperature of the environment and so on. I think by studying these things, one could perhaps help the clinician. It could give an indication how to change the environment of the preterm-born fetus, how to change the formula, in order to stimulate him to swallow, just as in utero.

R.M. Pitkin: I have not studied this myself, but there is some information from animal experimemts. Of course, such experiments don't give always information about physiological events. As far as I know, the pattern of swallowing is somewhat different from that of fetal breathing in that swallowing occurs very regularly. There does not seem any relation to either fetal breathing or other fetal activity.

NUTRITION AND METABOLISM OF THE FETUS AND INFANT

UMBILICAL UPTAKE OF SUBSTRATES AND THEIR ROLE IN FETAL METABOLISM

FREDERICK C. BATTAGLIA, M.D.*

INTRODUCTION

The nutrients which the mammalian fetus receives to meet both its growth requirements and its fuel requirements are represented by the umbilical uptake of carbohydrates, amino acids, and fats. This composite substrate flow into the umbilical circulation may be considered the "fetal milk" upon which the fetus grows and develops. In many respects this unique arrangement by which the fetus receives its nutrients through its umbilical cord permits far more precise studies of nutrition and metabolism in a growing organism than is possible in postnatal life when one must consider variations in gastrointestinal absorption to arrive at net substrate flow to the liver and other organs. One can measure the umbilical uptake of substrates by an application of the Fick Principle in which umbilical blood flow and the arteriovenous difference of whole blood concentrations of solutes are determined simultaneously. The product of these two measurements represents the net uptake of substrates by the fetus. A fairly complete description of the composition of this "fetal milk" has been provided for at least one mammalian fetus, the fetal lamb, under unstressed steady state conditions. Similarly, the fetal calf and horse have also been studied fairly extensively in terms of the composition of substrate flow into the fetal umbilical circulation. These data have recently been reviewed and a carbon and nitrogen balance sheet prepared for the ovine fetus based upon these direct measurements of carbon and nitrogen uptake (1, 4). For this reason, I shall not dwell upon these aspects of fetal nutrition and metabolism, but center the paper upon a consideration of the data stemming from several different sources supporting the fact that amino acids play a major role, not only as building blocks for protein synthesis, but as metabolic fuels as well.

* Department of Pediatrics, University of Colorado, 4200 East Ninth Avenue, Denver, Colo. 80262, U.S.A.

H.K.A. Visser (ed.), Nutrition and Metabolism of the Fetus and Infant, 83-91. All rights reserved.
Copyright © 1979 Martinus Nijhoff Publishers b.v., The Hague/Boston/London.

GROWTH AND FUEL REQUIREMENTS

My colleague, Dr. MESCHIA and I, have previously published a balance sheet for the total caloric requirements of the ovine fetus during the later third of gestation (2, 3), a time in which approximately 40% of the total caloric requirement is represented by tissue accretion and approximately 60% by the oxygen consumption. Earlier, it was pointed out that the oxygen consumption of mammalian fetuses differing widely in size and maturity at birth had remarkably similar oxygen consumptions per kilogram of fetal body weight (1). (See table 1.)

The caloric requirements of other mammalian fetuses may be calculated in a similar fashion assuming an oxygen consumption of approximately 7 ml/kg/min and using data for the fetal growth rate in each species. However, one must be cautious in extrapolating to interspecies comparisons from such calculations at this time for the following reasons:

Table 1. *Oxygen consumption rates of adults and fetuses in species of different size.*

Animal	O_2 Consumption, ml/min/kg body weight	
	Adult	Fetal
Horse	2.0	7.0
Cattle	2.2	7.4
Sheep	4.0	6–9.4
Rhesus monkey	7.0	7.0
Guinea pig	9.7	8.5

From: BATTAGLIA, F.C. and G. MESCHIA. (1978) Physiol. Rev. 58:502.

1. The caloric equivalents of fetal tissue have not been measured in species other than the sheep. It will certainly vary among species reflecting primarily differences in total body water content and body fat composition. In addition, for similar reasons, it will vary within the same species depending upon the gestational age.

2. Comparisons between species must consider the varying growth rates within a species at different stages of gestation (e.g. the human fetus may vary in its growth rate from > 3% at approximately 20–25 days gestation to < 1.0% at term). Thus, very different conclusions may be drawn at the two stages of gestation for the human fetus in terms of the percent of total caloric requirements devoted to new tissue accretion.

PRINCIPAL CARBON AND NITROGEN SUPPLY

The principal carbon and nitrogen sources of the ovine fetus have been described (4) and the data supporting these conclusions have been reviewed on several occasions (1, 5). Thus, I shall not discuss the studies leading to these conclusions concerning the principal substrates providing carbon and nitrogen to the fetus. I should emphasize, however, that in a number of mammalian species studied under chronic steady state conditions the glucose consumed by the fetus has been shown to be inadequate to meet the oxygen consumption of the fetus let alone provide additional carbon for growth. Another major source of carbon for the fetal lamb at least is provided by the umbilical uptake of lactate, a derivative of the high placental production rate of lactate under aerobic conditions. In the ovine fetus, these two carbohydrates could account for approximately 75% of the oxygen consumption. Earlier, a high rate of urea production by the fetal lamb has been described. Later, a series of studies confirmed the role of the amino acids as metabolic fuels in the ovine fetus. Since it is an important and in some ways unexpected characteristic of fetal metabolism, I should like to review the three lines of investigation which support this conclusion.

AMINO ACID CATABOLISM

The first evidence came from measurements of the urea production rate of the fetal lamb. This study represented the first time that measurements of placental clearance had been used not for studies of placental permeability alone, but for studies of fetal metabolism. Since the arteriovenous difference of urea across the umbilical circulation is too small to be measured with precision, independent measurements of urea clearance in the fetal lamb were made using a constant infusion technique for ^{14}C urea and simultaneous determinations of umbilical blood flow. The normal urea concentration difference which exists between the fetal and maternal bloods under chronic steady state conditions was determined and from the product of the clearance and arterial concentration difference the urea production rate of the fetus could be calculated (6). The study demonstrated a urea production rate of approximately 0.54 mg/min/kg per fetus, sufficient to account for approximately 25% of the oxygen consumption.

The next study lending support to the role of amino acids as fuels was that in which the umbilical uptake of amino acids in the fetal lamb was measured directly and comparisons with accretion rates for each of the amino acids in the fetus was made. The study clearly demonstrated that the umbilical uptake of most of the neutral amino acids was in considerable excess of that required for growth supporting their role as fetal fuels (7). An interesting point in this regard is a recent publication in which an attempt was made to quantitate the umbilical arteriovenous differences of amino acids in the fetal lamb under acute operative and anesthetic stress (8). Figure 1 presents a comparison of the umbilical arteriovenous differences in the two studies. It is clear that for most of

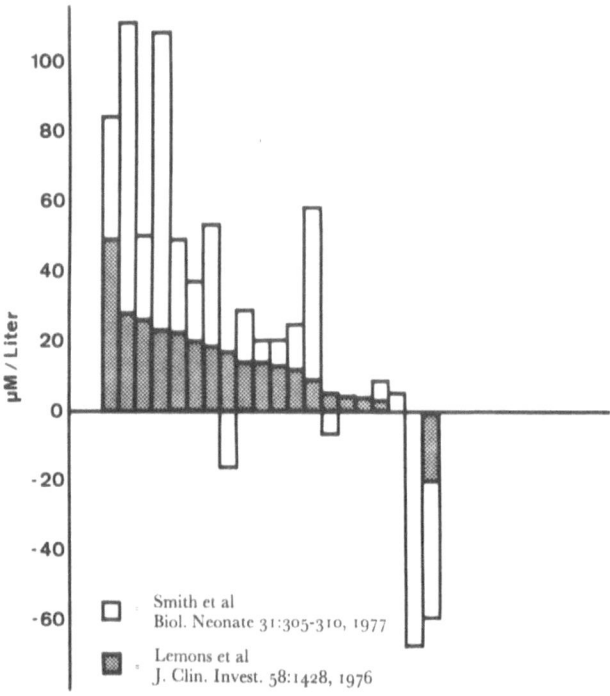

Fig. 1. A comparison of umbilical A-V differences in the fetal lamb under acute operative stress vs chronic steady state conditions.

the amino acids the arteriovenous differences were much larger in the animal study under acute operative stress implying a marked reduction in umbilical blood flow in those animals. Many other differences both qualitative and quantitative between the data from the two studies are apparent. This comparison points out once again the difficulties in attempting to describe placental and fetal metabolism characteristic of a *growing* organism under acute surgical conditions. In fact one has no basis for the presumption that the fetus is indeed capable of sustaining growth under such conditions of acute stress. This has been the principal difficulty in comparing data acquired in the smaller mammals with those in the large mammals; one is not only comparing species differences but also two sets of data collected in animals differing widely in biologic state.

A third study supporting the delivery of amino acids to the fetus in quantities exceeding the accretion requirements has recently been completed in our laboratories (9). In this study, the arteriovenous differences of amino acids across the uterine circulation has been measured along with simultaneous measurements of oxygen content differences. Thus, the quantity of nitrogen leaving the uterine circulation for each amino acid could be calculated in terms of its oxygen equivalents. Since the oxygen consumption of the pregnant ovine uterus has been measured in several different laboratories, one can then calculate the total nitrogen flow into the uterus. This estimate must be corrected for the ammonia production of the uterus (10). The study demonstrated an amino acid uptake by the uterus of $\geqslant$ 1.3 gN/day/kg fetal weight. The quantity of nitrogen representing umbilical uptake of amino acids is in good agreement in the two studies, both studies showing an amino acid uptake in excess of accretion.

CARBOHYDRATE TURNOVER RATES

I should like to complete this presentation by presenting some recent work in our laboratories directed at assessing turnover rate of glucose (12). There has been a great deal of recent work directed at the question of interpretation of glucose turnover rates measured with either ^{14}C or ^{3}H glucose at various positions in the glucose molecule (11). In fact the difficulties have, if anything, become more apparent as additional data have been collected in animals studied at various nutritional planes. I shall not comment upon this literature except to point out that these problems are present in studies during fetal and neonatal life as well and are not circumvented by the use of ^{13}C or deuteriated glucose.

However, even if one establishes that the turnover rate obtained with glucose labelled at a particular position with carbon or tritium provides the best reflection of total glucose entry (or total glucose utilization) within an organism, there are special problems in attempting to apply the technique to the mammalian fetus. Recently we have been studying the turnover rate of glucose in the fetal lamb (12). In a series of experiments ^{14}C and ^{3}H glucose labelled at various positions were infused simultaneously at a constant rate into the fetal circulation. The study was designed so that concentrations and specific activities of various compounds could be measured as arteriovenous differences across both the umbilical and uterine circulations. The first point that should be emphasized is that approximately 50% of the ^{14}C or ^{3}H-glucose infused into the fetal circulation leaves the fetus and enters the placenta and maternal circulation as glucose. Figure 2 presents these data diagrammatically. Clearly if one does not subtract the quantity of ^{14}C or ^{3}H-glucose which leaves the fetal circulation from the quantity infused one calculates a fetal

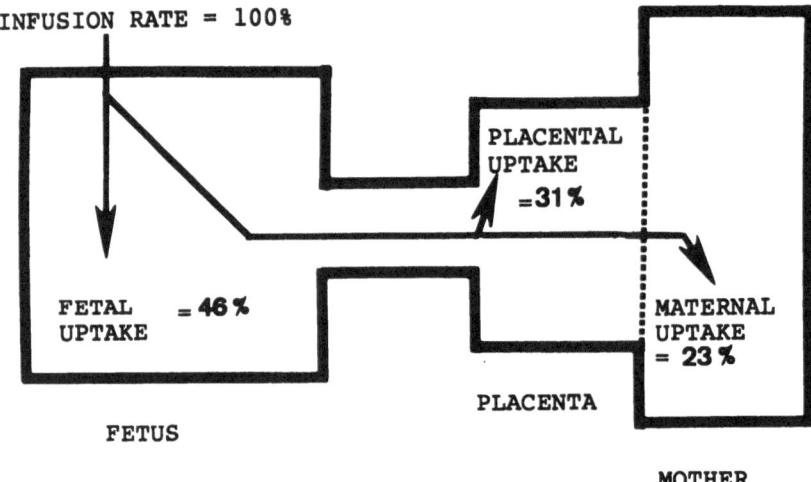

Fig. 2. Fate of radioactive glucose.

glucose turnover rate which has little metabolic significance. The correction for substrate infused which drains into the placental and maternal circulation must be made for any substrate when one attempts to calculate a turnover rate in the fetus which reflects metabolism of the compound, although the percentage which leaves may be more or less than the approximately 50% value for glucose. Several studies on glucose turnover rate in the fetal lamb have not made such measurements of net

¹⁴C glucose drain into the placenta. For this reason the turnover rates for glucose were high and should not be interpreted as reflecting the rate of glucose metabolism in the fetus (13, 14, 15).

Another relatively unique aspect of fetal metabolism concerns the exogenous glucose entry rate into the fetal glucose pool. Figure 3 presents the fetal glucose balance diagrammatically. Unlike postnatal life the exogenous glucose entry rate represented by the umbilical glucose uptake can be measured precisely even with the animal in the fed state. Thus, if umbilical glucose uptake and the glucose turnover rate are measured simultaneously, the total endogenous glucose entry rate can be calculated as the difference between umbilical glucose uptake and

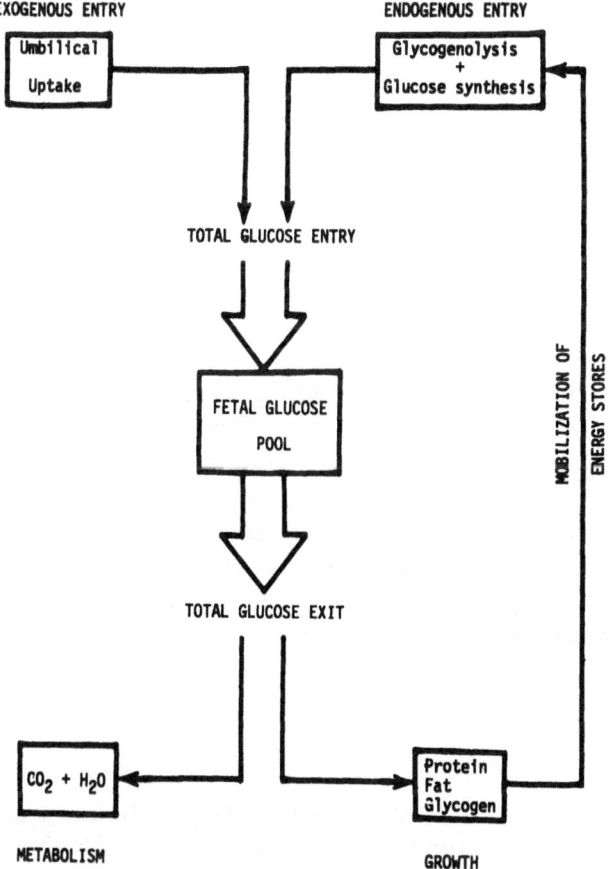

Fig. 3. Fetal glucose balance.

glucose turnover rate. The ability to determine glucose turnover rate and exogenous glucose entry rate enables one to assess the endogenous glucose production rate from all other sources; glycogenolysis, gluconeogenesis, and glucogenesis. In the lamb umbilical glucose uptake was 4.8 mg/min/kg. The glucose turnover rate determined with ^{14}C-1-glucose or ^{14}C-6-glucose was 5.2 mg/min/kg. The turnover rate measured with ^{3}H-2-glucose or ^{3}H-6-glucose was significantly higher, 8.8 mg/min/kg. This discrepancy between ^{14}C-glucose and ^{3}H-glucose turnover rates is not found in the adult sheep. At this time we cannot be certain which determination best approximates the true rate of fetal glucose utilization. It is likely, however, that the dual measurements effectively bracket the true value and that a small but significant endogenous glucose entry rate exists even with the mother in the fed state.

SUMMARY

The major carbon and nitrogen sources for growth and oxidative metabolism in the fetal lamb in the later third of gestation have been described. These consist primarily of carbohydrates (e.g. glucose and lactate) and amino acids. Amino acids are delivered to the fetus in amounts exceeding that required for nitrogen accretion and are used extensively as fetal fuels. The measurement of turnover rates of substrates in fetal life require the estimation of the radio labelled substrate loss from the fetal circulation into the placenta and maternal circulation. If this correction is made, the turnover rate will reflect the utilization rate of substrate. Exogenous substrate entry rate can be directly determined (e.g. umbilical uptake). The difference between the simultaneously determined turnover rate and the umbilical uptake represents an estimate of the endogenous entry rate of the substrate from all sources. Examples are given of the application of these concepts to studies of fetal glucose and fetal lysine balance in the lamb.

REFERENCES

1. BATTAGLIA, F.C. and G. MESCHIA. (1978) Physiological Reviews 58:499.
2. SCHREINER, R.L. et al. (1977) In: Circulation of the Fetus and Newborn, Longo, L. ed., Raven Press, New York, N.Y.
3. BATTAGLIA, F.C. (1978) Pediatric Research 12:736.

4. BATTAGLIA, F.C. and G. MESCHIA. (1973) In: Proceedings of the Sir Barcroft Centenary Symposium, Comline, K.S. and K.W. Cross eds., Cambridge University Press, London, p. 382.

5. BATTAGLIA, F.C. (In press) In: Pregnancy Metabolism, Diabetes and the Fetus. (Ciba Foundation Symposium 63), Elsevier Excerpta Medica / North-Holland, Amsterdam.

6. GRESHAM, E.L. et al. (1972) Pediatrics 50:372.

7. LEMONS, J.A. et al. (1976) J. Clin. Invest. 58:1428.

8. SMITH, R.M., I.G. JARRETT, R.A. KING, and G.R. RUSSELL. (1977) Biol. Neonate 31:305.

9. HOLZMAN, I.R., C. TENG, G. MESCHIA and F.C. BATTAGLIA. (In press) Amino acid arteriovenous differences across the uterine circulation during ovine pregnancy. J. Devel. Physiol., 1979.

10. HOLZMAN, I.R., J.A. LEMONS, G. MESCHIA and F.C. BATTAGLIA. (1977) Proc. Soc. Exp. Biol. Med. 156:27.

11. RAMBERG, C.F., JR. (1977) Federation Proc. 36 (2):225.

12. HAY, W.W., J.W. SPARKS, B.J. QUISSELL, F.C. BATTAGLIA and G. MESCHIA. (1978) Abstract: Society for Pediatric Research Annual Meeting, New York, N.Y., p. 394.

13. HODGSON, J.C. and D.J. MELLOR. (1977) Proc. Nutr. Soc. 36:33.

14. WARNES, D.M., R.F. SEAMARK and F.J. BALLARD. (1977) Biochem. J. 162:617.

15. PRIOR, R.L. and R.K. CHRISTENSON. (1977) Am. J. Physiol. 233 (6):E462.

16. This study supported by NIH grant # HD 00781-15.

THE ENERGY COST OF GROWTH ESTIMATED FROM SIMULTANEOUS DIRECT AND INDIRECT CALORIMETRY IN INFANTS OF LESS THAN 2500 G

P.J.J. SAUER[*], R.G. PEARSE[*], H.J. DANE[**] and H.K.A. VISSER[*]

Studies on the energy cost of growth in babies of less than 2 kg are few. Direct measurement of the energy cost of growth is not possible but the concept of the energy balance equation makes it possible to calculate the energy cost of growth in these babies. The energy balance equation has been written as follows (SPADY et al. (1), SINCLAIR (2)):

$$\text{Energy}_{in} = \text{Energy}_{excreted} + \text{Energy}_{expended} + \text{Energy}_{stored}.$$

E_{in} represents the energy in the food. The energy present in the food can be calculated from the constituents or can be measured using a bomb calorimeter.

$E_{excreted}$ occurs mainly via the faeces in the postnatal period because energy losses via the urine are quite small and via other routes are negligible.

$E_{expended}$ comprises (i) the energy used in maintenance (ii) the energy used for thermoregulation (iii) the energy used in activity (iv) the energy used for synthesis of new tissue.

E_{stored} is the energy inherent in the components of new tissue.

The energy cost of growth can be divided into two parts, the energy present in the components of new tissue and the energy necessary to organize these components into the new tissue. Both these parts of the energy cost of growth are stored in new tissue. It would therefore seem incorrect to use the term E_{stored} to mean only the energy present in the components of new tissue. We therefore suggest the following terms: the energy cost of growth (E_{cg}) equals the energy present in the components of new tissue ($E_{components}$) plus the energy necessary to organize these components into new tissue ($E_{synthesis}$).

[*] Department of Pediatrics, Academic Hospital Rotterdam/Sophia Children's Hospital and Neonatal Unit.
[**] Department of Applied Physics, Delft University of Technology, Delft.

H.K.A. Visser (ed.), Nutrition and Metabolism of the Fetus and Infant, 93-107. All rights reserved.
Copyright © 1979 Martinus Nijhoff Publishers b.v., The Hague/Boston/London.

$$E_{cg} = E_{components} + E_{synthesis}.$$

The energy balance equation can now be written:

$$E_{in} = E_{excreted} + E_{expended} + E_{components}.$$

$E_{expended}$ has been measured by both direct and indirect calorimetry. Since the studies of HOWLAND (3) in 1912 and DAY and HARDY (4) and DAY et al. (5) in 1942 and 1943 it has been assumed that both methods give identical results. This paper describes the results of measurements of $E_{expended}$ by simultaneous direct and indirect calorimetry in low birth weight babies during a phase of rapid growth. Possible causes for the difference between the results obtained by direct and indirect calorimetry will be discussed. The energy cost of growth for these children has been calculated using the energy balance equation.

MATERIALS AND METHODS

$E_{expended}$ was measured a number of times in 6 babies weighing less than 2 kg during a period when they were growing rapidly. All of the patients had been referred to our hospital for intensive care, however they were all healthy at the time of the study. The birth weight varied between 920 and 1400 g and the gestational age at birth from 29 to 33 weeks.

The babies' weight at the time of study varied between 870 and 2110 g and the age from 8 to 58 days. Further details are given in table 1. The

Table 1. *Data of subjects.*

N	b.wt.	g.a.	group	Period of study		Complications before measurement
				days	weight	
1	1280	33	s.g.a.	23–37	1500–1940	septicaemia
2	920	29	s.g.a.	8–58	870–2044	P.D.A.
3	1370	33	s.g.a.	9–30	1350–2048	–
4	1400	30	a.g.a.	31–45	1460–1987	R.D.S. P.D.A.
5	940	32	s.g.a.	20–43	938–1501	septicaemia
6	1320	30	a.g.a.	24–45	1325–2110	R.D.S.

b.wt.	birth weight
g.a.	gestational age
s.g.a.	small for gestational age
a.g.a.	appropriate for gestational age
P.D.A.	patent ductus arteriosus
R.D.S.	respiratory distress syndrome

patients were growing rapidly during the period in which the measurements were made, however their growth curve for weight was below but parallel to the – 2 SD growth curve of USHER and MCLEAN (6). These babies were therefore all small for gestational age at the time of study. 34 studies were made and the measurement period lasted from 4 to 24 hr in all cases and in 28 cases lasted 6 hr. A 6 hr period of study was chosen because the normal regime on our unit consists of 5 hr continuous feeding followed by a 1 hr feeding pause. During the weeks in which these studies were done and during the measurements themselves, the babies received 175 ml/kg/24 hr Nenatal as a continuous infusion into the stomach via a nasogastric tube. Nenatal is an adapted milk formula feed developed by Nutricia for feeding the preterm baby. The composition is given in table 2. The patients were nursed naked during the measurement period with the exception of a plastic covered nappy (Pamper) to prevent evaporation of urine and faeces. The figures given by HEY and KATZ (7) were

Table 2. *Composition of nenatal (Nutricia) per 100 ml formula.*

Milk fat	0.1 g
Vegetable fat	4.4 g
(Linoleic acid	1.4 g)
Protein	1.8 g
Whey-protein	1.1 g
Casein	0.7 g
Lactose	2.4 g
Glucose	2.2 g
Dextrin-maltose	2.9 g
Minerals	0.4 g

used as a guide to the initial temperature setting of the incubator, and this was adjusted when necessary taking account of the measured skin and oesophageal temperatures. The incubator temperature was adjusted during the period of nursing on the unit using the evidence obtained during the measurement periods.

It was assumed that the measurement period was representative of the whole day and in order to compare the results, all the data were calculated for a 24 hr period. A period of 6 hr is too short to be able to measure the increase in body weight due to growth accurately because of the influence of retention or passage of urine and faeces. Since it has been assumed that the measurement period was representative of a longer period, the babies were weighed regularly on the 2 days before and after each measurement period and the average growth velocity was calculated. This growth velocity was assumed to have been maintained during the measurement period. The energy loss via faeces and urine was not measured. It was assumed that 10% of the caloric intake was lost in the faeces and urine. This figure was chosen because the fat in Nenatal consist of a high proportion of medium chain triglycerides and unsaturated fatty acids which are well absorbed by preterm babies (ROY et al. (8), TANTIBHEDHYANGHUL and HASHIM (9).

APPARATUS

A new calorimeter was designed to measure the energy expenditure of babies below 2.5 kg. A detailed description of the apparatus will be published. A brief summary will be given here.

The calorimeter was designed by W.P.J. Holland and built in the central research workshop of the Erasmus University Rotterdam. Mr. Dane was responsible for a considerable number of improvements in the system and for maintenance and for the calculation of the results.

The calorimeter (fig. 1) is a closed system and consists of an incubator, which has a double gradient layer that makes it possible to measure the heat loss from radiation and convection even while the incubator temperature is changing. The incubator is so constructed that heat loss through conduction can be ignored. Water circulates between the double walls of the incubator and the temperature of the water can be altered rapidly and accurately. The air coming from the incubator is passed through a bacterial filter and goes into a dewpoint hygrometer where the amount of water which has been produced, is measured. Subsequently the carbon dioxide production is measured and then the CO_2 is absorbed out of the circulating air. The air then passes through a pump from which it goes to a bubble chamber and then a condensor so that it is brought to a dewpoint of 18 °C. The oxygen consumption is measured using 2 oxygen sensors and a reference vessel and the oxygen consumed is then replaced. The air passes through a flow meter, bacterial filter and a heater and thence back into the incubator.

The accuracy of the various measurements is as follows: Dry heat loss $\pm$ 0.1 W; wet heat loss $\pm$ 0.2 W; oxygen consumption $\pm$ 0.5 ml/min; carbon dioxide production $\pm$ 0.5 ml/min.

Calibration using an alcohol flame gave a maximum difference between direct and indirect calorimetry of 10 kJ/24 hr.

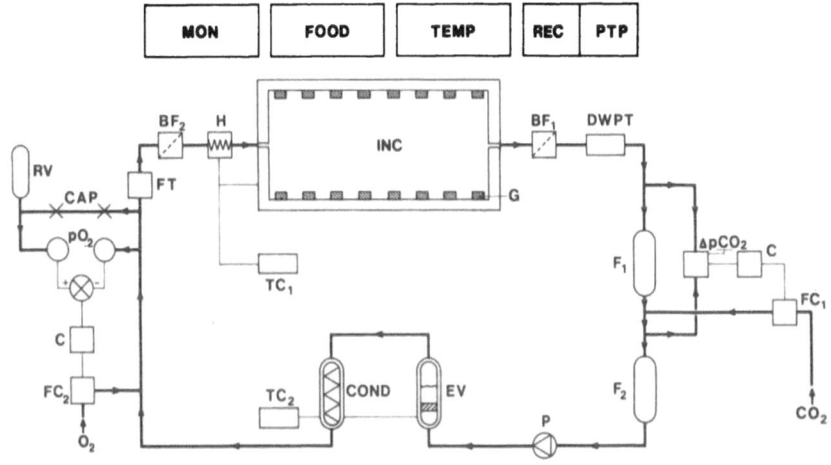

Fig. 1. Schematic diagram of the calorimeter.

INC	=	incubator
G	=	gradient layer
BF	=	bacterial filter
DWPT	=	dewpoint hygrometer
F_1 and F_2	=	CO_2 absorbers
ΔpCO^2	=	CO_2 partial pressure difference sensor
C	=	electronical controller
FC_1	=	flow controller CO_2
P	=	main circuit pump
EV	=	bubble chamber
COND	=	condensor
TC_2	=	temperature controller of condensor and bubble chamber
FC_2	=	flow controller O_2
PO_2	=	O_2 partial pressure sensors
RV	=	reference vessel
CAP	=	capillary
FT	=	main circuit flow sensor
H	=	heat exchanger
TC_1	=	temperature controller of incubator and heat exchanger
MON	=	heart beat and apnea monitor
FOOD	=	feeding system
TEMP	=	thermometer system
REC	=	recorder
PTP	=	paper-tape puncher

The formula:

$$M = \frac{4.2}{60} \, (3.8 \, V_{O_2} + 1.2 \, V_{CO_2}) \; (\text{OKKEN} \, (10)),$$

was used for the calculation of the indirect calorimetry. M denotes heat produced in watts, V_{O_2}-oxygen consumption in ml/min and V_{CO_2}-carbon dioxide production in ml/min.

During the measurements, the temperature was recorded continuously at 6 sites on the skin and in the mid oesophagus.

Continuous nasogastric feeding was given during the measurements via an air-tight port in the side of the incubator.

RESULTS

Direct and indirect calorimetry

The results of the 34 measurements are given in figure 2 and figure 3. As can be seen in figure 2 the metabolic rate increases linearly with increasing body weight when measured by both direct and indirect calori-

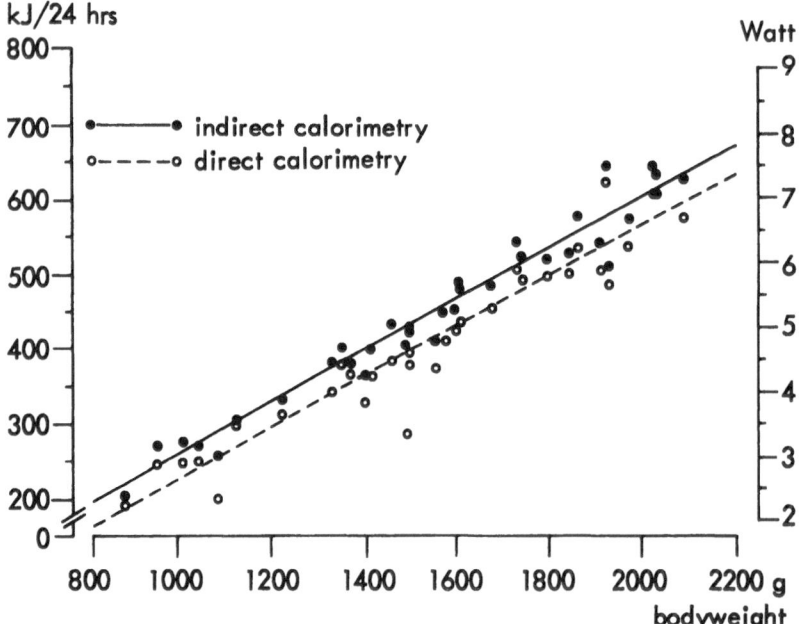

Fig. 2. Heat production as a function of body weight.

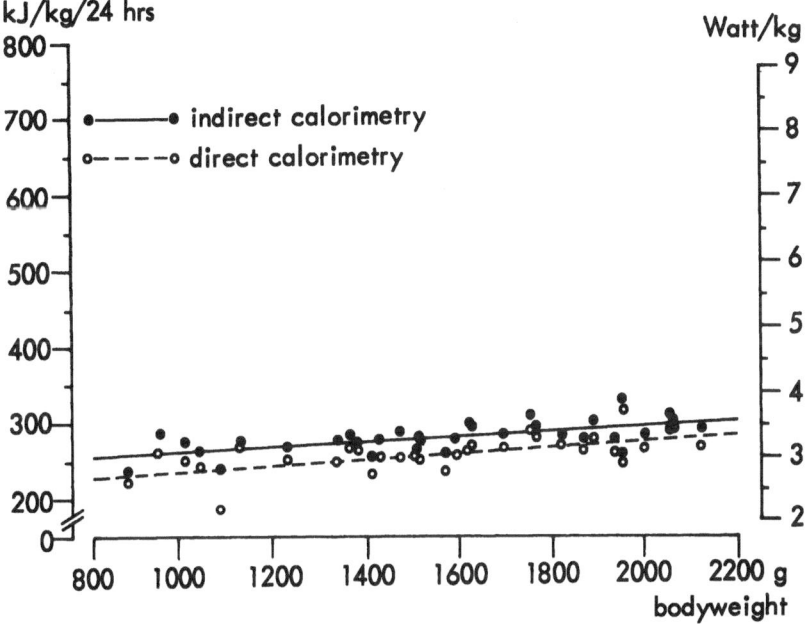

Fig. 3. Heat production per kilogram body weight as a function of body weight.

metry. The metabolic rate, expressed per kilogram body weight, remains virtually constant, increasing from approximately 250 kJ/kg/24 hr at 1000 g body weight to approximately 280 kJ/kg/24 hr at 2000 g. The heat production measured by direct calorimetry was lower in all measurements than the metabolic rate calculated from indirect calorimetry. This difference was on average 23 kJ/24 hr or 7.2% of the value obtained by indirect calorimetry.

Energy balance

The energy balance is given for 2 patients in figures 4 and 5 in the manner which was proposed in the introduction and using the results obtained. These patients were representative of the whole group. The whole column represents the energy available in the feeding given (E_{in}). The stippled area at the bottom of the column is the estimated energy loss via the faeces and urine. The lower, cross hatched area represents $E_{expended}$ calculated from direct calorimetry. The whole hatched area represents $E_{expended}$ calculated by indirect calorimetry. The upper white

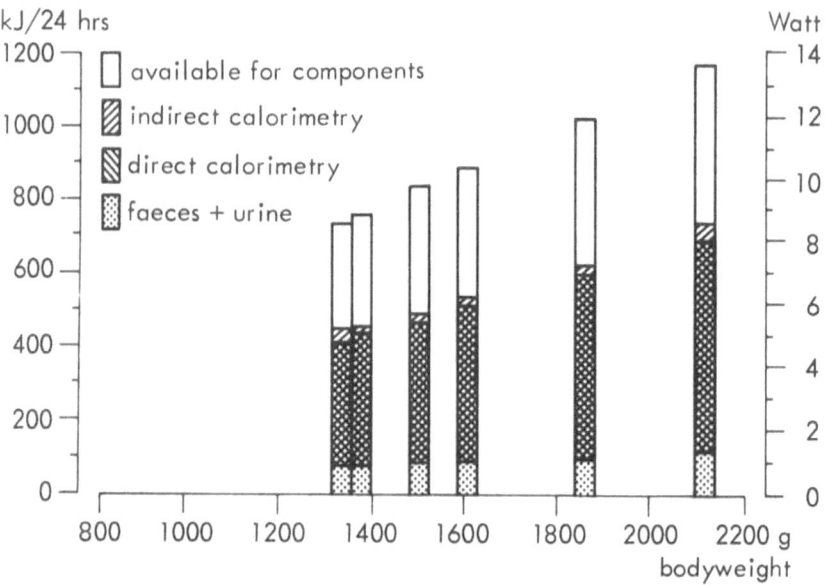

Fig. 4. Energy balance for a typical baby during growth.

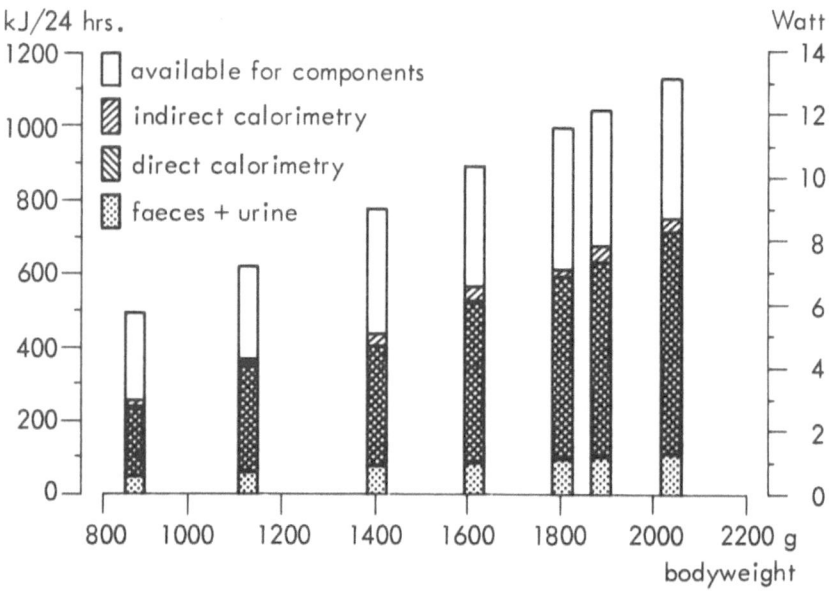

Fig. 5. Energy balance for a typical baby during growth.

part of the column represents that part of the feed which is absorbed but not oxidized. This is the energy which is stored in the components of new tissue ($E_{components}$). $E_{components}$ was calculated for all measurements and these results are given in figure 6. $E_{components}$ was 11.9 ± 4 kJ/g growth.

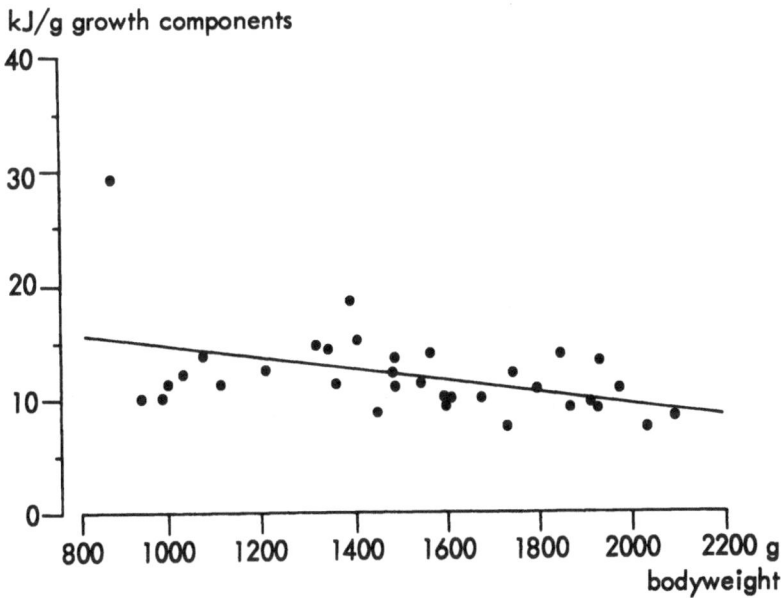

Fig. 6. Calculated energy costs of components of new tissue.

DISCUSSION

Energy expenditure

The energy expenditure of low birth weight infants at rest has been calculated in many studies of oxygen consumption in the literature. Many authors have shown that the oxygen consumption is lowest in the first few days after birth and that it increases slowly during the first 10 to 14 days (HILL and RAHIMTULLA (11), HILL and ROBINSON (12), MESTYAN et al. (13), SCOPES and AHMED (14), OKKEN (10), GENTZ et al. (15). Whether the oxygen consumption at rest increases after the first 2 weeks of life is not well known. HILL and ROBBINSON (12) found a large increase, while KARLBERG (16) found a small increase and HILL and RAHIMTULLA (11) found that the oxygen consumption remained constant. MESTYAN (17) and RUBECZ and MESTYAN (18) have measured oxygen consumption during a period of several hours (including periods of activity) in both preterm and small for gestational age infants. RUBECZ and MESTYAN showed a significant difference in oxygen consumption per kilogram body weight between the period when the small for gestational age infants were not growing (3–15 days) and the period when they were growing (16–39 days). During the non-growing phase, the metabolic rate was $\pm$ 210 kJ/kg/24 hr, whereas during the growth phase it was $\pm$ 290 kJ/kg/24hr. The authors suggested that this increase was due to both an increase in activity and an increase in resting oxygen consumption.

We have not done any studies during the period in which the babies were not growing. However, during the phase of rapid growth the metabolic rate (calculated from O_2 consumption and CO_2 production) rose from $\pm$ 250 kJ/24 hr at 1000 g to $\pm$ 560 kJ/24 hr at 2000 g; expressed per kilogram body weight from $\pm$ 250 to $\pm$ 280 kJ/kg/24 hr. These values are in reasonable agreement with those given by RUBECZ and MESTYAN. The reason for the small increase per kilogram body weight requires further study.

Difference of direct and indirect calorimetry

Since the studies of HOWLAND (3), DAY and HARDY (4) and DAY et al. (5) it has been assumed that direct and indirect calorimetry give identical results. Day did his studies on small children, however the duration of measurements was very short and the temperature of the children changed considerably during the study. It is not possible to make an accurate comparison of direct and indirect calorimetry from this study. PITTET et al. (19) have done simultaneous direct and indirect calorimetry on adults before and after a meal. In the fasting state the metabolic rate calculated from indirect calorimetry was lower than that measured by direct calorimetry. After a meal the result from indirect calorimetry was higher than that obtained by direct calorimetry, which remained constant. The rise in metabolic rate measured by indirect calorimetry was 8.5–16.5% of its original value, depending on the composition of the meal.

Indirect calorimetry is calculated using the oxygen consumption and the carbon dioxide production from the oxidation of the food. From these results the composition and quantity of the food metabolized can be calculated. The contribution of the metabolism of protein to the total heat production can be calculated by measuring nitrogen excretion.

Direct calorimetry measures the amount of heat produced by the body and lost via radiation, convection, conduction and evaporation. A correction must be made for any change in body temperature during the measurement period.

The results of direct and indirect calorimetry will be identical whenever all the energy produced by the combustion of foodstuffs is given off as heat. However, the energy produced by combustion, which is stored in the body without causing an increase in body temperature, will not be measured by direct calorimetry but will be measured by indirect calorimetry.

As discussed earlier, apart from the energy present in the components of new tissue, energy is also necessary to organise these components into new tissue ($E_{synthesis}$). Both parts are stored in new tissue. $E_{synthesis}$ is produced from the combustion of foodstuffs and thus uses oxygen and gives off carbon dioxide. Therefore the energy release calculated from

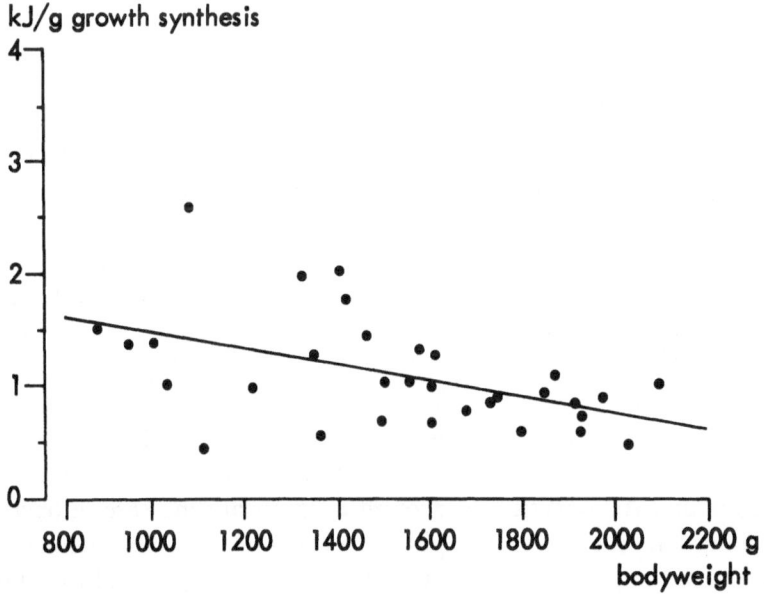

Fig. 7. Calculated energy costs of synthesis of new tissue.

oxygen consumption and CO_2 production (indirect calorimetry) contains $E_{synthesis}$, whereas the energy, measured by direct calorimetry, does not because $E_{synthesis}$ is not released as heat.

Thus, in a growing individual $E_{synthesis}$ is equal to the difference between $E_{expended}$ measured by indirect calorimetry and $E_{expended}$ measured by direct calorimetry. In our study the difference between the two measurements was 23 ± 7 kJ/24hr or 7.2% of the indirect calorimetry. $E_{synthesis}$ was calculated for all measurements and these results are given in figure 7. $E_{synthesis}$ was 1.1 ± 0.5 kJ/g growth.

Energy cost of growth

The estimated total energy cost of growth ($E_{cg} = E_{components} + E_{synthesis}$) from our studies is 13.0 ± 4 kJ/g growth.

Studies of the energy cost of growth of low birth weight infants have not been made previously due to the technical problems involved in measuring $E_{expended}$ during a long period. However, in the literature 4 methods are described for calculating the energy cost of growth in infants. These are given in table 3. Using the studies of WIDDOWSON (20) and ZIEGLER et al. (21) on the body composition of preterm babies who died in the immediate perinatal period, it is possible to calculate $E_{components}$ in the period of growth from 1000–2000 g. $E_{synthesis}$ can be calculated using the figures given by KIELANOWSKY (22) from animal studies.

HOMMES et al. (23) have calculated the E_{cg} in a term baby of 3900 g using Atkinson's metabolic price system. They calculated $E_{components}$ as 6.8 kJ/g growth and $E_{synthesis}$ as 1.3 kJ/g growth.

Many studies have been performed on malnourished children in the tropics during a phase of rapid catch-up growth in which the E_{cg} has been calculated using the energy balance equation given in the introduction. ASHWORTH (24) found that the E_{cg} was 23 kJ/g growth. She assumed that $E_{expended}$ was 1.5 times the metabolic rate measured at rest. SPADY et al. (1) have calculated $E_{expended}$ using heart beat counting. They calculated that E_{stored} was 13.8 kJ and $E_{synthesis}$ 4.6 kJ/g growth. BROOKE and ASHWORTH (25) showed a significant increase in oxygen consumption after a feed in rapidly growing children. This increase in oxygen consumption was proportional to the speed of growth. From their data it is possible to calculate the E_{cg}, which is 1.1 kJ/g growth.

In our study in small for gestational age infants with weights between

Table 3. *Energy cost of growth, data from literature.*

	(kJ/g growth)		
	Storage (components)	Synthesis	Total
Body composition			
WIDDOWSON (20), KIELANOWSKI (22)	6.0	2.5	8.5
ZIEGLER et al. (21) KIELANOWSKI (22)	6.4	3.0	9.4
Metabolic price system			
HOMMES et al. (23)	6.8	1.3	8.1
Balance in recovering from malnutrition			
ASHWORTH (24)			23
SPADY et al. (1)	13.8	4.6	18.4
Specific dynamic action			
BROOKE and ASHWORTH (25)			1.1
This study	11.9	1.1	13.0

870 and 2110 g, we calculated that the E_{cg} was 13.0 kJ/g growth. The energy present in the components ($E_{components}$) was 11.9 kJ/g and the energy cost of tissue synthesis ($E_{synthesis}$) was 1.1 kJ/g.

These figures are higher than those calculated from body composition, however they are lower than the results given by ASHWORTH (24) and SPADY et al. (1). Our results are in reasonable agreement with the values calculated by HOMMES et al. (23).

To check the validity of our results we are planning to do a simultaneous study of the changes in body composition with study of the energy cost of growth. From both methods it is possible to estimate the energy cost of growth in the same baby and then a comparison of the results obtained by these two different approaches will be made.

SUMMARY

A new calorimeter has been developed in which it is possible to do both direct and indirect calorimetry simultaneously over long periods in babies below 2.5 kg. Thirty four studies were performed on 6 healthy babies during rapid growth while they weighed between 870–2110 g. The total heat production increased proportionately to the increase in body weight from 250 kJ/24 hr at 1000 g to 560 kJ/24 hr at 2000 g. Expressed per kilogram body weight there was only a very small increase, from 250 kJ/kg/24 hr to 280 kJ/kg/24 hr. The total heat production measured by direct calorimetry was always less than that calculated from indirect calorimetry, the difference was 23 ± 7 kJ/24 hr. From the energy balance equation the energy cost of the components of new tissue was calculated as 11.9 ± 4 kJ/g growth.

In our study there is a marked difference between the metabolic rate measured by direct and indirect calorimetry; we postulate that this difference is due to the energy cost of tissue synthesis. We calculated $E_{synthesis}$ as 1.1 ± 0.5 kJ/g growth. The total cost of 1 g growth in our study was on average 13 ± 4 kJ. Within the accuracy of the measurement technique this agrees well with the energy cost of growth calculated by other methods.

REFERENCES

1. SPADY, D.W., P.R. PAYNE, D. PICOU and J.C. WATERLOW. (1976) Am. J. Clin. Nutr. 29:1073.
2. SINCLAIR, J.C. (1978) In: Growth and Development of the Full-Term and Premature Infant, Jonxis, J.H.P. ed., Excerpta Medica, Amsterdam-Oxford, p. 19.
3. HOWLAND, J. (1912) In: Tr. 15th Internat. Cong. Hyg. and Demog. ii, p. 438.
4. DAY R. and J.D. HARDY. (1942) Am. J. Dis. Child. 63:1986.
5. DAY, R., J. CURTIS and M. KELLY. (1943) Am. J. Dis. Child. 65:376.
6. USHER, R. and F. MCLEAN. (1969) J. Pediatr. 74:901.
7. HEY, E.N. and G. KATZ. (1975) Arch. Dis. Child. 45:328.
8. ROY, C.C., M. STE-MARIE, L. CHARTRAND, A. WEBER, H. BARD and B. DORAY. (1975) J. Pediatr. 86:446.
9. TANTIBHEDHYANGHUL, P. and S.A. HASHIM (1975) Pediatrics 55:359.
10. OKKEN, A. (1976) Warmtehuishouding van pasgeborenen met een laag geboortegewicht, Thesis, Groningen.
11. HILL, J.R. and K.A. RAHIMTULLA. (1965) J. Physiol. 180:239.
12. HILL, J.R. and D.C. ROBINSON. (1968) J. Physiol. 199:685.
13. MESTYAN, J., M. FEKETE, G. BATA and I. JÁRAI. (1964) Biol. Neonate 7:11.
14. SCOPES, J.W. and I. AHMED. (1966) Arch. Dis. Child. 41:407.
15. GENTZ, J., M. GELLUM and B. PERSSON. (1976) Acta Paediatr. Sand. 65:445.
16. KARLBERG, P. (1952) Acta Paediatr. Scand. 41 suppl. 89:67.
17. MESTYAN, J., I. JARAI and M. FEKETE. (1968) Pediatr. Res. 2:161.
18. RUBECZ, J. and J. MESTYAN. (1975) Acta Paediatr. Acad. Sci. Hung. 16:335.
19. PITTET, Ph., P.H. GYGAX and E. JÉQUIER. (1974) Brit. J. Nutr. 31:343.
20. WIDDOWSON, E. (1974) In: Scientific Foundations of Paediatrics, Davis, J.A. and J. Dobbing eds., Heinemann Medical Books, London, p. 154.
21. ZIEGLER, E.E., A.M. O'DONNELL, S.E. NELSON and S.J. FOMON. (1976) Growth 40:329.
22. KIELANOWSKI, J. (1965) In: Energy Metabolism, Blaxter, K.L. ed., Academic Press, London, p. 13.

23. HOMMES, F.A., Y.M. DROST, W.X.M. GERAETS and M.A.A. REIJENGA. (1975) Pediatr. Res. 9:51.
24. ASHWORTH, A. (1969) Brit. J. Nutr. 23:835.
25. BROOKE, O.G. and A. ASHWORTH. (1972) Brit. J. Nutr. 27:407.

FATTY ACID METABOLISM BEFORE
AND AFTER BIRTH

D. HULL*

Changes in fatty acid metabolism during development might be predicted knowing that before birth the fetus is probably on a low fat diet,
that the birth experience is a powerful stimulant of sympathetic nervous
activity, that after birth the infant experiences acute total starvation
probably for the first time, and that subsequently the infant grows
rapidly on milk, a relatively high fat diet. But it is difficult to gather
evidence of what is actually happening and to know whether or not any
particular infant is making an inadequate or inappropriate response. As
in many areas of fetal and neonatal research, animal studies have proven
to be very instructive; but their use in the translation of the situation
relating to fatty acid metabolism in man is limited due to wide and
fascinating species variations.

Important factors which will influence an individual infant's metabolic adjustment after birth are his experiences in late fetal life. In this
brief review I shall concentrate on these factors as they relate to two
questions. What sort of "fat diet" might an infant receive before birth?
To what extent does the fetus supply his own fatty acids?

FAT "DIET" DURING DEVELOPMENT

BATTAGLIA and MESCHIA (1) have recently written a detailed review on
the principle substrates of fetal metabolism. Much of our present understanding of fetal nutrition rests on the fine series of investigations that
they and others have made on chronically catheterized sheep (2, 3, 4, 5).
BATTAGLIA (6) concludes that "fetal milk" in the ovine fetus consists
essentially of the two carbohydrates, glucose and lactate, and amino-
acids. He goes on to speculate that a baby may well receive his first fatty
meal with his first milk feed. If this is the case then there would be a major

* Department of Child Health, University of Nottingham, Medical School, Nottingham, England.

H.K.A. Visser (ed.), Nutrition and Metabolism of the Fetus and Infant, 109-122. All rights reserved.
Copyright © 1979 Martinus Nijhoff Publishers b.v., The Hague/Boston/London.

change of direction in fatty acid metabolism in man at birth. However, evidence is accumulating to suggest that this is not so.

The fetus needs fatty acids for structure and storage and possibly also for energy. In theory, he may make his own fatty acids, or alternatively he may draw them from the mother across the placenta. There is no doubt that fetal tissues have a considerable capacity for fatty acid synthesis (7, 8, 9, 10). It has been demonstrated in fetal adipose tissue in early gestation (11). The activities of the enzymes of fatty acid synthesis in adipose tissue fall after birth (12). In general, fatty acids synthesized from carbohydrate are even chain saturated fatty acids, the major component being palmitic acid ($C16:0$). There is no evidence that the fetus can make essential fatty acids, so if *all* fatty acids were made by the fetus, the fetus would be deficient in essential fatty acids. If *most* of the fatty acids are made by the fetus then what essential fatty acids there are would be used in structure and very little would be left over for storage. This, in fact, is the case in the lamb (13, 14, 15) but it is not the situation in many non-ruminant mammals including man (16) (fig. 1). The presence of around 2.5% linoleic acid in fetal adipose tissue stores in man at term argues strongly that fatty acids cross the placenta in sizeable amounts.

Before trying to estimate how much, it is important to consider some of the mechanisms which might be involved. For example, are fatty acids selectively transferred across the placenta? In theory it might be expected that fatty acids of different chain lengths, and with differing numbers of unsaturated bonds and thus with differing solubilities in lipids and water would cross the membranes and cells of the placenta at different rates. Similarly differing affinities to albumin, and the amount of albumin in the vascular compartments on either side of the placenta would also influence the net flow in any direction. Measurements that have been made so far would suggest that the effects of these factors are small. Thus in the anaesthetized pregnant rabbit, fatty acids are transferred across the placenta in generous amounts and it is relatively easy to measure the percentage fatty acid composition of the venous-arterial difference in the umbilical blood free fatty acid compartment. It was found to mirror that of the maternal circulating free fatty acids (17) (fig. 2). Arachidonic acid (20:4) is a notable exception. There is evidence that the placenta elongates linoleic acid (18:2) to arachidonic acid (20:4) in a number of species including man (18, 19, 20, 21).

Studies on the isolated perfused human placenta suggested initially

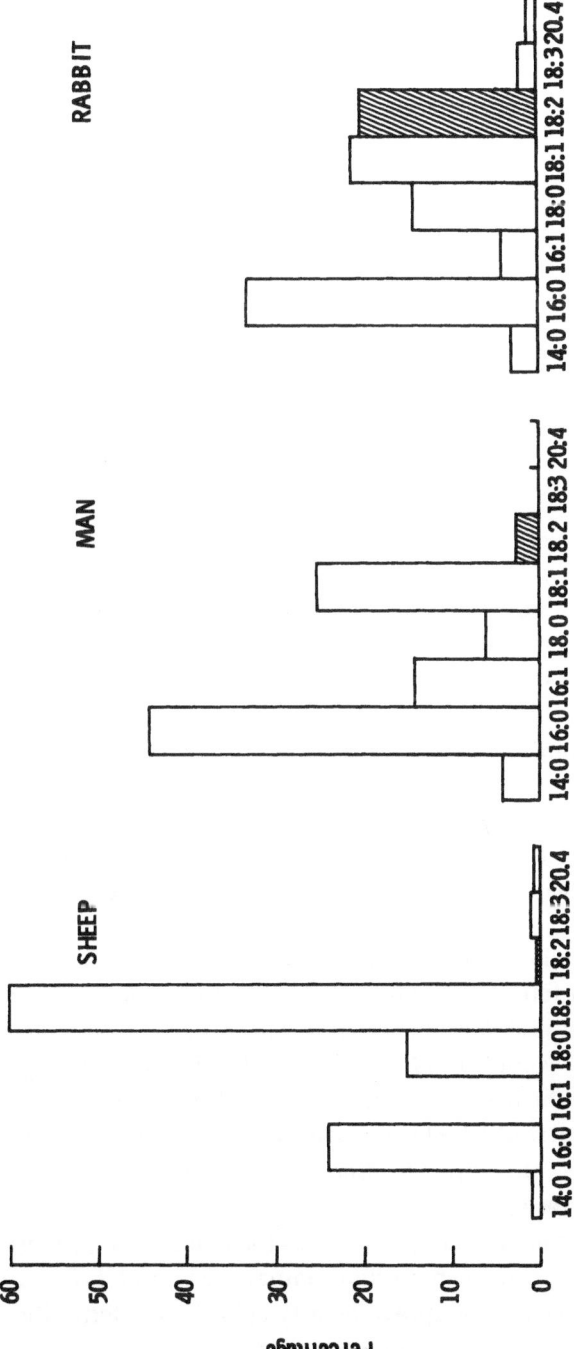

Fig. 1. Fatty acid composition of fetal adipose tissue triglyceride in late gestation.

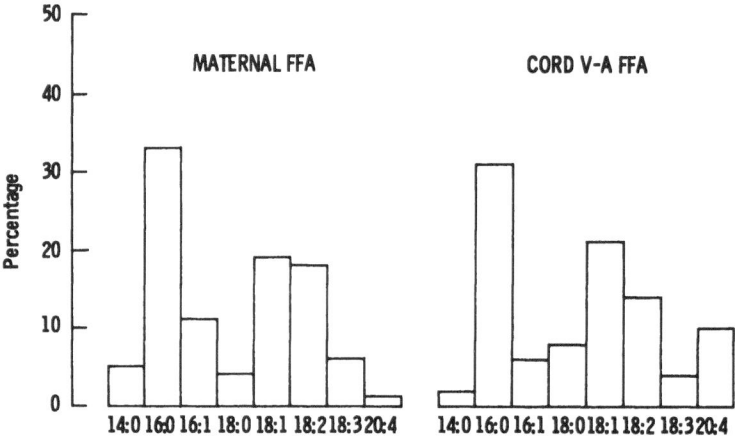

Fig. 2. Fatty acid composition of maternal circulating free fatty acids and of the umbilical venous-arterial free fatty acid difference in rabbits immediately prior to delivery by Caesarean section.

that there might be selected transfer (22) but subsequent studies showed that the observed differences could be explained on the relative affinity of the different fatty acids for albumin (23). From these investigations there is no doubt that fatty acids can cross the perfused human placenta. The net flow from maternal to fetal side is directly related to the concentration of free fatty acids in the perfusate on the maternal side (24). This is consistent with the view that the flow of each fatty acid across the placental cells and membranes is in relation, amongst other things, to its concentration in the free fatty acid compartment in the maternal circulation.

The umbilical blood venous-arterial differences in free fatty acid in the human fetus are small compared to those found in the rabbit, but nevertheless under certain circumstances they reach a magnitude which if sustained would supply the fetus with all his needs (25, 26, 27, 28). Analysis of the percentage composition of this difference is difficult. We attempted to study this by analysing blood collected at elective caesarean section (29) (fig. 3). The findings were again consistent with non-selective transfer.

If we assume that fatty acids cross the placenta in proportions close to those in the supplying maternal compartment, and if we also assume that there is non-selective uptake of fatty acids by the fetus, then analysis of the fetal triglyceride stores for the relative amount of essential fatty acids

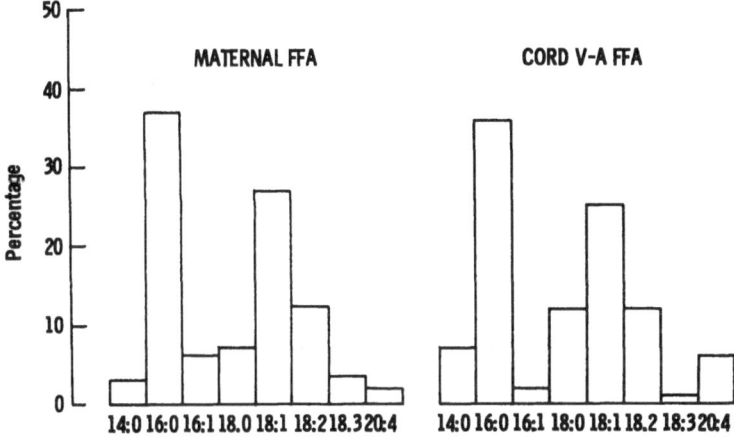

Fig. 3. Fatty acid composition of maternal circulating free fatty acids and of the umbilical venous-arterial free fatty acid difference in women and their infants immediately prior to delivery by elective Caesarean section.

present give us some clue as to where they all come from. Detailed analyses have not been made on any mother infant couples. Calculations based on averages taken from the literature suggest that if material free fatty acids are the only supply of fatty acid to the placenta then on average around 15-20% of fetal lipid is derived from the mother.

This estimate could be improved if matching samples were taken from a mother infant pair. But before such a study is undertaken the assumptions on which the calculation is based must be examined more closely. Firstly, is the use of fatty acids by the fetus non-selective? Fatty acids might be used for structure or energy. Structural lipids, particularly phospholipids require relatively more of the unsaturated fatty acids, the basic units of which are linoleic (18:2) or linolenic acid (18:3). In this respect it is relevant to note, that despite high cord venous arterial differences of arachidonic acid, very little is found in adipose tissue stores. The extent to which the fetus can and does use fatty acids for cellular energy is uncertain. The activity of enzymes concerned with fatty acid oxidation measured in fetal tissue in vitro have been found to be low in some species (30) and high in others (31, 32) and there appears to be a delay, at least in some circumstances and in some tissues, in oxidizing fatty acids after birth. The enzyme activities in tissue studied in vitro increase postnatally (33). If the fetus does oxidize fatty acid, then from the evidence available it would appear likely that linolate will be more readily oxidized (34, 35). Thus is adipose tissue stores those fatty acids not used for structure or energy, it will contain relatively less linoleic acid (18:2) than the fatty acid mixture which crossed the placenta even if there were no fatty acid synthesis in fetal liver and adipose tissue.

Secondly, is the maternal blood free fatty acid compartment the only source of fatty acid available to the placenta? The answer is probably no. There is some evidence in the sheep and rabbit that maternal phospholipid fatty acids may enter the placenta and be transferred to the fetus (36, 37, 38). There is far more evidence in animals and man that the placenta takes up fatty acids from the triglycerides of chylomicron and very low density lipoprotein and that these fatty acids enter the fetal circulation (39, 40, 41). Fatty acid uptake from circulating triglyceride by peripheral tissue, adipose tissue, mammary tissue etc., depends on the activity of a lipoprotein lipase which is situated in the lining of the endothelial cells of the capillaries. This poses an interesting question with regard to placental tissues for in many species maternal capillaries are not present. There does appear to be a lipoprotein lipase present in placental tissue (42) although there have been no studies on changes in activity under different circumstances.

The evidence that triglyceride fatty acid crosses the placenta in animals is based on measurements made after endogenous triglyceride became labelled after injection of labelled fatty acids or after infusion of labelled chylomicron or Intralipid (Vitrum, Stockholm). The latter is an artificial product in which between 45–50% of the fatty acid is linoleic acid ($C18:2$). We took the opportunity to study the cord lipids in infants born by caesarean section who were given Intralipid prior to the birth (40). Not only did the venous-arterial difference of the cord blood free fatty acids show the imprint of Intralipid, but there was also a large and highly significant venous-arterial difference in triglycerides also containing a high content of linoleic acid. Many years ago significant venous-arterial differences in concentrations of triglyceride were reported (43) and we from time to time have found this also, but it is not a consistent finding. However it does raise the possibility that the placenta might under certain circumstances release triglyceride as well as free fatty acids into the fetal circulation. These observations need confirmation. In a more controlled experimental situation we were unable to detect a similar phenomenon in either rabbit or sheep.

Even if maternal triglycerides are an important supply of fatty acids to the fetus it will not invalidate the crude calculation made above because under usual conditions the fatty acid composition of the free fatty acids are on average likely to resemble dietary lipids, though it is true that they will tend to obtain a lower percentage of linoleic acid (18:2).

It was demonstrated long ago that in guinea pigs and man the fatty acid composition of fetal lipids varied with the fatty acid composition of the diet given to the mother (44, 45, 46, 47). An interesting variation of this approach is to feed an unusual lipid, say corn oil, to pregnant rabbits for two days only before delivery. In this short period the maternal source of free fatty acids, adipose tissue triglyceride, will change little, so the fatty acid profile in free fatty acids will differ considerably from those in circulating chylomicron. In a preliminary study using this approach it was found that the mixture of fatty acids in fetal lipid stores resembled those in the diet. (HULL and ELPHICK, unpublished.)

The amount and mix of fatty acids received by a particular fetus will be different depending upon the circumstances.

Most of the observations on fat transfer to the fetus in man relate to conditions operating at the time of birth and this will tend to emphasize the contribution from maternal free fatty acids for maternal blood concentrations of free fatty acids are increased by exercise, fear, pain and surgery, so whether the baby is born by elective Caesarean section or vaginally after a normal labour the trend will be for the baby to receive a "fatty meal" from maternal free fatty acids during the birth. The pregnancy state itself augments this phenomenon for towards term the lipolytic response in adipose tissue to given stimuli is greater and more prolonged. The effect will be further magnified if the birth is proceeded by a period of starvation, as it may well be for elective Caesarean section or after a prolonged labour.

During the course of a day the circulating concentrations of free fatty acids fluctuate (48, 49) and the net flow of fatty acid to the fetus will presumably vary accordingly. Circulating free fatty acids may be low, and therefore the contribution from this compartment to the fetus may be small, in well fed mothers on a high plane of nutrition. If the diet is rich in fat then presumably the fetus will receive those fatty acids present in the mother's diet, if the diet is rich in carbohydrate then the fetus will make fatty acids locally. There is no evidence to indicate whether this should be viewed as response to "excess" glucose or as an inherent drive in developing adipose tissue to lay down triglyceride.

The amount and mixture of fatty acids received by any one newborn

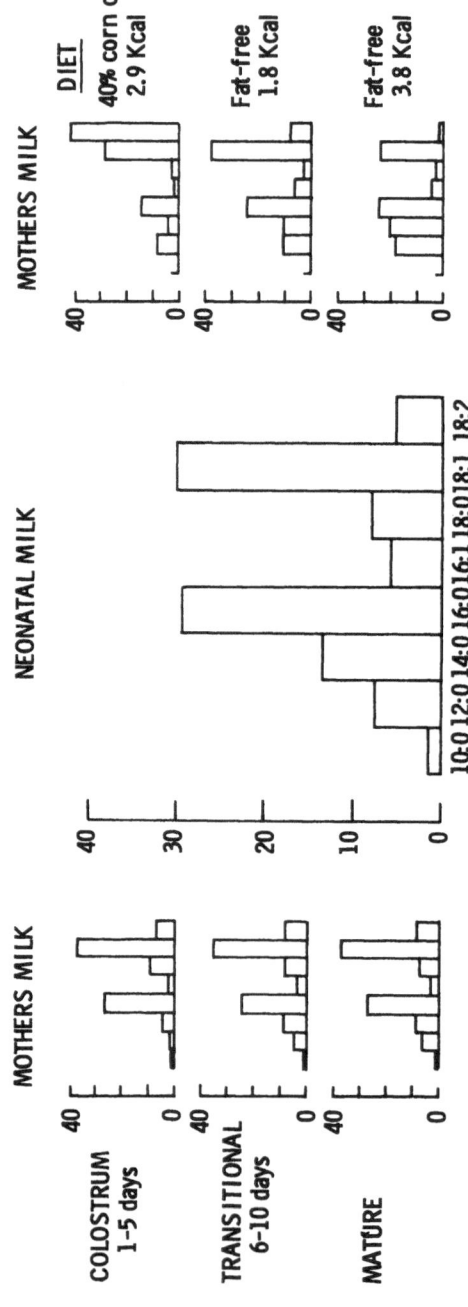

Fig. 4. Fatty acid composition of human milk. The values for colostrum, transitional and mature are averages taken from WIDDOWSON (50), the values on the different diets are those from INSULL et al. (51), the figures on neonatal milk are the average of 23 analyses taken from infants in the first four weeks of life (McKIERNAN, J., M.C. ELPHICK and D. HULL, unpublished).

infant will depend on conditions remarkably similar to those operating in the fetus, namely the diet and plane of nutrition of the mother. True, the amounts will be greater but then the demands for energy and growth are greater. Milk lipids may be derived by fatty acid synthesis in the mammary cells, or the cells may take up fatty acids from the free fatty acids or triglycerides in the maternal blood stream. The mixture of fatty acids in the milk will reflect the source. The average values for colostrum, transitional and mature milk indicate a mixed source (50). The possible extremes are beautifully illustrated in the study by INSULL et al. (51). When the mother studied was on a high fat diet, then the milk reflected the fatty acid mixture in the diet; when she was on a low calorie fat free diet it reflected the fatty acids in her adipose tissue stores; when she was on a high calorie fat free diet the fatty acids in the milk were mainly those one might expect from fatty acid synthesis. Under these conditions many of the shorter chain fatty acids $C10:0$, $C12:0$, $C14:0$ are produced. In rabbits there appears to be a special enzyme system which develops in the breast during pregnancy which interferes with the normal sequence in fatty acid synthesis to produce $C8:0$ and $C10:0$ fatty acids (52, 53, 54). These midchain fatty acids may be more readily digested and oxidized.

The newborn infant, male as well as female, is also able to produce milk and the fatty acid mixture is interesting. There are relatively large fractions of $C12:0$ and $C14:0$ indicating considerable fatty acid synthesis.

FREE FATTY ACID SUPPLIES DURING DEVELOPMENT

The human fetus differs from the other mammals whose fetal and neo-natal biology has been investigated in that he stores considerable amounts of lipid in adipose tissue during late fetal life and has sufficient energy stores at term to support his energy metabolism for 3 or 4 weeks (55, 56). Furthermore in mouse, rat, rabbit, guinea pig and lamb most of the lipid is stored in the brown adipocytes (57, 58). The pig has very little fat anywhere. In human infants at term most of the fat is in sub-cutaneous white adipocytes with smaller deposits in the deeper brown adipocytes. The biochemical behaviour of the white adipocyte in the newborn differs from that in the adult (59, 60, 61, 62). It is generally a more active tissue, with a greater vascularity and higher rates in enzymic activities for lipolysis and oxidation. Theoretically it might be that these differences represent the behaviour of tissues passing through a stage in development, an explanation which on principle I am not happy to accept, or they might reflect a biological response of a tissue to the needs of the organism. The high activity of adipose tissue in the immediate newborn period raises the possibility that fetal adipose tissue is active before birth. Rabbit fetal brown adipocytes in vitro behave like those of the newborn, they respond to lipolytic agents by release of fatty acids and glycerol and by an increase in cellular oxidation (32). The extent to which the FA released by lipolysis in the brown adipocyte enters the circulation depends on the availability of oxygen. If little oxygen is available by virtue of either low blood saturations or limited tissue perfusion then fatty acids will be released. With good perfusion they will be oxidized and the resultant energy released as heat (63).

Attempts to demonstrate lipolysis in vivo in experimental fetal animals has not been too successful (64, 65, 66). However the explanation may lie in the experimental approach rather than poor rates of release. It is difficult to deliver the lipolytic agent directly to the adipose tissue mass and to collect the effluent. JONES (67) observed a rise in fetal free fatty acids with maternal hypoxia towards the end of gestation. The rise was directly related to catecholamine levels. These findings suggest that the fatty acids are mobilized from fetal tissues in vivo. However in these experiments the maternal free fatty acid concentration also increased and the possibility that placental permeability to fatty acids was changed by hypoxia was not excluded.

There is some indirect evidence that adipose tissue releases free fatty acids. The fetal liver takes up free fatty acids, some it stores as triglyceride, (and it may lay down a sizeable store), and some it releases as endogenous triglyceride. This the body clears rapidly in much the same way as chylomicron are cleared after birth. Now if we overlook the possibility and I am not sure that we should, that "exogenous" triglyceride enters the fetal circulation from the placenta, then cord triglyceride concentrations will indicate the flow of free fatty acids to the liver over the previous hours. Thus during maternal starvation, energy stores are mobilized from adipose tissue, more fatty acids cross the placenta, the stores of lipid in the fetal liver increase and the concentration of circulating triglyceride rise. In experimental animals all the steps in the above sequence, have been demonstrated (68, 69, 70). In women, an association between food intake over the hours prior to birth and high cord triglyceride concentrations has been found (71).

But high cord triglyceride concentrations have also been found in asphyxiated infants and in infants who are under size (72, 73, 74).

Experimental hypoxia in fetal animals, and clinical asphyxia in the human newborn causes a rise in free fatty acids (75). In the "under-nourished" fetus challenged by the birth experience there is a greater rate of mobilization of its limited reserves of fat. After birth free fatty acid concentrations in undersized infants on average rise faster than those of normal infants. It is interesting that in the infant of the diabetic mother, where the balance is more set for storage rather than mobilization, the free fatty acids rise at a slower rate than normal after birth.

So in answer to the question "are fatty acids released by fetal adipose tissue?" the answer would appear to be yes and to degrees that vary considerably according to circumstances.

There are a number of studies on fatty acid concentrations after birth (76, 77, 78, 79, 80, 81, 82). Under usual conditions they rise. If the birth is easy, asphyxia is minimal and cold exposure is avoided the rise is likely to be less. But there is wide variation between apparently similar babies. We found this again recently in a group of healthy infants at five days of age in a study aimed at evaluating the variability due to warm or cool environments (83). Because so many factors initiate mobilization and because the half life is so short, single measurements of free fatty acid concentrations are unlikely to be very instructive. Circulating concentrations in the other lipid compartments (excluding chylomicron) rise fairly steady after birth. This is also true for the first week or so of life of those infants with congenital bowel anomalies which preclude oral feeding (84). There does not appear to be any difficulty after birth in mobilizing the fat reserves.

After birth the demands for energy increase. Partly due to a general rise in the minimal metabolic rate, and partly due to increased activity and the need to maintain thermal control. Rabbits can double or even treble their metabolic rate given a cold stimulus within minutes of birth; most of the increase is due to oxidation of fatty acids to produce heat. In the human infant an increase in heat production in response to a cool environment within minutes of birth has not been demonstrated. The response appears to develop over the first few hours of life (85). This may reflect adjustments in central control, but it might also be due to initial limitation in the enzyme capacity for fatty acid oxidation. As the fatty acids are already in the cell there is no limit in supply of fuel.

SUMMARY

Before birth the amount and fatty acid composition of fat received by the fetus varies with maternal experiences, plane of nutrition and diet. After birth the amount of fat available to the newborn in the mother's milk are greater but both quantity and composition still vary with maternal experiences, plane of nutrition and diet.

Before birth the fetus lays down triglyceride in adipose tissue and appears to be able to mobilize free fatty acids on demand. The birth experience is likely to accelerate fatty acid mobilization, the extent to which it occurs might be expected to vary according to many factors few of which have been investigated. After birth the human newborn appears to have no difficulty supplying fatty acids to meet the increased energy demands.

REFERENCES

1. BATTAGLIA, F.C. and G. MESCHIA. (1978) Physiol. Rev. 58:499.
2. MESCHIA, G., J.R. COTTON, C.S. BREATHNACH and D.H. BARRON. (1965) Quart. J. Exptl. Physiol. 50:185.
3. JAMES, E.J., J.R. RAYE, E.L. GRESHAM, G. MAKOWSKI, G. MESCHIA and F.C. BATTAGLIA. (1972) Pediatrics 50:361.
4. MORRIS, F.H. Jr., R.D.H. BOYD, E.L. MAKOWSKI, G. MESCHIA and F.C. BATTAGLIA. (1974) Proc. Soc. Exptl. Biol. Med. 145:879.
5. SILVER, M. (1976) In: Fetal Physiology and Medicine, Beard, R.W. and P.W. Nathanielsz, eds., W.B. Saunders, London, Philadelphia, Pa.
6. BATTAGLIA, F.C. (1978) Pediat. Res. 12:736.
7. VILLEE, C.A. and J.M. LORING. (1961) Biochem. J. 81:488.
8. ROUX, J.F. and T. YOSHIOKA. (1970) Clin. Obstet. Gynec. 13:595.
9. JONES, C.T. and W. FERMIN. (1976) Biochem. J. 154:159.
10. VILLEE, D.B. (1975) In: Human Endocrinology, W.B. Saunders, Philadelphia, Pa., p. 81.
11. DUNLOP, M. and J.M. COURT. (1978) Early Human Development 2/2:123.
12. NOVAK, M., P. HAHN, D. PENN, E. MONKUS and L. KIRBY. (1973) Biol. Neonate 23:19.
13. LEAT, W.M.F. (1966) Biochem J. 93:598.
14. LEAT, W.M.F. (1978) Proc. Nutri. Soc. 37:52A.
15. ELPHICK, M.C. and D. HULL. (1978) J. Physiol. 276:65P.
16. BAKER, L., P. PODHIPLEUX and M.L. WILLIAMS. (1964) Abstracts Soc. Pediat. Res. 34th annual meeting, Seattle, Washington, p. 126.
17. ELPHICK, M.C., D.G. HUDSON and D. HULL. (1976) J. Physiol. 252:29.
18. ELPHICK, M.C. and D. HULL. (1977) J. Physiol. 264:751.
19. ROBERTSON, A.F. and H. SPRECHER. (1968) Acta Paediat. Scand., Supplement 183.
20. CRAWFORD, M.A., A.G. HASSAN, G. WILLIAMS and W.L. WHITEHOUSE. (1976) Lancet 1:452.

21. FILSHIE, G.M. and M.D. ANSTEY. (1978) Brit. J. Obstet. Gynecol. 85:119.
22. DANCIS, J., V. JANSEN, H.J. KEYDEN, H. SCHNEIDER and M. LEVITZ. (1973) Pediat. Res. 7:192.
23. DANCIS, J., V. JANSEN and M. LEVITZ. (1976) Pediat. Res. 10:5.
24. ELPHICK, M.C., J.L. EDSON, and D. HULL. (1978) IRCS Med. Sci. 6:114.
25. SABATA, V., H. WOLF and S. LAUSMANN. (1968) Biol. Neonate 13:7.
26. TOBIN, J.D., J.F. ROUZ and J.S. SOELDNER. (1969) Pediatrics 44:668.
27. PERSSON, B. and R. TUNNELL. (1971) Acta Pediat. Scand. 60:385.
28. SHEATH, J., J. GRUNWADE, K. WALDRON, M. BICKLEY, P. TAFT and C. WOOD. (1972) Amer. J. Obstet. Gynec. 113:358.
29. ELPHICK, M.C., D. HULL and R.R. SAUNDERS. (1976) Brit. J. Obstet. Gynecol. 83:539.
30. WARSHAW, J.B. (1972) Devel. Biol. 28:537.
31. VILLEC, C.A., D.D. HAGERMAN and N. HOLMBERG. (1958) Pediatrics 22:953.
32. HUDSON, D.G. and D. HULL. (1977) Biol. Neonate 31:316.
33. SCHMIDT-SOMMERFELD, E., M. NOVAK, D. PENN, P.B. WIESER, M. BUCH and P. HAHN. (1978) Pediat. Res. 12:660.
34. LINDSAY, D.B. (1975) Proc. Nutr. Soc. 34:241.
35. HAVEL, R.J., L.A. CARLSON, L.G. EKELUND and A. HOLMGREN. (1964) J. Appl. Physiol. 19:613.
36. BODY, D.R., F.B. SHORLAND and Z. CZOCHANSKA. (1970) J. Sci. Food Agri. 21:220.
37. SHORLAND, F.B., D.R. BODY and J.P. GLASS. (1966) Biochem. Biophys. Acta 125:217.
38. BIEZENSKI, J.J., J. CAROZZA and J. Li. (1971) Biochem. Biophys. Acta 239:92.
39. HUMMEL, L., A. SCHWARTZ, W. SCHIRRMEISTER and H. WAGNER. (1976) Acta Biol. Med. Germ. 35:1635.
40. ELPHICK, M.C. and D. HULL. (1977) J. Physiol. 273:475.
41. ELPHICK, M.C., G.M. FILSHIE and D. HULL. (1978) Brit. J. Obstet. Gynecol. 85:610.
42. MALLOV, S. and A.A. ALOUSI. (1965) Proc. Soc. exp. Biol. Med. 119:301.
43. BOYD, E.M. and K.M. WILSON. (1935) J. Clin. Invest. 14:7.
44. SODERHJELM, L. (1953) Acta Soc. Upsaliensis 58:239.
45. SATOMURA, K. and L. SODERHJELM. (1962) Texas Reports on Biology and Medicine 20:671.
46. WIDDOWSON, E.M., M.J. DAUNCEY, D.M.T. GAIRDNER, J.H.P. JONXIS and M. PELIKAN-FILIPKOVA. (1975) Brit. Med. J. 1:653.
47. PAVEY, D.E. and E.M. WIDDOWSON. (1975) Proc. Nutr. Soc. 34:107a.
48. PERSSON, B. and N.O. LUNELL. (1975) Am. J. Obstet. Gynec. 122:737.
49. GILLMER, M.D.G., R.W. BEARD, N.W. OAKLEY, F.M. BROOKE, M.C. ELPHICK and D. HULL. (1977) Brit. Med. J. 2:670.
50. WIDDOWSON, E.M. (1974) In: Scientific Foundations of Pediatrics Davis J., and J. Dobbing eds., Heinemann, London, p. 153.
51. INSULL, W., JR., J. HIRSCH. T. JAMES and E.H. AHRENS, Jr. (1959) J. Clin. Invest. 38:443.
52. CHIVERS, L. and R.R.A. DILS. (1977) Biochem. Biophys. Acta 487:361.
53. CLARK, S. and R.R.A. DILS. (1976) Biochem. J. 160:683.
54. DILS, R.R.A. and S. CLARK. (1977) Comparative aspects of milk fat synthesis. In: Comparative aspects of lactation, Academic Press, London, p. 43.
55. JONXIS, J.H.P. (1976) In: Early Nutrition and later development, Wilkinson, A.W. ed., Pitman Medical, London, p. 79.
56. HULL, D. (1976) In Early Nutrition and later development, Wilkinson, A.W. ed., Pitman Medical, London, p. 49.

57. Hull, D. (1973) In: Comparative physiology of thermoregulation, Whitton, G.C. ed., Academic Press, New York, p. 167.
58. Alexander, G. (1975) Brit. Med. Bull. 31:62.
59. Hahn, P. and M. Novak. (1975) J. Lipid res. 16:79.
60. Novak, M. and E. Monkus. (1972) Pediat. Res. 6:73.
61. Novak, M., E. Monkus, H. Wolf and U. Stave. (1972) Pediat. Res. 6:211.
62. Novak, M., D. Penn and E. Monkus. (1973) Biol. Neonate 22:451.
63. Hardman, M.J. and D. Hull. (1970) J. Physiol. 206:263.
64. Comline, R.S. and M. Silver. (1972) J. Physiol. 222:233.
65. Elphick, M.C., D.G. Hudson and D. Hull. (1975) J. Physiol. 252:29.
66. Harding, P.G.R. and E.D. Ralph. (1970) Am. J. Obstet. Gynecol. 106:907.
67. Jones, C.T. (1977) J. Physiol. 265:743.
68. Edson, J.L., D.G. Hudson and D. Hull. (1975) Biol. Neonate 27:50.
69. Edson, J.L. and D. Hull. (1977) Pediatric.Res. 11:793.
70. Elphick, M.C., J.L. Edson and D. Hull. (1978) Biol. Neonate 34:231.
71. Elphick, M.C., A.T. Harrison, J.P. Lawlor and D. Hull. (1978) Brit. J. Obstet. Gynecol. 85:303.
72. Tsang, R., C. Glueck, G. Evans and P.M. Steiner. (1974) Amer. J. Dis. Child. 127:78.
73. Anderson, G.G. and B. Friis-Hansen. (1976) Intensive Care of the Newborn, Stern, L. and B. Friis-Hansen eds., Medical and Technical Publishers, New York and London, p. 88.
74. Cress, H.R., R.M. Shaher, R. Laffin and K. Karpowicz. (1977) Pediat. Res. 11:19, 1977.
75. Sabata, V., S. Lausmann and H. Wolf. (1969) In: Metabolism of the Newborn, Ed. Joppich, G. and H. Wolf eds., Hippokrates Verlag Stuttgart, p. 163.
76. Melichar, V. and H. Wolf. (1967) Biol. Neon. 11:50.
77. Persson, B. and J. Gentz. (1967) Acta Paed. Scand. 55:353.
78. Pribylova, H. and M. Novak. (1970) Biol. Neon. 15:315.
79. Gentz, J., M. Kellum and B. Persson. (1976) Acta paed. Scand. 65:445.
80. Persson, B., D. Copher and R. Tunell. (1969) In: Metabolism of the Newborn, Joppich, G. and H. Wolf eds., Hippokrates Verlag Stuttgart, p. 9.
81. Hardman, M.J.R. and D. Hull. (1969) J. Physiol. 201:685.
82. Alexander G., A.W. Bell and J.R.S. Hales. (1972) Biol. Neonate 20:9.
83. Smales, O.R.C. and D. Hull. (1978) Arch. Dis. Childh. 53:407.
84. Elphick, M.C. and A.W. Wilkinson. (1973) Personal communication.
85. Smales, O.R.C. and R. Kime. (1978) Arch. Dis. Childh. 53:58.

THE FATTY ACID COMPOSITION OF BROWN AND WHITE FAT IN NEWBORN INFANTS AND THE INFLUENCE OF THE INGESTED FAT ON THE FATTY ACID COMPOSITION OF THEIR BODY FAT

J. H. P. JONXIS[*]

The appreciation of the average clinician of fat as a major component of our food and of the human body is generally rather negative. Tasty food is often fattening, and many of us are too fat. A high fat intake, moreover, is likely one of the causes of arteriosclerosis, the most common finding in elderly people in the Western world.

Some fatty acids, however, are essential nutrients, and particularly these fatty acids are major constituents of the cellular membranes and precursors of the prostaglandins. Fat is by far the most important form of energy storage and subcutaneous fat forms our main protection against heat losses and is thereby very important for thermoregulation.

Sixteen percent of the body of the full term infant consists of fat. It is accumulated during the last 12 weeks of life in utero. In a fetus of 28 weeks with a weight of $\pm$ 1000 g the total fat content is only 1%. Of these 10 g an unknown, but likely significant part is localized in the cellular membranes and central nervous system and the amount of fat available as energy reserve is still negligible. Since the amount of glycogen that can be mobilized for covering the needs of the premature infant who experiences its first period of acute starvation after birth, is very limited, already soon after birth the 1000 g infant is dependent on energy supplied by food, nowadays mainly administered intravenously in the form of glucose. The amount of fat accumulated by the fetus during the last 12 weeks of intrauterine life is considerable (in the order of 550 g).

The presence of the essential fatty acid C18:2 in the fetal subcutaneous fat proves that fatty acids can cross the placental wall. Perfusion experiments (1) make it likely that this transfer across the placenta is limited compared with that of glucose and that at most 20% of the fat of the fetus is derived from fatty acids which have crossed the placental wall. The C18:2 content of the subcutaneous fat of the full term infant

* Groningen

H.K.A. Visser (ed.), Nutrition and Metabolism of the Fetus and Infant, 123-129. All rights reserved.
Copyright © 1979 Martinus Nijhoff Publishers b.v., The Hague/Boston/London.

born in the Groningen University Hospital proved to be at an average of 3%, that in the subcutaneous fat of Groningen youngsters ±13% and in milk from Groningen women ±15%. When fatty acids or fat would cross the placental wall in such amounts that all fat accumulated by the fetus would be supplied by the mother, one might expect a C18:2 level in the subcutaneous fat of the newborn baby at about the same level as that of the mother. The C18:2 level, however, is only 20–25% of that of young adults. The major part of the fat formed by the fetus in utero is derived from glucose.

The free energy of long chain fatty acids is considerably higher than that of glucose. The synthesis of these fatty acids from glucose by the fetus requires therefore energy to be derived from the oxidation of extra glucose. Dr. Hommes has calculated for me the amount of glucose and oxygen necessary for the synthesis of 1 mol of palmitic acid. Dependent on the possibility whether only the NADH involved in the reaction is oxidized to generate the necessary ATP or that all NADH involved in the metabolic process is reoxidized to generate ATP, 1.36 resp. 8 mol of oxygen are consumed, while 15 mol of CO_2 are produced in both variants. 4.03 mol (725 g) or 5.16 mol (1260 g) of glucose are metabolized for the synthesis of 1 mol (256 g) of palmitic acid. ±2 g of fat per kilogram of body weight are daily newly formed by an infant of ±3000 g during intrauterine life. For the synthesis of this amount of fat from glucose 200, resp. 1400 ml of oxygen and 5.6 or 9.7 g glucose are needed, the total oxygen need per kilogram of body weight per 24 hr of the premature infant in utero being ±7200 ml.

In 1974 WIDDOWSON et al. and our group compared the fatty acid composition of the subcutaneous fat of British and Dutch newborn babies and the changes in the fatty acid composition of their subcutaneous fat in the months following birth (2). The British babies were fed on a formula whose fat was cow's milk fat, the Dutch ones on a formula with fat on the basis of maize oil (Almiron). At birth, the C18:2 content of the subcutaneous fat of the British babies was 1%, that of the Dutch ones 2.9% (table 1). There was a marked difference in the fatty acid composition of the subcutaneous fat depending on the fatty acid composition of the formula. In the months following birth the C18:2 content of the subcutaneous fat of the Dutch infants rose considerably to ±25%, dropping again to ±8% when the children were on a mixed diet some months later. In the British babies there was practically no rise in the C18:2 content as long as they were formula-fed, their C18:2 percentage rising to 3.5% when they were 6–12 months old and on a mixed diet.

Since, we have repeated these investigations from time to time to see whether, owing to changes in diet, there were changes in the fatty acid composition of the subcutaneous fat of the children in the northern part of the Netherlands, between 1974 and 1977/78. For the newborn babies no changes have been found, the amount of linoleic acid in the subcutaneous fat of prematurely born infants being slightly lower than that of full term infants (table 1). In older children, however, the C18:2 content of the subcutaneous fat increased from 10.2% in 1974 to 13.7% in 1978. The children were out-patients of the Pediatric Department of

Table 1. *Fatty acid composition (as %) of the subcutaneous fat of newborn infants.*

	C14	C16	C16:1	C18	C18:1	C18:2
English 1974 (n = 19)	3.8	49.6	12.6	4.1	29.6	1.0
Dutch 1974 (n = 14)	3.3	45.8	15.2	3.8	29.0	2.9
Low b.w. 1978 (n = 14)	2.9	54	15.6	3.5	30.5	2.3
Dutch 1978 full-term (n = 7)	4.1	45.5	14.6	3.6	28.0	3.2

Groningen University Hospital and were in good health (table 2). They did not follow a special diet. The increased C18:2 percentage reflects probably a further rise in the consumption of vegetable oils in our population.

Since values have become available of the fatty acid composition of the milk of British mothers (3) we made determinations of values of

Table 2. *C18:2 content (%) of subcutaneous fat of Dutch children, out-patients of the Pediatric Department, University Hospital, Groningen, the Netherlands, 1974, (n = 9), age 1–8 yr. 1977–1978, (n = 16), age 3–19 yr.*

	C12	C14	C16	C16:1
1974	3.4	3.7	22.3	11.9
1977/78	1.4	3.9	21.0	8.2

	C18	C18:1	C18:2
1974	3.1	43.7	10.2
1977/78	5.7	44.7	13.7

corresponding human milk in the northern part of the Netherlands. In our study the milk was collected 5 days after the confinement. Table 3 gives the results. The $C_{10:0}$ and $C_{12:0}$ contents are higher in the milk from British mothers, while the $C_{18:2}$ content of the Groningen women was twice as high as that of their British colleagues. These data reflect likely differences in the fatty acid composition of the dietary fat of British women and of women from the northern part of the Netherlands.

We may assume that the optimum growth rate of the premature infant is the same as the normal intrauterine one and that the child should accumulate as much fat as it might have done in utero over the same

Table 3. *Fatty acid composition (as %) of human milk. English mature pooled milk, 1977. Dutch (Groningen), 5 days after confinement, ($n = 25$), 1977.*

	$C_{10:0}$	$C_{12:0}$	$C_{14:0}$	$C_{16:0}$
English	1.4	5.4	7.3	26.5
Dutch	0.7	3.8	6.2	24.5

	$C_{16:1}$	$C_{18:0}$	$C_{18:1}$	$C_{18:2}$
English	4.0	9.5	35.5	7.2
Dutch	3.2	9.3	34.5	15.1

period. For an infant of 2500 g this amounts to 1.8 g/kg body weight/day.

Even when we keep the child's metabolic rate near to its basal metabolic rate by nursing it at its neutral temperature, a high food intake is necessary to allow such growth rate and fat accumulation. The absorption rate of fat of the low birth weight infant, however, is less than that of the full term baby (4). Losses of fat or fatty acids with the faeces may reduce the energy uptake considerably. By adding medium chain triglycerides (MCT) to the formula the fat absorption rate increases. Not only the medium chain triglycerides are well absorbed, but they improve the absorption of the saturated and unsaturated long chain fatty acids (5). Medium chain fatty acids, therefore, have been recently added to formulas which are especially designed for the very low birth weight infants.

One of these formulas, Nenatal, differs mainly from Almiron in its fatty acid composition. In the latter the fat is mainly maize oil; in Nenatal it consists of 40% of MCT and 60% of maize oil. The total fat percentage is

4.5% in Nenatal, and 3.5% in Almiron. For the fatty acid composition of both formulas, see table 4.

The fatty acid composition of the subcutaneous fat of a number of low birth weight infants (birth weights 1200–1800 g) was determined when

Table 4. *Fatty acid composition (as %) of Almiron and Nenatal.*

	C8	C10	C12	C14	C18
Almiron	trace	trace	trace	trace	trace
Nenatal	17.5	14.7	1.0	trace	8.3

	C18	C18:1	C18:2	C18:4
Almiron	2.0	27.2	58.2	1.6
Nenatal	1.5	17.4	39.1	0.7

the children had reached the age of 6–8 weeks, being fed either on Almiron or on Nenatal. Table 5 shows the results. Only traces of $C10:0$ and $C12:0$ were found to be present in the subcutaneous fat of the infants who had received the Nenatal formula. The $C18:2$ content of their subcutaneous fat is only slightly lower than that of infants with the

Table 5. *Fatty acid composition (as %) of subcutaneous fat of 6–8 weeks old full-term and low birthweight (LWB) babies, fed on Almiron (Alm.) and Nenatal (Nenat.).*

	C10	C12	C14	C16
Alm. full-term (n = 7)			2.1	29.1
Alm. LBW (n = 20)			3.3	25.9
Nenat. LBW (n = 14)	1.0	0.25	3.0	29.9

	C16:1	C18	C18:1	C18:2
Alm. full-term (n = 7)	11.9	3.4	30.2	22.1
Alm. LBW (n = 20)	10.2	2.8	30.5	29.5
Nenat. LBW (n = 14)	8.0	3.2	24.9	28.6

same birth weight, but who were fed on Almiron, although the $C18:2$ content of Almiron is 50% higher. If the C8:0 and C10:0 present in the formula would have been converted into long chain saturated or mono-unsaturated fatty acids, we might expect a lower $C18:2$ concentration in the subcutaneous fat of the Nenatal fed infants. These results make it likely that the main part of the medium chain fatty acids enters directly the pathway of energy metabolism and are neither stored in the subcutaneous fat nor converted into long chain fatty acids.

Whereas 10–20 mg of subcutaneous fat are easily obtainable by simple needle biopsy, brown fat can only be obtained at autopsy or occasionally during major intrathoracal surgery. Table 6 gives the $C18:2$ composition of brown and white fat of full term and premature infants who died soon after birth. The values for the white fat do not differ from those we found

Table 6. *$C18:2$ content (as %) of white and brown fat in premature and full-term babies who died soon after birth.*

	1000–2000 g	2000–3000 g	3000–3500 g
White	2.7	3.7	2.1
Brown	5.0	6.1	5.8

earlier in newborn babies. The $C18:2$ level in the brown fat is about twice as high as in the white fat. Its amount is about equal both in the premature and the full term baby. Small quantities of $C20:4$ (arachidonic acid) (0.4–1.5%) turn out to be present in the brown fat.

Up till now we could obtain only 5 samples of brown and white fat from infants whose ages varied from 2 to 8 weeks. Table 7 gives the $C18:2$ levels. Except for the 8 weeks old infant who was fed on Almiron and died a sudden death, the four remaining children were fed on Nenatal. In all

Table 7. *$C18:2$ content of white and brown fat in babies fed on Nenatal.*

Age	2 weeks	4 weeks	8 weeks
white	2.0	4.5	29.6
brown	9.9	21.2	49.6
white	10.5	7.8	
brown	21.9	24.3	

cases the rise in the $C18:2$ content in the brown fat proved to be more rapid than in the white fat. In the 8 weeks old infant the $C18:2$ percentage in the brown fat had reached an exceptionally high level. The few values we were able to collect should be interpreted with care. They indicate that in the weeks following birth the $C18:2$ content of the brown fat rises much more rapidly than that of the subcutaneous fat. As the fat intake of these babies over the short period of their extrauterine life was quite low, it is more likely that the increase of the $C18:2$ percentage in the brown fat is due to a decrease in the amount of non-essential fatty acids than to the accumulation of $C18:2$. Metabolism is very active in the brown adipose tissue during cold stress after birth and the non-essential fatty acids may be broken down preferentially during this period of high metabolic activity.

The rise of the $C18:2$ content in the 8 weeks old baby who died of cot death and who had gained weight very fast in the previous weeks is on the other hand likely, at least partly, due to a preferential storage of $C18:2$ in the brown adipose tissue. It may be of interest to mention that the $C20:4$ levels in the brown adipose tissue remained at the newborn level.

REFERENCES

1. DANCIS, J., V. JANSEN, H.J. KAYDEN, H. SCHNEIDER and M. LEVITZ. (1973) Pediatr. Res. 7:192.
2. WIDDOWSON, E.M., M.J. DAUNCEY, D.M.T. GAIRDNER, J.H.P. JONXIS and M. PELIKAN-FILÍPKOVA. (1975) Brit. Med. J. 1:653.
3. The composition of mature human milk. (1977) Department of Health and Social Security, Report on Health and Social Subjects, 12, London.
4. KATZ, L. and J.R. HAMILTON. (1974) J. Pediatr. 85:608.
5. TAUTIBHEDHYANGKUL, P.L. and S.A. HASHIM. (1975) Pediatrics 55:359.

SUBCUTANEOUS FAT MEASUREMENT AS AN INDICATION OF NUTRITION OF THE FETUS AND NEWBORN

ANDREW WHITELAW, MD, MRCP*

INTRODUCTION

Although subcutaneous fat is the tissue that adults are most keen to lose, to the newborn, it is an important energy store and insulating coat. Both these functions are important to the young infant as gastro-intestinal disease, failure of the milk supply and exposure to cold are all common threats. Subcutaneous fat is mobilised in calorie deprivation and a reduction in fat is a central feature of prolonged energy deprivation.

MEASUREMENT OF ADIPOSE TISSUE

In general, increased body weight means increased fat, but body weight does not necessarily indicate the amount of fat in the body. Individuals may be heavy without being fat if they are long, have heavy bones, big muscles or water retention. In newborns, differences in head size may appreciably affect body weight. One can attempt to estimate the fat content of the body by the total body water or total body potassium estimations. However, total body water is unstable in the neonatal period (1) and the relationship between whole body potassium and lean body mass is inconstant (2). Whole body fat has been measured in adults using gases soluble in fat e.g. cyclopropane (3), radiokrypton (4) and nitrogen (5). Recently, METTAU et al. (6) have measured body fat in newborns using xenon absorption. However, the methods are very complicated and expensive. Since triglyceride has a lower density (0.901) than lean tissue (1.097), measurement of body density can be used to calculate percentage body fat (7). Body density is usually determined in the adult by weighing the subject in air and then immersed in water, with corrections for air in the lung and intestine. Immersion is not suitable for

* Division of Perinatal Medicine, The Hospital for Sick Children, 555 University Avenue, Toronto, Ontario M5G 1X8, Canada.

H.K.A. Visser (ed.), Nutrition and Metabolism of the Fetus and Infant, 131-143. All rights reserved.
Copyright © 1979 Martinus Nijhoff Publishers b.v., The Hague/Boston/London.

young infants. However, body volume (and therefore body density) can be determined in newborn infants without discomfort by plethysmography (8). Unfortunately, the density of the lean body mass in newborns of different gestational ages is not known with certainty and this method needs further development. Standardised antero-posterior radiographs of the left lower leg show separate shadows for muscle and subcutaneous tissue. Garn (9) used the subcutaneous layer on X-ray as an indication of fat in the newborn. However, the radiation exposure, although small, makes this method now unacceptable for routine use in healthy infants. Furthermore, X-rays differentiate poorly between fat and oedema.

Most of the adipose tissue in the body is subcutaneous and skinfold measurements provide a non-invasive method of assessing subcutaneous fat. The technique has been used extensively in nutritional surveys in children and in adults and the Harpenden skinfold caliper has been vigorously evaluated and meets internationally agreed criteria (10).

TECHNIQUE OF SKINFOLD MEASUREMENT IN NEWBORNS

I have used 4 skinfold sites. The biceps site is over the biceps muscle with the arm partly extended, the fold being vertical and about 1 cm proximal to the skin crease at the elbow (11). The triceps site is on the back of the arm, directly above the olecranon, at a level measured with a paper tape measure halfway between the acromion and the olecranon, the elbow being extended and by the side of the body (12). The subscapular site is just below the inferior angle of the scapula with the fold being either in a vertical line of slightly inclined, in the natural cleavage line of the skin (12). The suprailiac site is in the mid-axillary line, with the fold horizontal about 1 cm above the iliac crest (modified from (11)). Obsessional attention to detail is necessary in selecting the sites, picking up the skinfolds and applying the caliper. As newborns have a variable degree of oedema, the caliper must be left on the skinfold long enough to sink through the oedema and measure the fat layers when the reading is stable. Usually the reading stabilises within 15 s but in some oedematous or pre-term infants the reading may not stabilise until 60 s. Table 1 shows the mean differences between duplicate readings at individual sites. For most purposes, it is sufficient to measure triceps and subscapular skinfolds on the left side of the body. For research purposes, I used the sum of all four skinfolds on each side, 8 skinfolds in all, as this figure gave better reproducibility than individual skinfolds and represented, in one figure

Table 1. *Reproducibility of skinfold readings.*

Skinfold site	Mean skinfold of 16 infants mm	Mean difference of duplicate readings			
		Separate sides mm	% mean	Both sides together mm	% mean
Biceps	2.72	0.12	4.3%	0.095	3.5%
Triceps	3.51	0.16	4.5%	0.13	3.7%
Subscapular	3.68	0.21	6.0%	0.17	3.7%
Suprailiac	2.87	0.19	6.5%	0.13	4.6%
Sum of 8 skinfolds	25.2			0.77	3.0%

both trunk and limb fat. When two experienced observers each measured the same 20 infants, independently, the difference in reading between the 2 observers on any one skinfold was never more than 0.3 mm.

FACTORS INFLUENCING FAT AT BIRTH

Sex

Table 2 shows size at birth in 326 full term infants. The girls had significantly lower birth weight, length and head circumference but significantly greater skinfolds. Thus at birth, females show the same anthropometric differences as at all other ages.

Table 2. *Sex and size at birth.*

	Males	Females	
No. of infants	161	165	
Birth wt. kg	3.43 ± 0.7	3.26 ± 0.7	$p < 0.001$
Length cm	52.8 ± 2.7	51.6 ± 3.6	$p < 0.001$
Head circ. cm	35.0 ± 1.8	34.4 ± 1.6	$p < 0.01$
8 Skinfolds mm	27.6 ± 6.5	29.0 ± 6.3	$p < 0.05$

Gestational age

Table 3 shows the sum of 8 skinfolds in 439 random newborn infants measured within 48 hr of birth, with mean ± SD at each week of gestation from 26 weeks to 42 weeks. There is a clear trend for skinfold

Table 3. *Gestational age and skinfold thickness.*

Gestational age		Sum of 8 skinfolds Mean ± 1 SD mm
Weeks	No	
23	1	10.4
26	6	10.93 ± 2.47
27	2	13.95
28	5	14.85 ± 3.47
29	3	14.00
30	6	14.98 ± 3.98
31	9	16.27 ± 2.62
32	13	17.25 ± 2.69
33	10	21.37 ± 3.19
34	19	20.74 ± 3.98
35	14	23.61 ± 4.23
36	25	24.11 ± 5.18
37	25	25.96 ± 7.22
38	36	26.30 ± 5.62
39	77	29.57 ± 6.06
40	117	30.30 ± 6.34
41	56	29.20 ± 5.44
42	15	29.36 ± 6.31
Total	439	
Preterm	113	
Term	326	

thickness to increase from 23 weeks to 40 weeks after which there is no further increase. This is in agreement with WIDDOWSON's (2) finding of a rapid increase in total body fat (by direct chemical analysis) from 23 weeks gestation to term.

Small for gestational age infants

Figure 1 shows skinfolds for a group of small for gestational age (SGA) infants (below 10th centile for birthweight (13) plotted against the reference mean ± SD derived from the 439 infants. Most of the SGA infants were more than one standard deviation below mean skinfold for gestational age. However, not all the SGA infants were thin. Nine of them were within one standard deviation of the mean. Most of these were light, but not thin, infants below mean length for gestational age (13). Two infants with Down's Syndrome (D), one with trisomy 18 (T) and one with cystic fibrosis (C) were within one standard deviation of

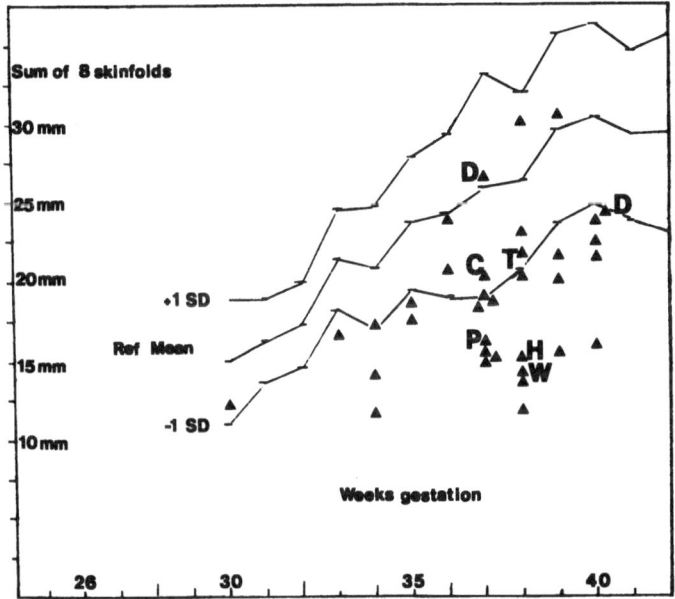

Fig. 1 Skinfold thickness at birth in light-for-gestational age babies.

the mean. One infant born to a mother on high dose prednisone therapy (P) and one infant with hydrocephalus were well below one standard deviation below the mean. One infant (W), nearly 3 standard deviations below the mean, was the only one to develop hypoglycaemic convulsions.

Reduced skinfold measurements may enable one to differentiate between 2 types of small-for-gestational-age infants – a) constitutionally small, short infants with familial short stature, chromosomal abnormalities, intrauterine infections or multiple malformation syndrome, or – b) thin, starved infants suffering from undernutrition and at risk of neonatal hypoglycaemia. Oakley (14) has shown a positive, though moderate, correlation between neonatal skinfold thickness and blood glucose 4 hr after birth.

INFLUENCE OF MATERNAL ADIPOSITY

Do fat mothers tend to have fat babies? When I discussed skinfold measurements with each mother, I measured the mother's triceps skinfold to show her the procedure was harmless and painless. This enabled me to classify the mothers into 3 groups a) obese, if the triceps skinfold was over the 90th centile for young adult females, b) normal, if the triceps skinfold was 10th to 90th centile and c) thin, if the triceps skinfold was below the 10th centile. Table 4 shows the size at birth in the full term babies of these 3 groups of mothers. At all skinfold sites the obese mothers had babies with significantly greater skinfolds than the babies of the normal mothers and these were in turn significantly greater than the

Table 4. *Size at birth in full term infants of obese, normal and thin mothers (mean $\pm$ 1 SD).*

	Maternal triceps skinfold centile		
	> 90th Obese	10th–90th Normal	< 10th Thin
N	65	234	27
Birth weight kg	3.59 ± 0.60[1]	3.31 ± 0.59[4]	3.05 ± 0.64
Length cm	52.76 ± 2.75	52.19 ± 4.20	50.65 ± 3.55
Head circ. cm	35.05 ± 1.41[2]	34.62 ± 1.59	34.28 ± 1.77
Biceps SFT mm	3.30 ± 0.69[1]	3.00 ± 0.60[5]	2.67 ± 0.46
Triceps SFT mm	4.37 ± 0.91[1]	3.91 ± 0.79[4]	3.50 ± 0.93
Subscapular SFT mm	4.65 ± 1.15[1]	4.01 ± 1.01[4]	3.57 ± 0.98
Suprailic SFT mm	3.72 ± 0.95[1]	3.24 ± 0.69[5]	2.83 ± 0.66
Sum of 8 SFT mm	32.1 ± 6.09[1]	28.43 ± 5.61[5]	25.13 ± 5.79
No. of smokers	6 (9%)	66 (28%)	16 (59%)
No. of primiparae	38 (58%)	117 (50%)	8 (30%)

[1] Significantly greater than the mean for infants of normal mothers. $p < 0.001$.
[2] Significantly greater than the mean for infants of normal mothers. $p < 0.05$.
[3] X^2 for trend 96.5. $p < 0.001$.
[1] Significantly greater than the mean for infants of thin mothers. $p < 0.05$.
[1] Significantly greater than the mean for infants of thin mothers. $p < 0.01$.

babies of the thin mothers. Obese mothers tend to smoke less and to be of greater parity than non-obese mothers but increased fatness of the infants was still found when allowance is made for these 2 factors. When the data were examined as continuous variables, by linear regression there was a significant positive correlation $r = 0.33$ ($p < 0.001$) between the sum of the infant's skinfolds and maternal triceps skinfold. Increased placental transfer of free fatty acids from the obsese mother is one possible explanation. It is also possible that blood glucose levels may be slightly higher in obese pregnant women than in non-obese pregnant women although thresholds for the diagnosis of diabetes mellitus were not reached. Other possible explanations include inherited differences in metabolic rate and differences in physical activity in-utero between fetuses.

INFLUENCE OF MATERNAL BLOOD PRESSURE

Table 5 shows size at birth in full term infants of – a) mothers whose blood pressure was below 140/90 mmHg throughout pregnancy and – b) mothers who had a blood pressure of 140/90 mmHg or more for a period of more than 2 weeks of the pregnancy (prolonged hypertension). Obese mothers and mothers who smoked were excluded because both these factors are known to affect birth weight. Table 5 shows a significant reduction in the babies' weight and skinfold thickness when the mother had prolonged hypertension, and this suggests some reduction in fetal nutrition. Reduced placental blood flow has been demonstrated in hypertensive pregnancy (15) and DIXON and ROBERTSON (16) showed histologically obliterative vascular changes in the placental bed in severe hypertensive pregnancies. It seems possible that such vascular lesions with reduced perfusion could result in a reduction in supply of nutrients to the fetus.

Table 5. *Size at birth (mean $\pm$ 1 SD) in full term infants of non-obese, non-smokers. Effect of blood pressure.*

	Normal BP	Prolonged raised BP
N	119	30
Birth wt kg	3.41 $\pm$ 0.60	3.12 $\pm$ 0.7[1]
Length cm	52.3 $\pm$ 3.7	52.1 $\pm$ 4.7
Head circumference cm	34.8 $\pm$ 1.6	34.3 $\pm$ 2.1
8 Skinfolds mm	28.5 $\pm$ 5.4	26.2 $\pm$ 6.1[1]

[1] Significantly less than the mean for infants of mothers with normal BP. $p < 0.05$.

INFLUENCE OF MATERNAL SMOKING

Table 6 shows the effect of smoking on size at birth in full term infants of non-obese, non-hypertensive mothers. The infants of smokers had significantly lower birth weight, length and head circumference, but there was no significant reduction in skinfold thickness. It seems unlikely that the changes in infants of mothers who smoke are mainly due to under-nutrition although a small effect may be present. Hypoxia from carbon monoxide might well stunt growth without depriving the fetus of calories. Fetal carboxyhaemoglobin in smoking mothers may reach 21%

Table 6. *Size at birth (mean ± 1 SD) in infants of smokers and non-smokers (obese and thin mothers and those with raised BP excluded).*

	Non-smokers	Smokers	t test
N	111	50	
Birth wt kg	3.44 ± 0.61	3.07 ± 0.63	p < 0.001
Length cm	52.5 ± 3.61	50.0 ± 3.5	p < 0.001
Head circumference cm	34.9 ± 1.6	33.9 ± 1.6	p < 0.001
Sum of 8 skinfolds mm	28.9 ± 6.1	28.1 ± 6.1	Not significant
Maternal triceps skinfold mm	16.3 ± 3.9	15.3 ± 3.9	Not significant
No. of primiparae	46 (41%)	13 (26%)	

(17). McGarry and Andrews (18) suggested that cyanide in tobacco smoke reduces the availability of vitamin B_{12} and impairs fetal growth as a result.

INFLUENCE OF MATERNAL DIABETES

Poorly controlled diabetes in pregnancy is associated with heavy, chubby infants. Skinfold thicknesses were measured in 40 newborn infants of diabetic mothers. Round-the-clock blood glucose monitoring had been carried out on these mothers for varying periods in the third trimester. Figure 2 shows the skinfold thickness of these 40 infants plotted against the reference ranges for gestational age. Many of the infants were several standard deviations above the mean. All the infants with a mean maternal blood glucose above 6 mmol/l (108 mg/100 ml) were at least one standard deviation above the mean. Whereas, 16 out of 30 of the infants with mean maternal blood glucose below 6 mmol/l (108 mg/100 ml) where within one standard deviation of the mean. Figure 3 shows the infants divided according to mean maternal fasting blood glucose. Sixteen out of 17 infants with a fasting maternal blood glucose above 5 mmol/l (90 mg/100 ml) had skinfold thicknesses one standard deviation or more above the mean. Whereas, only 6 out of 20 of the infants with maternal fasting blood glucose levels below 5 mmol/l (90 mg/100 ml) were more than one standard deviation above the mean. Expressing each infant's skinfold thickness as a percentage of the reference mean for gestational age enabled infants of different gestational age to be compared. Figure 4 shows skinfold thickness as a percentage of mean plotted against maternal fasting glucose. There was a highly

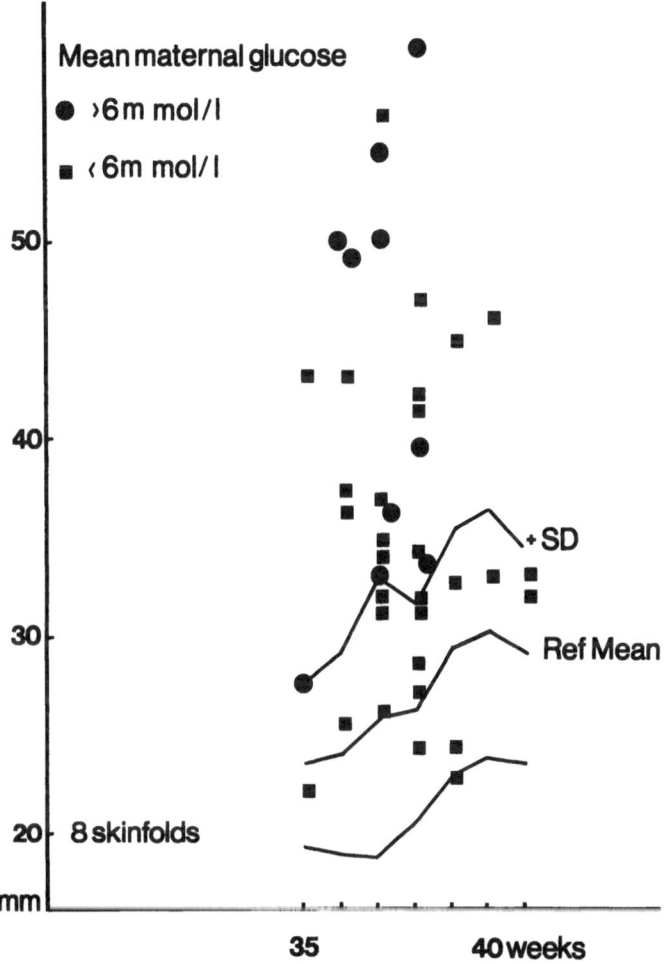

Fig. 2. Skinfold in infants of diabetics.

significant positive correlation r = 0.57 (p < 0.001). These findings are consistent with PEDERSEN's hypothesis (19) that fetal hyperglycaemia results in fetal hyperinsulinism which stimulates lipogenesis in adipose tissue. To put it simply, the fetus is like a child who eats too many sweets. The excess sugar not required for growth, activity and basal metabolism is laid down as fat. The finding that neonatal skinfold thickness correlates better than birth weight with maternal blood glucose suggests that

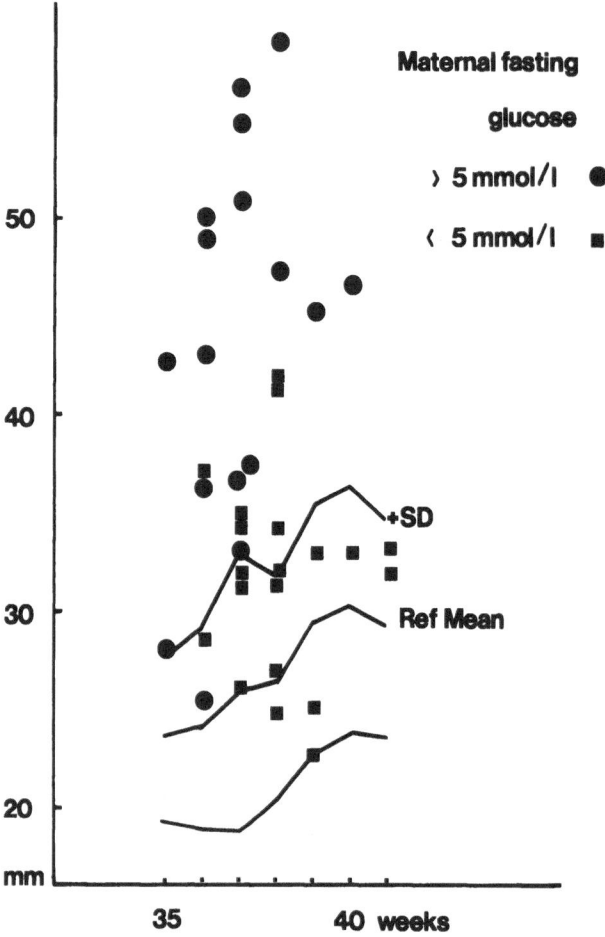

Fig. 3. Skinfold in infants of diabetics.

neonatal skinfold measurements may be a better criterion than birth weight by which to judge diabetic control in pregnancy. If one aims for metabolic normality in the fetus, mean maternal blood glucose should be below 6 mmol/l (108 mg/100 ml) and mean fasting blood glucose below 5 mmol/l (90 mg/100 ml).

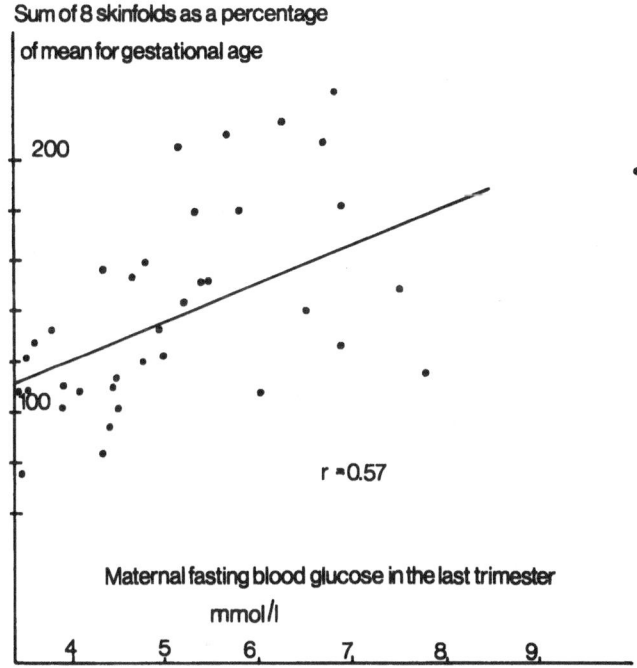

Fig. 4. Neonatal skinfold thickness in infants of diabetic mothers.

PRACTICAL USES OF NEONATAL SKINFOLD MEASUREMENTS

Skinfold measurements are harmless, cheap and reproducible. They increase from 26 weeks to 39 or 40 weeks. They are increased if the mother is obese or diabetic. They are decreased if the mother has prolonged hypertension and are unchanged if the mother smokes.

Skinfold measurements are useful in:

a) Assessing the small for gestational age infant for evidence of calorie undernutrition. We now have centile charts for triceps and sub-scapular skinfolds for each week from 37 to 42 weeks, derived from 1293 newborns (20).

b) Assessing the metabolic normality of the infant of the diabetic mother (21).

c) Assessing and comparing different feeding regimes. We all like to see a baby putting on weight but we also like to know where the increased weight is. A combination of weight, length, head circumference and two skinfolds can indicate if the growth is in brain, bone and/or subcutaneous fat.

SUMMARY

To the newborn, adipose tissue is an imporant energy store and insulating coat. Subcutaneous fat is mobilised during calorie deprivation and a reduction in subcutaneous fat is a central feature of prolonged energy nutrition.

Skinfold thickness measurements are a convenient and reproducible method of assessing subcutaneous fat if the caliper is left on the skinfold until the reading is stable. Skinfold thicknesses were measured at the biceps, triceps, subscapular, and suprailiac sites on both sides in 439 newborn infants. Mean and standard deviation were calculated for the sum of all skinfolds at each week of gestation and there was a progressive increase from 26 weeks until 40 weeks after which there was no further increase. Not all light-for-gestational age infants were thin for gestational age, some being constitutionally small and short. It is suggested that in light-for-gestational age infants, skinfold thickness may differentiate the undernourished, thin infant, at risk from hypoglycemia, from the constitutionally small infant.

The effects of several maternal factors on subcutaneous fat at birth were investigated. Maternal hypertension (if prolonged for more than 2 weeks of the pregnancy) was associated with reduced neonatal skinfold thickness. Maternal adiposity (triceps skinfold) had a moderate positive correlation with neonatal skinfold. Maternal smoking was found to have no significant effect on neonatal skinfold thickness, despite there being reduced birth weight. Maternal diabetes mellitus was associated with increased neonatal skinfold thickness and the infants' skinfold thickness correlated well with maternal blood glucose levels in a group of 40 infants of diabetic mothers. It is suggested that neonatal skinfold thickness may be a useful parameter by which to assess the adequacy of diabetic control in pregnancy.

Another application of skinfold measurements is in comparing different feeding regimes. It is desirable to know if weight gain is associated with brain growth, bone growth and/or accumulation of subcutaneous fat. Length, head circumference and skinfold measurements help to elucidate this.

For most purposes, triceps and subscapular measurements are adequate. Centiles for these two skinfolds, compiled from 1293 infants are available for female and male infants at each week of gestation from 37 to 42 weeks.

REFERENCES

1. MacLaurin, J.C. (1966) Arch. Dis. Childh. 41:286.
2. Widdowson, E.M. (1974) In: Scientific Foundation of Paediatrics, Davis, J.A. and J. Dobbing, eds., Heinemann, London, p. 153.
3. Lesser, G.T., W. Perl, and J.M. Steele. (1960) J. Clin. Invest. 39:1791.
4. Davidsson, D., I. MacIntyre, A. Raport and J.E.S. Bradley. (1956) Biochem. J. 62:34p.
5. Behnke, A.R. (1945) Medicine 24:359.
6. Mettau, J.W., H.J. Degenhart, H.K.A. Visser and W.P.S. Holland. (1977) Pediat. Res. 11:1097.
7. Forbes, G.B. (1962) Pediatrics 29:477.
8. Pearse, R.G. (1975) St. Thomas' Hospital, London. Personal communication.
9. Garn, S.M., G.R. Greaney and R.W. Young. (1956) Human Biology 28:232.
10. Edwards, D.A., W.H. Hammond, M.J.R. Healy, J.M. Tanner and R.H. Whitehouse. (1955) Brit. J. Nutr. 9:133.
11. McGowan, A., M. Jordan and J. MacGregor. (1975) Biol. Neonate 25:66.
12. Tanner, J.M. and R.H. Whitehouse. (1975) Arch. Dis. Childh. 50:142.
13. Gairdner, D. and J. Pearson. (1971) Arch. Dis. Childh. 46:783.
14. Oakley, J. (1977) Arch. Dis. Childh. 52:81.
15. Brown, J.C. McC. and N. Veall. (1953) J. Obstet. Gynaec. Brit. Cwlth. 60:141.
16. Dixon, H.G. and W.B. Robertson. (1958) J. Obstet. Gynaec. Brit. Cwlth. 65:803.
17. Cole, P.V., L.H. Hawkins and D. Roberts. (1972) J. Obstet. Gynaec. Brit. Cwlth. 79:782.
18. McGarry, J.M. and J. Andrews. (1972) Brit. Med. J. 2:74.
19. Pedersen, J. (1954) Acta Endocrin. 16:330.
20. Oakley, J.R., R.J. Parsons and A.G.L. Whitelaw. (1977) Arch. Dis. Childh. 52:287.
21. Whitelaw, A. (1977) Lancet 1:15.

DISCUSSION

(Chairman: E.M. Widdowson)

PAPER BY F.C. BATTAGLIA

M. Young: You know the data obtained by Dancis and his colleagues, recently, from the isolated lobule of the human placenta perfused closed circuit? They started with the same concentrations of amino acid on the maternal and fetal sides and measured the fetal:maternal (F:M) concentration ratios over an hour. This ratio rose for lysine, alanine and glycine, indicating concentrative transport, but fell for aspartic and glutamic acid, whilst glutamine and asparagine accumulated in the fetal perfusate, suggesting production of these substances by the placental tissue. Do you agree with their interpretation?

F.C. Battaglia: I have trouble with extrapolating from perfusion experiments to in vivo transfer rates. I think you will find that in sheep, in the latter part of gestation, there is an uptake of glutamine from the uterine circulation into the placenta (uterine A-V difference of glutamine ~ 9.3 μM). We have not done simultaneously umbilical uptake to uterine release of amino acids. It is a mammoth undertaking. So that I'm being cautious in saying I feel our data prove that there is no "glutamine-glutamate" cycle. The reason I have to be cautious is that it is very dependent on the uterine flow to umbilical flow ratio's, which are normally two to one in the sheep, but can vary considerably. We have to be cautious about it but at least I can tell you that we find no data that would support the necessity of postulating a glutamine-glutamate cycle. By that I mean that the evidence does not support the hypothesis that all of the glutamine received by the fetus reflects placental synthesis. There is an appreciable glutamine uptake from the uterine circulation, and no significant uterine uptake of glutamate. Of course, this does not preclude some synthesis of glutamine within the placenta in vivo. In fact, I think that is likely.

M. Young: You suggested that you didn't have a big percentage uptake of glutamine from the maternal circulation.

F.C. Battaglia: No, we don't have, the uterine A-V difference is ~ 9.0 μM. To find out how much you must know flow times the A-V difference. What I am saying is that we have never undertaken the study, nor has anyone else that I know of, where uterine and umbilical flows and A-V differences of amino acids were measured simultaneously. So I'm hedging, because we have done a study of umbilical uptake (J. Clin. Invest. 58:1428, 1976) and seven years later did a study of uterine uptake, (HOLZMAN, I.R., J.A. LEMONS, G. MESCHIA, and F.C. BATTAGLIA. Uterine uptake of amino acids and placental glutamine-glutamate balance in the pregnant ewe. J. Devel. Physiol. In press.) But if I take a flow ratio of two to one, then there is no need to postulate that there is insufficient amount of glutamine entering from the uterus.

M. Young: But on the other hand, I think that does demonstrate that there must be some glutamine production by the human placenta.

F.C. Battaglia: Yes, in the perfused placenta in vitro, glutamine is coming out. In vivo, our data support the hypothesis of placental glutamine synthesis as well.

R.M. Pitkin: Does the swallowing of amniotic fluid and potential recycling of any isotope labeling enter into these considerations at all?

F.C. Battaglia: No. When we calculate the substrate flow into the umbilical vein, we're expressing that in quantities per kilo per minute. And this is why I raised the question earlier this morning; if you cleared all the amniotic fluid as substrate how long could you support the fetal requirements? At least for glucose I've done that calculation and you won't do it for more than some minutes. Certainly not for days.

C.T. Jones: I was rather concerned about your interpretation of the radio-active turnover experiments. One thing we have found using various isotopes labeled with fetal tissues is that in many of the tissues where there are high rates of activity of pentose-phosphate pathway (a characteristic of many fetal tissues) there are phenomenal rates of glucose recycling. Secondly, and particularly with the use of [2-^{3}H] glucose, another characteristic of fetal tissues (particularly the fetal liver) is that the rate of ^3H_2O-production from $[2\text{-}^3H]$ glucose, which you used to estimate glucose-phosphorylation rate, is about half the rate of glucose phosphorylation as measured by glucose uptake. So I would think that for both of those and other reasons, it is very difficult to make quantitative assessments of glucose consumption by the fetus, using these various ^3H-labeled glucoses.

F.C. Battaglia: I don't follow you to that last step, because the errors are in different directions – the ^{14}C and tritium. I didn't have time to go into that, but for instance tritiated glucose at the sixth position and ^{14}C at the sixth position have the same differences as ^{14}C at the first position and tritium at the second position. (HAY, W.W., J.W. SPARKS, B.J. QUISSELL, F.C. BATTAGLIA and G. MESCHIA. (1978) Pediatr. Res. 12:394.)

C.T. Jones: The sixth position is a bit more difficult.

F.C. Battaglia: You're right. And from the substrate flow into the uterine circulation, we made similar calculations of turnover rates in the adult sheep which agreed very nicely with the data in the literature. So I don't think it's an error in methodology.

C.T. Jones: But the trouble is that you're making assumptions about the way in which these compounds are metabolized. And the closer you look at the metabolic pathways of the metabolism of glucose in the tissues, the more you realize that they are inadequate, particularly to explain the release or redistribution of label. So I think one has to be extremely careful in quantitating such data.

F.C. Battaglia: I want to make clear to the rest of the audience what I said. I believe the ^{14}C and tritium data labeled at those four positions effectively bracket the true glucose turnover rate. I did not make a value judgement on which is closer to this true value, but I do believe they effectively bracket the utilization rate of glucose.

B.S. Lindblad: We have studied uptakes in a different organ, the brain, of infants. (SETTERGREN, S., B.S. LINDBLAD and B. PERSSON. (1976) Acta Paediatr. Scand. 65:343.) I was interested to see the close correlation demonstrated by you between uptake and arterial level, as there is also such a correlation across the brain. However, we have found no correlation with blood flow. Would you comment upon that? Another thing is the difficulty we have even with the modern ion-exchange chromatography method to demonstrate what we should call "significant" A-V differences. I wonder how you would define significance there?

F.C. Battaglia: You are bringing up a very good point. I would certainly agree with you that when the coefficient of utilization is under 5 or 6%, there is no way to arrive at a good estimate of uptake with column chromatography. And we were sufficiently concerned about that with glutamine and glutamate, since glutamine flux is so large in a fetus, that we set up the enzymatic method and compared the two on a large series of samples. (HOLZMAN, I.R., J.A. LEMONS, G. MESCHIA and F.C. BATTAGLIA. Uterine uptake of amino acids and placental glutamine-glutamate balance in the pregnant ewe. In press).

I quite agree with you that the problem we showed for estimating urea production rate is not restricted to urea. We cannot apply the Fick principle when the coefficients of utilization are very low. Whatever the methodology, you're going to exceed your ability to measure differences that small. In fact that comes out: because if I showed you the variance of each A-V difference, you would find a very large variance for glycine which is there in very high concentration. I think the explanation is exactly that.

PAPER BY P.J.J. SAUER

A. Okken: I like your work very much, but it also gives me a lot of trouble because, from a theoretical point of view, the heat output of a baby measured by means of direct calorimetry should be greater than that measured by indirect calorimetry. This is because there is heat produced during the process of hydrolysis, which is not represented in oxygen uptake or carbon-dioxide production. You do find that heat production measured by direct calorimetry is less than the heat production calculated from indirect calorimetry. How do you calculate heat production from O_2 and CO_2. You will know that the accuracy of the calculation of heat production really depends on what you are using in the calculation. Are you calculating heat production from O_2 or are you calculating it from O_2 and CO_2? Or are you using O_2, CO_2 and nitrogen in your calculation? In addition to this it is also possible that there is a difference in heat production measured from indirect and direct calorimetry when a baby is gaining heat during the experiment, when heat is stored in the body. Did you measure such heat storage? Did you heat up the food you supplied to the baby–because, if this food was at room temperature, this may account for half a kilo-calorie for the period of 6 hours at the infusion rate you mentioned.

P.J.J. Sauer: To answer the first question: we used both oxygen and carbon dioxide for calculating indirect calorimetry. We did not use nitrogen. We calculated the kind of mistake we would make if we did not use nitrogen and we came to less than 1% for the RQ ratio most infants have. The second point about gaining heat of the infant, we corrected for the warming up during the experiment, it was very little, 0.1° or 0.2°. We measured both the skin temperature and the oesophageal temperature and we made a correction for this warming-up in our direct calorimetry. As to the last question: the incubator is in a room of 30° to 31°. We heated the food up to 37 C, then it cooled down to 31° (room temperature), but it was a long time in the incubator before it reached the infant – in the incubator the temperature is 33°–34° – so the error was small.

J.C. Sinclair: We are then left with this very perplexing difference between the results calculated from direct and indirect calorimetry. I did not understand the postulation that you made in explanation of this difference. If I understood what you said, you postulate that the energy oxidized in support of – what you call – arrangements of molecules laid down in new tissues would show up in oxygen consumption and CO_2 production, but not in the elaboration of heat. I am having difficulty with that concept.

A. Okken: As far as I understand – but I may have a very simplistic view on it – the conversion from ADP to ATP is measured with oxygen uptake. Thus, part of the energy necessary to arrange tissue is measured with your oxygen uptake, I think.

PAPER BY D. HULL

F.C. Battaglia: I have a comment more than a question, because Professor Hull and I have discussed this enough that I don't think we are in disagreement. He's always very cautious to express the quantity of fat, free fatty acids, entering the umbilical circulation as a percentage of the fat store, and that comes in the human to approximately 20 or 30% of the fat store.

Now, when we are talking about differences between species, the differences in fact may be very deceptive ones. I should be perfectly prepared to accept – since no one can measure that value with precision – that 30% of the fat stored in a lamb fetus may also be delivered from the maternal circulation. It is only 1% of body weight. So, if you calculate that in terms of umbilical flows, it's not something we would be able to measure. I guess what I am asking here is that when we talk about substrate flow, we keep the same reference points in our discussion. If we mean total carbon requirements, that is one reference point. If we mean total caloric requirements, that is another reference point. Thus, if one assumes that 20% of fat stores from free fatty acids in the human fetus, that will not come up to a very large percentage of the total caloric requirement in the human fetus. So, I think there are more similarities than differences.

D. Hull: Yes, if I follow that, I was only talking about what sort of conclusions you can make from the evidence that we have available. I do not think there is any evidence in man of net uptake by the fetus of calories in carbon in the form of fatty acids. However, from studies on the chronic sheep preparation, the placenta seems to be relatively impervious to fatty acids.

F.C. Battaglia: My point is that in both the human and the lamb one must still build the rest of the fat-free body and this is not coming from fatty acids.

A.G.L. Whitelaw: I was most interested in the diets that you're feeding your mothers in Nottingham and I wonder if you could tell us a little bit more about giving intralipid prior to delivery and what this abnormal fatty acid was that you could use as a marker?

D. Hull: The intralipid contains about 45% linoleic acid. It is a strange mixture. Normally the chylomicrons and free fatty acids have more like 5 to 10% linoleic acid.

A.G.L. Whitelaw: Was it given for any particular reason? And how long was it given before delivery?

D. Hull: It has been given in Australia with the idea that it would nourish the fetus, as a deliberate way of trying to get fat across to nourish an infant with fetal growth failure. We had certain misgivings about doing this because it has not been demonstrated firstly that fatty acids go across and secondly that it's a good thing for fatty acids from intralipid to cross. We decided to look if they did get across and if so in what form. A word of warning: there is some evidence that intralipid might induce uterine contractions. It didn't happen in our series.

A.G.L. Whitelaw: I am interested because in Toronto, recently, we had a lady that was on total parenteral feeding for two months prior to delivery because of intractable vomiting. She had a liter a day of 10% intralipid for two months before delivery.

   We are at the moment, in fact, analyzing the adipose tissue fatty acid composition of the baby. Did you give it to your mothers for only a few days?

D. Hull: No, no. Our mothers had a single twenty-minute injection prior to delivery by section.

M. Orzalesi: I do not quite understand your concept of non-selective transfer. Do you mean that there is no active transport, or do you mean that all free fatty acids will cross the placenta equally well. I think we have physical-chemical evidence that this does not happen because of the differences in molecular weight, PK, solubility constant and so on of the various free fatty acids. So when you say that all essential fatty acids are transferred through the placenta and are not synthesized by the fetus, how do you end up with the calculation of 20 to 30% – which is a wide range – of free fatty acids being transferred in that way? Did you take into account the different permeability – at least theoretically – of the placenta for the different fatty acids?

D. Hull: Yes, in my text I have worded it very carefully. I don't really want to be stuck with the 20 to 30%. What I mean by non-selective is that linoleic acid does not go across by itself, the other fatty acids cross the placenta as well.

You're right the relative solubilities of the various fatty acids in water, their affinity for the transfer albumin in the placenta on the two sides, will affect their rate of transfer across the placenta membrane.

M. Orzalesi: Is there any evidence, because of those physical-chemical properties, that linoleic acid is transferred more rapidly, more efficiently?

D. Hull: The evidence from studies with the perfused, isolated human placenta is that there is a relatively higher rate of linoleic acid transfer, which is explained, as I understood it, by the relative amount and affinity for albumin on the two sides of the membrane. If you look at the cord venous-arterial differences, the magnitude of this effect doesn't appear to be large. If you look at it in general, then the mixture of fatty acids that comes across the placenta is similar to the mixture of the maternal source. So that if these factors, i.e. affinity for albumin are working, they are working to a relatively small effect rather than to a large effect.

PAPER BY J.H.P. JONXIS

A. Ballabriga: I should like to give some comments concerning the paper of Professor Jonxis. We know that by manipulation of the different milk formulas, especially the content of linoleic acid, you can change the composition of the subcutaneous fat. The extent in which we can change the composition of the subcutaneous fat is in direct correlation with the quantity of linoleic acid in different milk formulas. That means that in different countries, the composition of the subcutaneous fat in the new-born, specially at the age of ten weeks, may be correlated with the kind of milk that the infant is consuming. You can change the composition of the subcutaneous fat considerably, for instance the concentration of linoleic acid may vary from 4% to 24%.

But we really don't know what the meaning of these findings is. Is it important, is it not important? It will be important to know if there are changes in the composition of other tissues. We have studied the composition of the red cell lipid stroma: concentrations of ethanolamine phosphoglyceride and choline phosphoglyceride. The composition of the red cell's lipid stroma is different after the infant has been fed for three weeks with different formulas. An infant that has been fed only a formula with a very low content of linoleic acid, can develop normally from the clinical point of view, but from the chemical point of view you may find increase of the 20:3 (ng) fatty acid, that is the fatty acid that is involved in linoleic acid deficiency, as was shown in experimental studies with animals.

So, we can manipulate now with different formulas not only the composition of the subcutaneous tissue, but also the composition of the membranes in red cells. This is someting to be more afraid of. May be with further study it will be possible to show that we also can manipulate the composition of the phosphoglycerides in brain. But the brain is an organ that is very resistant. However, we have now the experience of using intravenous nutrition with large quantities of fat, for instance intralipid, during more than two weeks and have found that you can also change the composition of the phosphoglycerides of the brain. And we do not know in the long term, what that means.

J.H.P. Jonxis: I suppose no one knows for certain. Firstly, we all know one thing: that human milk has not at all a fixed composition of fatty acids. The milk of an African woman may contain a rather high concentration of medium-chain fatty acids. In the milk of Dutch women and perhaps of women in other countries, the amount of linoleic acid is rising. There is no fixed composition and we have no reference point for human milk. We know that the fatty acid composition of human milk reflects mainly that of the food of the female.

We also made some studies on the fatty acid composition of the membrane of the erythrocyte. We found little changes in our group of prematures. We found that the fatty acid composition of the red cell membrane was not altered to the same degree as that of the subcutaneous fat. I am not at all sure how far the membranes – let us take mitochondrial membranes on which we did some work – are changed to a major extent, except when the animal or the woman has been under circumstances of linoleic acid shortage. Further investigations in this field are surely necessary.

R.D.G. Milner: I was very interested in the slides that you showed of the babies of 1.1 to 1.3 kg who were fed on the two diets and who had a 76 and a 86% fat absorption. Can you tell us anything about the rate of weight gain of the two groups of babies? Did those who have the better absorption grow more quickly?

J.H.P. Jonxis: No. The weight gain was just the same. I could show you the balances of absorption of the different fatty acids. You would see that the absorption of even the stearic acid increases by the addition of medium chain fatty acids. But it had no influence on the weight of the child over the period of 15 days the special formula was given. But we did not study the body composition and the fat percentage might differ in the two groups.

E.R. Boersma: With the help of Professor Jonxis, we did some investiga-tions on subcutaneous fat of children born in Tanzania. It was very interesting to see that, when you give Dutch infants a feeding that contains quite a high percentage of medium-chain fatty acids, this will not be reflected in their subcutaneous fat. On the other hand, in Tan-zanian infants, you do see a relatively high content of C_{12} and C_{14} in their body fat. Although we have not yet determined the composition of the fatty acids in the breast milk, there is good evidence to expect that the concentration of C_{12} and C_{14} in breast milk of these women is high. (BOERSMA E.R. (1979) Changes in the fatty acid composition of body fat before and after birth in Tanzania. An international comparitive study in relation to dietary patterns. Brit. Med. J.: in press.)

J.H.P. Jonxis: You have pointed out, as far as I see, that in your African children's subcutaneous fat you do find medium-chain fatty acids, while we with our formula which is quite rich in medium-chain fat, we don't find it. But I believe your babies in Africa, while they surely were not starved, had a moderate caloric intake. Our babies were on a high caloric diet. I believe that may be the reason for the differences in our two observations.

B. Friis Hansen: I would like to return to the comments made by Professor Ballabriga, because I think that it is important to realize if we are possibly doing any harm by giving a lot of linoleic acid. I think that the answer is also given by Professor Ballabriga's observation that the composition of the membranes seems to change in a few weeks. It has been postulated that individuals who have taken a very high content of unsaturated fatty acids as prevention of atherosclerosis have an increased risk of malignancies.

Later, however, it has been said that this was not the case. Even if there is a slight risk, I think that it is important that our babies only get a formula with a high content of linoleic acid for 6 months or less. Then they start to get a large proportion of other fatty acids, and the membranes will return to a – let's call it – "normal" composition, regardless of what we have given before. If malignancies take, say, 20 or 40 years to develop then we are not doing any harm and presumably we are doing something good with a moderately high content of linoleic acid. I would like to hear your comment.

J.H.P. Jonxis: I am somewhat worried about this talk of malignancies. When you go through the literature, you see that, according to some authors, practically every food component can cause malignancies. So I think we better eat nothing. The linoleic acid intake of the Dutch population is now rather high. Up till now we have not seen any harm. What to do? Tell the people to eat butter again? But then you get another group of people alarmed. So, when we combine these different advices, we all should starve and die very early and don't get malignancies.

I am making a joke. I have, however, followed the literature on this point carefully. There is surely reason for caution. Practically every substance, when given in excessive amounts, can be harmful. As long as the human race exists, for many people nuts and seeds rich in vegetable oils and linoleic acid have been the main source of energy. After all, cow's milk is not a normal food for man. It is a relatively recent acquisition. Cow's milk fat is very low in linoleic acid. For this reason one might object taking butter. The coastal population of Holland lived in former days mainly on fish (herring) with all its "dangerous" oils. However, many of those people became quite old and the population had the advantage of not getting rickets. As long as we have no reliable data we should be very careful in giving statements about supposed risks.

PAPER BY A.G.L. WHITELAW

E.M. Widdowson: The paper is open for discussion, and I wonder if I could ask one question first. How much does the mere fact of a baby being smaller affect the skin folds? If you've got two babies with the same percentage of fat in their bodies and one is smaller than the other, the fat will have to be spread over a larger area because the small baby will have a larger surface in proportion to its weight and it will of necessity have to have a smaller skin fold.

A.G.L. Whitelaw: Yes, indeed. I take that point, Dr. Widdowson. I think that the scheme which was used by Dauncey and Gardner to calculate total body fat may help to answer that. (DAUNCEY, M.J., G. GANDY and D. GAIRDNER. (1977) Arch. Dis. Childh. 52:223.)

This does take account of small stature, because you have to measure the length of various bits of the baby, the length of the arms, the length of the legs and so on. One works out from these geometrical simplifications of the body, what the fat volume must be and by taking this into account, one does arrive at an estimate of total body fat which would compensate to some extent for differences in length and therefore differences in surface area. I have used this scheme for working out total body fat, but I do feel that it needs to be standardized. I think at the moment we don't know what the norms are and it is difficult to interpret one's results. At least with skin folds one has got some kind of standard.

F.C. Battaglia: I think the idea that skin fold thickness measurements might help sort out this very heterogeneous group of small-for-gestational age (SGA) babies is a very nice one. Do you have any data to support that idea, other than the data you showed us?

A.G.L. Whitelaw: Only the babies I mentioned – the ones that are SGA but not starved, the chromosomal problems, the babies with constitutional problems.

F.C. Battaglia: That was three of nine. What about the other six?

A.G.L. Whitelaw: They all had reduced lengths and mothers whose maximum height was 155 cm, in that group, which is rather low for the British population. I would suggest, tentatively, that there was familial and short stature in that group.

M. Orzalesi: Dr. Battaglia asked exactly the same question I wanted to ask you. And the other six babies? Do you have any evidence that there was increased incidence of chronic hypoxia, perinatal asphyxia, or fetal heart-rate abnormalities as a justification for SGA?

A.G.L. Whitelaw: No. They did not have any evidence of either acute or chronic hypoxia. I think one has to bear in mind that I was dealing with babies below the tenth centile. Ten percent of the population has to be below the tenth centile and it's possible that, in fact, there was nothing wrong with them. They just happened to be at the end of a distribution without having really any pathology.

F.C. Battaglia: Using skinfold thickness measurement as the only parameter, you cannot differentiate between SGA babies who are below the tenth centile. It is a heterogenous group.

A.G.L. Whitelaw: No. But I think that it's one more piece of evidence: that you want to try and convince me that a baby has had caloric undernutrition. After all, this is what we do with nutritional surveys in older children. It's one piece of evidence that is used. I agree, you don't depend on just one piece of evidence.

B.S. Lindblad: When we were studying the small-for-date babies of mothers with hypertension (LINDBLAD, B.S. and R. ZETTERSTRÖM. (1968) Acta Paediatr. Scand. 57:195.), we found a very poor correlation of all measurements of the infants, or biochemical data, with the severity of the maternal condition. I wonder, did you subdivide your material into essential hypertension before pregnancy and during pregnancy?

A.G.L. Whitelaw: Yes. I made no distinction between women who had been hypertensive before pregnancy and women who developed hypertension during pregnancy. But note that I excluded smokers and obese mothers, I found that over 50% of them had hypertension in pregnancy and that if you looked at the obese hypertensive women, they had normal-size babies. In other words, the effect of the hypertension sort of seemed to cancel out the effect of the obesity and you ended up with a normal-size baby. In fact, in one or two cases, you could get a small-for-gestational age baby, because, for some reason, the hypertension had been particularly severe.

G.J. Kloosterman: How do you compute the mean maternal glucose level? How many estimations per 24 hour did you perform? And why did you do it only in the last trimester? I have the impression that these women with diabetes were rather poorly controlled during the whole pregnancy, because there was such a large number of very heavy babies. It is our experience that especially the first part of pregnancy is much more important than the last weeks.

A.G.L. Whitelaw: I would remind you that Dr. Widdowson's data show that there is very, very little fat until twenty weeks. So, it's rather difficult to see how insulin and glucose, before 20 weeks, could affect deposition of fat although I'm aware that it will affect a lot of other things, it will affect almost everything else.

Now, to answer your first question: the mothers were customarily admitted to the hospital several weeks before the planned date of delivery for blood-glucose monitoring, adjustment of insulin dosage, ultra-sound measurements of the fetus and general obstetric management. Many of the mothers had indwelling intravenous canulae and had blood-glucose measurements done every one to two hours throughout the 24 hours. I refer you to the work of Dr. Gilmer, St. Mary's Hospital, where I studied most of these babies (GILMER, M.D.G., R.W. BEARD, F.M. BROOKE and N.W. OAKLY. (1975) Brit. Med.J. 3:399.). Those that didn't have one to two hourly blood samples mostly had them every four hours around the clock. There were one or two mothers who didn't have blood samples done during the night. This is unfortunate, because it means that their data is not so reliable, but this is just one of the difficulties of working with human beings.

GENERAL DISCUSSION

M. Young: Dr. Battaglia, could you tell us of what importance you consider the intra-cellular concentration of free amino acid in the placenta, in relation to the placental transfer of amino acids? You have a recent publication on their values in the human placenta (PHILIPS, A.F., I.R. HOLZMAN, C. TENG and F.C. BATTAGLIA. (1978) Amer. J. Obstet. Gynec. 131:881.).

F.C. Battaglia: I think if we're talking about the net umbilical uptake of amino acid, I don't think those measurements have any relevance. Because we're not really asking whether they're coming, over a short period of time an hour's collection for example, from release of amino acids from the placenta or represent transfer from the uterine circulation.

I think where it becomes important – and what prompted our study – is when you begin to look at placenta in vitro, that is, either with placental perfusion experiments or with incubations of villi. Because then you're obligated to look at whether glutamine efflux could be accounted for by a decrease in the glutamine pool, either as free amino acid or in the acid hydrolysate of the placental protein.

There's one other thing, we were talking at the tea break about interpreting umbilical A-V differences on the cord blood in the delivery room. I would like to point out that there are both qualitative and quantitative differences in amino acid A-V differences. If the only effect of a collection in a delivery room were alterations in umbilical flow, then I would expect all A-V differences to double as the flow fell 50%. That isn't the case and so I have to think that there is some other factor entering in and it could be, again, release of amino acids either from the free amino acid pool or from protein breakdown in the placenta. I think that's another situation where it could be entering in.

G.J. Kloosterman: I should like to know whether I understood you right. If I remember your words well, than we can conclude that the placenta uses almost one-third of the total mass of energy that the mother is sending to the fetal-maternal unit. Is that right or is it a complete misinterpretation of your words?

F.C. Battaglia: I commented about glucose alone, it's only with glucose and lactate that we have measured simultaneously, in the same animal, the uterine release and the umbilical uptake. We don't have such data for the amino acids. I wish we could do that. But for glucose, it's true that only a third of the glucose that leaves the uterine circulation could be accounted for by glucose entry into the umbilical circulation. That is correct in the latter third of gestation. The rest is being consumed and used within the placenta. Half of that glucose which goes into the placenta we account for as carbon delivered as lactate into the umbilical and uterine circulations. So it is returned to the fetus, but as lactate. We're now having some lively discussions, where I am on sabbatical, why there's an advantage to the mammalian fetus of delivering the carbon as lactate rather than glucose. That's not immediately apparent to me, but I believe it is a feature that is quite general in fetal metabolism, since the human placenta, the sheep placenta, the rat placenta, the cow placenta all produce lactate in large amounts under aerobic conditions.

F. Widdowson: Can you give us any idea of the result of your discussions in Paris?

F.C. Battaglia: No.

C.T. Jones: On that question, Dr. Battaglia, you obviously have convincing data for the sheep whose placenta produces lactate. But I presume all the data from the other species is from in vitro studies. Are you convinced that those are suitable models to infer that placental lactate production in vivo is a consistent feature across the species.

For instance, if you isolate all of them, one of the first things that happens is you get substantial glycogenolysis producing a lot of lactate.

F.C. Battaglia: Obviously, it would be nice to have direct measurements of lactate uptake for the human fetus. I feel confident about it because since the first demonstration of lactate production by the rat placenta in the 1920's it has been shown for the placenta of many other species. No, I can't say that from studies in vitro on the placenta which show a high aerobic production of lactate, it must follow that this occurs in vivo. However, in all instances where umbilical A-V differences of lactate have been measured in different species, a large umbilical uptake of lactate has been demonstrated. I would point out that that is a characteristic of tumor tissue as well. For tumors, it can also be demonstrated with A-V differences across the tumor in vivo. So there are a lot of reasons to think placentas are producing lactate in a number of mammals.

C.T. Jones: It doesn't really prove your argument, for every perfused organ investigated can be a net lactate producer.

F.C. Battaglia: I never implied that organs other than the placenta are producing lactate, although I believe that there is a fetal production of lactate as well.

C.T. Jones: That is not necessarily true for the perfused muscle.

A. Okken: I've still got two questions for Dr. Sauer. The first one is about the energy used for synthesis. Simplistically spoken, what we are talking about is the "glue" necessary to "glue" the bricks together – if I can say that components for tissue synthesis are glued together. As far as I understand, the energy equivalent of this glue is reflected in oxygen uptake. I think it's very difficult to say that you can calculate the energy used for synthesis from the differences in heat production measured with direct and indirect calorimetry.

The second question is about the indirect calorimetry again. As far as I know, equations used for calculating heat production are only valid when the respiratory quotient is between 0.7 and 1.0.

If it's less than 0.7 and greater than 1.0 think we are getting into trouble. From our studies, I do know that frequently babies have respiratory quotients of greater than 1.0.

P.J.J. Sauer: I completely agree with Dr. Okken. I tried to explain that for the "glue" you need oxygen and food. The components plus the "glue" are stored. To get "glue", you need conventional food, you need oxygen, so you can measure it with indirect calorimetry. But this process cannot be measured with direct calorimetry, because no heat is given off. That is my explanation for the difference between direct and indirect calorimetry.

The respiratory quotients of our patients were between 0.8 and 1.0 in our studies, which were at least 6 hours long. There may have been some minutes when the quotient was higher than 1.0. During the whole period of time, every 16 seconds we printed out the oxygen consumption and carbon dioxide production and it was only during some minutes that it was more than 1.0.

D. Hull: Dr. Sauer, I was interested in your data. You said that you determined thermal environment from the data that Edmund Hey has produced.

I am not sure he gives too good a guide for babies under 1.5 kg. So I would be interested to know exactly what thermal environment you are using, particularly for babies under two weeks of age?

P.J.J. Sauer: I agree with you that the data of Hey on the thermoneutral environment of very small babies are not very accurate. We carefully controled skin and esophageal temperatures, because in prior studies we had seen that before the oxygen uptake rose, the skin temperature was falling. Then the esophageal temperature was falling and after that the oxygen uptake was increasing. So we adjusted the temperature of the incubator to the skin temperatures.

D. Hull: In some of the babies, the skin temperature might be low because of the high trans-epidermal water losses, particularly those under two or three weeks of age of that gestation.

Do you not set the incubator according to the thermal environment rather than the baby?

P.J.J. Sauer: Now you enter into a very difficult problem: How to nurse such a baby in a thermoneutral environment. Is it the baby or the environment that is the most important? We looked at both the eso-phageal temperature and the skin temperature at six places. We indeed saw that when a baby was sweating then the temperature of the forehead was falling and the temperature of the abdomen was rising. When the temperature of the environment was low and that of the hand and feet was falling, then only after some time the abdominal temperature was falling.

D. Hull: I think that's very interesting. It has been reported that babies of this gestation do not sweat at all. I'm sure you're right that they do.

A. Okken: I have a question for Dr. Whitelaw. He has measured double skin thickness at several sites. How was the distribution of skin thickness in the normal babies and how was the distribution in the small-for-dates babies? Could you say whether there is any site which is specially sensi-tive to a low-calorie intake?

A.G.L. Whitelaw: I would say that the most sensitive site for either deficiency or excess is the subscapular skin fold. If you are going to do just one site, I think that's the one that goes up or goes down the most. The biceps is probably the least variable; it's very unusual to get very, very thick fat over the biceps. Does that answer your question?

G.E. Gaull: I want to comment just for a moment about changeable fatty acids and the very interesting data of Professor Ballabriga.

I think the fact that these changes can be brought about at an early age in a group of membranes that, later, turnover rather slowly has particu-larly more significance than the changes they may have in the depot fat. There is an increasing amount of concern, I understand from some of my friends who are interested in lipids and membranes, that the fatty acid composition will very much alter the stiffness of the membrane and there are concerns in some quarters about not just the nutritional effect, but the potential for interaction with viruses. There was an interesting paper three or four years ago by Agranoff and Goldberg (Lancet Nov. 2, 1974, p. 1061.) about the correlation of disseminated sclerosis throughout the world with the ingestion of cow's milk. I think now that we're reaching a point in nutrition where we're beginning to think about the later implications of early nutrition. I don't think we can necessarily take comfort in the fact that we don't see at the moment any significance in particular changes, that maybe really are significant.

J.H.P. Jonxis: It's very difficult to answer. In the Netherlands, for about fifteen years, the majority of the Dutch infants have had formulas high in linoleic acid. Many of those are now youngsters. As far as I see, our youngsters are quite normal and not different from other ones. That's the only answer I can give. My problem in the whole affair is: what is the normal food of the human? Being interested in history I believe there is none. Everything would be so simple about fats and fat intake if we knew what is the normal food of a human. We have no reference point. It makes the whole situation, for me, very intriguing but very uncertain. You see my point?

G.E. Gaull: I agree about the uncertainty.

C.A. Canosa: I would like to address myself to Professor Jonxis. It seems that the main data for body composition in subcutaneous tissue is coming from artificially fed infants in the newborn period. I wonder if you are willing to comment about the possible implications of changing the mother's diet in regard to changes in the free fatty acids and triglycerides in the composition of subcutaneous fat of the newborn baby.

J.H.P. Jonxis: If I understand your question well, you're asking what's happening in babies that are breast fed.

C.A. Canosa: Yes.

J.H.P. Jonxis: The number of breast-fed babies in this country is increasing again, but it is quite difficult to get samples of subcutaneous fat. Perhaps Dr. Boersma can tell you something about what he has seen. He has studied breast-fed babies, not in Holland but in East Africa.

E.R. Boersma: In the breast-fed children in Tanzania the linoleic acid composition at birth was approximately the same as that which was found here, in Holland (WIDDOWSON E.M., M.J. DAUNCEY, D.M.T. GAIRDNER, J.H.P. JONXIS and M. PELLIKAN-FILIPKOVA (1975) Brit. Med. J. I:653).

From birth on, you see an increase of linoleic acid and a remarkable increase of the "smaller-chain" fatty acids, of C_{12} and C_{14}. You see a rise from, let us say, 3% to about 8% of linoleic acid, and when the children are weaned, you will find a further increase to about 9%. So that at the age of about 1½ years, the children in Tanzania will have a linoleic acid concentration in their body fat ranging from 7 to 12% (BOERSMA, E.R. (1979). Changes in the fatty acid composition of body fat before and after birth in Tanzania. An international comparitive study in relation to dietary patterns. Brit. Med. J. : in press).

A. Ballabriga: In our babies fed with mother's milk, the composition of subcutaneous fat after three weeks of lactation will depend on the diet of the mother, and the content of linoleic acid in breast milk will vary widely. Some levels will be as low as 3%, some as high as 15%. It will also depend on the economic situation of the family, i.e. the kind of oil the family consumes. Is the consumption of the mother corn oil or maize oil, or is it peanut oil, or olive oil? Now that olive oil in our country is more expensive, the concentration of linoleic acid in the breast milk is higher than before, because families are using more maize oil.

E. Widdowson: Thank you very much. It is quite clear that you can alter the composition of the fat of the baby by altering the composition of the breast milk and the latter is altered by the diet of the mother. But you cannot produce such big changes as you can by feeding, say, corn oil directly to the baby. I think this is now becoming evident.

J.C.L. Shaw: I would like to refer to Professor Jonxis's question, "What is the normal food for humans?" It seems to me that the search for the normal or perfect food is rather like the search for the Philosophers Stone. The human gene pool has enormous heterogeneity and presumably we can adapt to a wide variety of diets. But, when we look at diets in detail we find that some are ideal for only a proportion of a population. The world wide distribution of lactase deficiency and the widespread use of cows milk is an example. In an atherogenic environment where there is an abundance of ice cream, the fat person may die early, but in an environment with periodic famine a fat person will survive longer. Surely our investigations will not lead us to a "normal food" but will teach us how we may, to our greater advantage, adapt our eating habits to the ever changing variety of food stuffs at our disposal.

E.M. Widdowson: I think this is a rather good note on which to finish. Professor McCance, do you want to make a closing comment?

R.A. McCance: This conundrum about the perfect food was really solved for us by one of the music-hall stars round about the close of the last century – Marie Lloyd I believe – "a little of what ye fancy does ye good".

NUTRITION OF THE PRETERM INFANT

BODY COMPOSITION OF THE FETUS AND INFANT

E.M. WIDDOWSON*, D.A.T. SOUTHGATE** and E.N. HEY***

At the Nutricia Symposium in Groningen in 1973 Professor VISSER et al. gave a paper on "Parenteral nutrition in low birth weight infants" (1). In the discussion afterwards the question was raised as to whether the low birth weight infant should receive an amino acid mixture corresponding to human milk, or to fetal plasma, and it was suggested that the best mixture might be one corresponding to that of the baby's body itself. At that time there were no figures for the amino acid make-up of the protein in the body of the human fetus. I promised that such information would be forthcoming, and this is the main subject of our paper today.

In all the older work on the composition of the human fetus, which was reviewed by KELLY et al. (2), the gestational ages of the fetuses analysed were not accurately known and this was true also of the fetuses analysed by us long ago (3, 4). Moreover, while water, nitrogen, fat and a number of inorganic constituents were determined, methods for the quick and accurate determination of amino acids and fatty acids were not then available, and in the early 1970's the time seemed to be ripe for a more detailed study of the chemical and biochemical development of the human fetus than had hitherto been made. The material was collected in Newcastle by E.N. Hey who made all the initial measurements and dissected the bodies. D.A.T. Southgate was responsible for the analyses in Cambridge. These are not yet all completed, nor have the results been thoroughly assessed. Those appearing in the final report may not be exactly the same as those presented here, but any differences will be minor rather than major ones.

Thirty-eight fetuses of accurately known gestational age which presented as abortions, fresh still-births or which had died just after birth were included in the series, and placentae, membranes and cords of most

* Department of Medicine, Addenbrooke's Hospital, Cambridge.
** Dunn Nutritional Laboratory, Milton Road, Cambridge.
*** The Princess Mary Maternity Hospital, Newcastle upon Tyne.

H.K.A. Visser (ed.), Nutrition and Metabolism of the Fetus and Infant, 169-177. All rights reserved.
Copyright © 1979 Martinus Nijhoff Publishers b.v., The Hague/Boston/London.

of them were also studied. Babies dying as a result of an haemolytic disease or a congenital abnormality were excluded. Of the 38 fetuses the weights of 31 were considered "normal", that is they were above the 10th percentile fetal growth curve of THOMSON et al. (5). The remaining 7 were below the 10th percentile and 3 of them were below the 5th; these 7 were considered "light for dates". Only the 31 fetuses of "normal" weight will be considered here (fig. 1).

The fetus was first weighed and crown-rump and crown-heel length measured, as were the circumference and the anterio-posterial and bi-parietal diameters of the head. The circumference of the chest was recorded, the fetus photographed, and an X-ray film of the body taken. In some fetuses skinfold measurements were made.

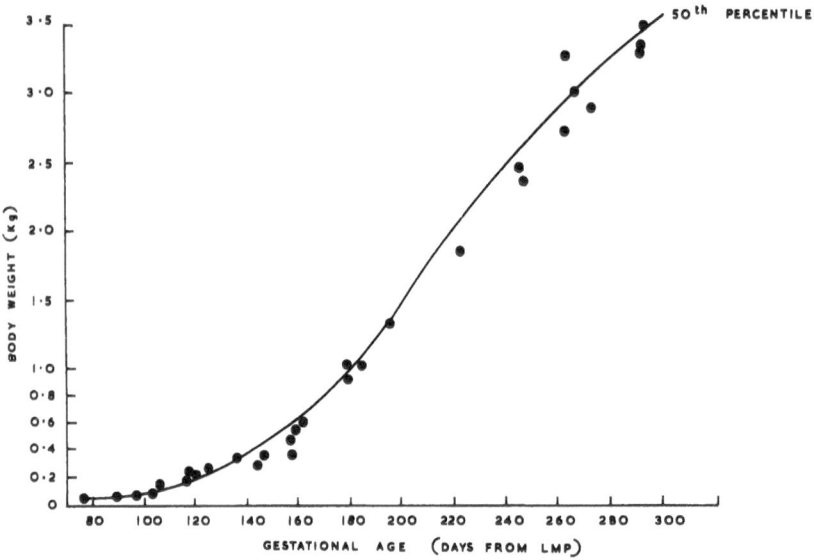

Fig. 1. Body weights of fetuses included in study compared with 50th percentile growth curve of THOMSON et al. (5).

The body was dissected according to standard autopsy procedure and the organs weighed and stored at $-20°$ for separate analysis. Samples of skeletal muscle, skin, white and brown adipose tissue, parietal bone, and left femur and humerus were also removed for analysis, and specific teeth were extracted from the jaw. The skin, with its subcutaneous fat, was separated from the remainder of the body, which contained the deep body fat. Fetuses weighing less than 100 g were not dissected, but the whole body was frozen at −20° for analysis.

The material was all transported from Newcastle to Cambridge in insulated containers in a frozen state where it was put into a deep freeze until it was analysed. Two parts of the body travelled further, to experts in the analysis of these particular organs, the brains to Professor J.W.T. Dickerson at the University of Surrey and the teeth to Dr. M.V. Stack at the University of Bristol. The skins, carcasses, organs, placentae, membranes and cords were freeze dried and portions taken for the measurement of water, nitrogen, protein, amino acids, fat, fatty acids, DNA, sodium, potassium, calcium, magnesium, phosphorus, iron, copper and zinc.

It is clearly impossible for me to present the results of all these analyses today, but they will be published in detail as a supplement to Acta Paediatrica. Many of the results, particularly those on the inorganic constituents, confirmed in general those we had previously obtained (3, 4). I shall confine myself mainly to an aspect of the work that is new – that is the incorporation of the separate amino acids into the body of the developing fetus. I shall also say something about the deposition of fat.

AMINO ACIDS IN THE DEVELOPING FETUS

The body and organs of each fetus were homogenised and freeze dried and most of the amino acids were measured in samples after hydrolysis with HCl as described by SOUTHGATE (6). Cystine, tryptophan and hydroxyproline required special methods and the results for these amino acids are not yet available. The values included the small amounts of amino acids present as such together with the much larger amounts originally in the form of protein. It became clear when the results for all the fetuses were examined that the contribution of each amino acid to the total amino acids in the body did not change appreciably throughout the period of gestation covered by this investigation – that is between 79 days and term. This made the calculation and presentation of the results much easier than they would otherwise have been.

Table 1 shows the amino acids in the body of the fetus expressed as mg of amino acid per g of total amino nitrogen. It has been assumed that 90% of the nitrogen in the whole body is present as amino nitrogen, which may not be exact, but is near enough for the present purpose. For comparison the results of VELASQUEZ et al. (7) for free amino acids in fetal

Table 1. *Amino acids expressed as mg amino acid per g total amino N.*

Amino acid	Free and bound in fetal body	Free in fetal plasma		Free and bound in	
		Artery	Vein	Breast milk	Cows' milk
ILE	237	212	223	320	350
LEU	511	270	267	580	640
LYS	489	533	540	430	510
MET	134	118	180	90	180
CYS		572	734	120	60
PHE	282	197	238	230	340
TYR	199	274	227	180	280
THR	283	606	672	275	310
TRP		147	208	140	90
VAL	322	380	348	415	460
ARG	523	462	362	230	250
HIS	178	358	494	145	190
ALA	492	1005	903	245	240
ASP	617	102	141	535	530
GLU	888	671	384	1076	1440
GLY	806	188	231	150	140
PRO	574	437	322	575	590
SER	299	370	395	255	370

plasma at term have been recalculated to the same method of expression, and values are also given for the total amino acids, both free and bound as protein, in breast milk and cows' milk (8). The relative contribution of isoleucine, lysine, methionine, phenylalanine, tyrosine and valine to the total amino acids in the body is similar to that for the free amino acids in the plasma, although the body contains a greater proportion of leucine and a smaller one of threonine. For these amino acids the contribution to the total in the fetal body is more like that in milk than it is in fetal plasma.

On the whole the same is true for the non-essential amino acids. Glycine, however, which is the second most plentiful amino acid in the fetal body, is not one of the major ones either in plasma or in milk. There seemed to be no correlation between the plasma AV difference and the amino acid composition of the fetal body, but we had no figures for blood flow as LEMONS et al. had for the sheep (9).

These values, which show the distribution of amino acids in the body, give no information about the total amounts incorporated into the fetal body during growth. In order to calculate this it is necessary to know the

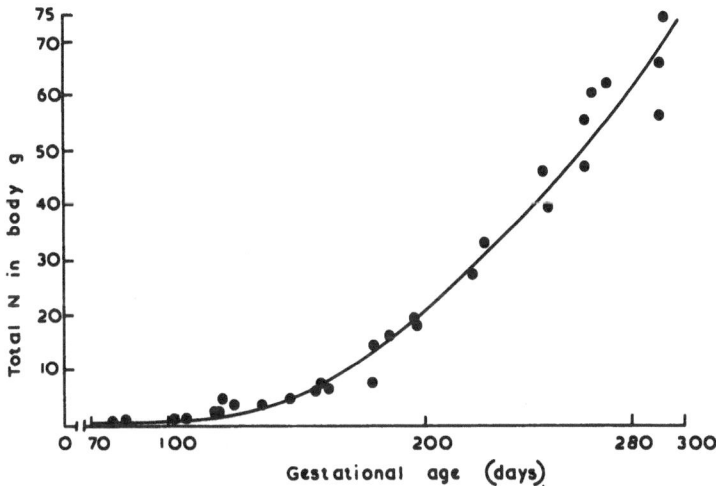

Fig. 2. Total nitrogen in body of fetus.

total amount of nitrogen in the body at different ages and this is shown in figure 2. Nitrogen does not begin to increase rapidly until about 160 days gestation and thereafter, as the fetus begins to gain weight faster, the deposition of nitrogen and of protein takes place at an increasing rate.

Table 2 shows the increments of amino acids in the body, as mg per day over 20 day periods, between 160 and 280 days gestation, that is between approximately 0.5 and 3.4 kg in weight. The amounts of the amino acids provided by 200 ml of breast milk are also shown to give some indication of the adequacy of this volume of milk say for a 1000 g baby. Isoleucine and leucine appear to be provided in ample amounts by breast milk but phenylalanine is more marginal. Tyrosine is not generally considered an essential amino acid, since it can be formed from phenylalanine, but if phenylalanine is in short supply, the amount of tyrosine becomes more important. The amount in 200 ml breast milk is again just about enough for the infant weighing 1 kg, but there is not much to spare. Of all the essential amino acids in breast milk, methionine seems to be most inadequate for the low birth weight infant, but until we have the values for cystine we cannot be sure.

So far as the so-called inessential amino acids are concerned, glycine, which is synthesised from other amino acids and incorporated very rapidly into the fetal body, appears to be inadequately supplied by breast milk on any showing. In view of its role as part of the molecule of

Table 2. *Increments of amino acids in body mg/day*

Age range days	160-180	180-200	200-220	220-240	240-260	260-280	Amino acid in 200 ml breast milk mg
Weight range kg	0.5-0.9	0.9-1.4	1.4-1.9	1.9-2.4	2.4-2.9	2.9-3.4	
ILE	59	71	85	102	119	140	134
LEU	127	153	184	220	256	301	240
LYS	122	147	176	210	245	289	180
MET	34	40	48	58	67	79	38
CYS							50
PHE	71	85	102	121	141	166	96
TYR	49	60	72	86	100	117	76
THR	71	85	102	122	142	167	116
TRP							60
VAL	81	97	116	138	161	190	174
ARG	130	157	188	225	262	309	98
HIS	45	53	64	77	89	105	62
ALA	123	148	177	212	246	290	104
ASP	154	185	222	265	309	364	220
GLU	222	266	320	382	444	524	450
GLY	202	242	290	347	403	476	64
PRO	144	172	207	247	287	339	240
SER	75	90	108	129	150	176	108
Total N	275	325	400	475	550	650	400

glutathione, of the porphyrin ring of hemoglobin, and of the nucleic acids perhaps particular attention should be paid to it in designing food for the low birth weight infant.

FAT

Up to 180 days there is very little fat in the fetal body, and what there is is divided approximately equally between subcuteanous and deep body sites (10). Thereafter the distribution changes and almost all the fat deposited in the body during the last part of gestation is in the subcutaneous tissues. At term 80% of the body fat is subcutaneous.

Fatty acid analyses of brown and white fat were made on a larger number of fetuses than those included in the detailed measurement of body composition (11). The fat becomes more saturated during gestation, and in particular the concentration of the polyunsaturated fatty acid, linoleic acid, in it decreases. Brown fat contains more linoleic acid than white (12), but in both types of fat the percentage of linoleic acid falls. This has been interpreted by some as indicating that synthesis of fat from glucose and amino acids by the fetus has taken the place of placental transport, which is the way the fetus gets all its fatty acids during the first months of gestation. The fetus cannot synthesise linoleic acid, so any of this fatty acid found in its body at any age must have come from its mother's circulation through the placenta. From the figures for total fat in the fetal bodies (10), and the percentage of linoleic acid in it at different ages (11) the approximate rate of deposition of linoleic acid in the depot fat of the whole body has been calculated. Table 3 shows the total amount of depot fat, and the amount of linoleic acid in it that are deposited in the body of the fetus per day between 160 days and term. Placental transport of linoleic acid continues throughout, and the fall in percentage of it in the fat is entirely accounted for by its dilution due to the increasing rate of synthesis of fat by the fetus. The rate of incorporation of linoleic acid into the fat does not fall, but increases. These calculations do not take account of the phospholipids in the brain and other tissues. The essential fatty acids in the brain are mainly long chain

Table 3. *Increments of linoleic acid in the body fat (British)*

Gestation days	Total fat in body g	Linoleic acid		
		as % total fatty acids	in total body fat g	gain per day mg
160	6	5.3	0.33	
180	23	4.8	1.10	38.5
200	49	4.2	2.06	48.0
220	97	3.6	3.49	71.5
240	165	3.0	4.95	73.0
260	265	2.4	6.36	70.5
280	476	1.8	8.57	111.0

derivatives of linoleic and linolenic acids, of which arachidonic acid is quantitatively important. We do not know how the arachidonic in the brain reaches it, whether by transfer across the placenta from the mother's circulation, or by conversion from linoleic acid in the fetal liver, or even in the placenta. If it is made from linoleic acid by the fetus then considerably more linoleic acid must be reaching the fetus than the amounts appearing in the body fat.

In collaboration with Professor Jonxis analyses have been made of the fatty acid composition of white fat of fetuses of Dutch mothers. The reason for this was that there was a suggestion from an earlier study (13) that at term the composition might be different from that for British infants. The slope of the linear regression was less steep for the Dutch fetuses, and their fat at term contained a significantly higher proportion of linoleic acid (3.6 ± 0.4%) than that of the British infants (1.8 ± 0.1%) (11). As far as we know no analyses have been made of the total amount of fat in the bodies of fetuses in Holland but, assuming that fat deposition were to go on at the same rate in Groningen as in Newcastle, then the increments of linoleic acid in the body fat of fetuses of Dutch mothers would be as shown in Table 4. The amount of linoleic acid incorporated into the fat each day is more than in U.K., suggesting that placental transport is higher, possibly because the concentration of this fatty acid in the plasma is higher in Dutch than in British women, though the two have not been compared. We know that Dutch people have a higher intake of polyunsaturated fatty acids than British people because they use soft margarine as their spreading fat whereas the British use butter.

We have known for a long time that fat is quantitatively the most variable constituent in the human body at any given age. It now seems that the same is true of its composition.

Table 4. *Increments of linoleic acid in the body fat (Dutch)*.

Gestation days	Linoleic acid		
	as % total fatty acids	in total body fat g	gain per day mg
160	5.3	0.33	
180	5.1	1.17	38.5
200	4.8	2.35	59.0
220	4.5	4.37	101
240	4.2	6.93	128
260	3.9	10.34	171
280	3.7	17.61	264

REFERENCES

1. VISSER, H.K.A., W. BLOM, J.F. VAN GILS, and T. ZURCHER. (1973) In: Therapeutic Aspects of Nutrition. Fourth Nutricia Symposium, Jonxis, J.H.P., H.K.A. Visser and J.A. Troelstra eds., H.E. Stenfert Kroese, Leiden, Holland, p. 272.
2. KELLY, H.J., R.E. SLOAN, W. HOFFMAN and C. SAUNDERS. (1951) Human Biol. 23:61.
3. WIDDOWSON, E.M. and C.M. SPRAY. (1951) Arch. Dis. Childh. 26:205.
4. WIDDOWSON, E.M. and J.W.T. DICKERSON. (1961) In: Mineral Metabolism, vol. 2A, Comar, C.L. and F. Bronner, eds., Academic Press, New York, p. 1.
5. THOMSON, A.M., W.Z. BILLEWICZ and F.E. HYTTEN. (1968) J. Obstet. Gynaec. Brit. Cwlth. 75:903.
6. SOUTHGATE, D.A.T. (1971) Biol. Neonat. 19:272.
7. VELASQUEZ, A., A. ROSADO, A. BERNAL, L. NORIEGA and N. AREVALO. (1976) Biol. Neonate 29:28.
8. PAUL, A.A. and D.A.T. SOUTHGATE. (1978) McCance and Widdowson's The Composition of Foods, ed. 4, Spec. Rep. Ser. med. Res. Coun. No. 297. H.M.S.O., London.
9. LEMONS, G.A., E.W. ADCOCK, III, M.D. JONES, M.A. NAUGHTON, G. MESCHIA and F.C. BATTAGLIA. (1976) J. Clin. Invest. 88:1428.
10. SOUTHGATE, D.A.T. and E.N. HEY. (1976) In: The Biology of Human Fetal Growth, Roberts, D.F. and A.M. Thomson eds., Taylor and Francis, London, p. 195.
11. PAVEY, D. (1978) In: Proceedings of the XIth International Congress of Nutrition. (In Press).
12. JONXIS, J.H.P. (1979) In: Nutrition and Metabolism of the Fetus and Infant, Fifth Nutricia Symposium, H.K.A. Visser ed., Martinus Nijhoff, The Hague, p. 123.
13. WIDDOWSON, E.M., M.J. DAUNCEY, D.M.T. GAIRDNER, J.H.P. JONXIS and M. PELIKAN-FILIPKOVA. (1975) Brit. Med. J. 1:653.

THE ABSORPTION OF MAGNESIUM, COPPER, ZINC AND IRON BY PRETERM INFANTS IN RELATION TO BODY COMPOSITION OF THE FOETUS

J. C. L. SHAW, MRCP*

The elements magnesium, zinc, copper and iron are essential nutrients for all living organisms. Since they play important roles at many levels of intermediary metabolism, a deficiency of any of these substances in the preterm infant will have an adverse effect on growth and development. The mechanism of the late iron deficiency anaemia of preterm infants is now well understood and routine prophylactic iron is given to all such babies. Deficiencies of magnesium, copper and zinc are not so easily detected and their existence has only been recognised comparatively recently. It is the purpose of this paper to present the results of measurements of magnesium, copper, zinc and iron absorption in preterm infants, and to relate the results to changes in body composition of the foetus.

RECOGNISED DEFICIENCY SYNDROMES

Iron deficiency is so well-known it need not be described here.

Magnesium

Magnesium plays an essential role in numerous biochemical processes from photosynthesis to oxidative phosphorylation. Magnesium ions activate numerous enzymes particularly those concerned in reactions involving ATP, they are associated with phosphate groups on DNA in the cell nucleus, and with RNA in the ribosomes where they are involved in protein synthesis. The deficiency syndrome in man includes tremor and involuntary movements, tetany, seizures, delirium and muscular weakness (1, 2). Hypomagnasaemia in association with symptoms has been reported in low birth weight infants (3) but a distinct nutritional deficiency syndrome has not been described in these babies.

* Department of Paediatrics, University College Hospital, Gower Street, London, WCI.

H.K.A. Visser (ed.), Nutrition and Metabolism of the Fetus and Infant, 179-194. All rights reserved.
Copyright © 1979 Martinus Nijhoff Publishers b.v., The Hague/Boston/London.

Zinc

Zinc is a component of at least seventy metallo-enzymes. It is, for example, a component of DNA and RNA polymerase and as such plays a central role in the replication and transcription of DNA during cell division (4). In the foetal rat, and perhaps also in man, zinc deficiency produces congenital malformations, particularly anencephaly and spina bifida (5, 6). In man the features of severe deficiency are those of Acrodermatitis Enteropathica, a formerly fatal condition shown to be due to a recessively inherited disorder of zinc absorption (7, 8). The features include alopecia, extensive vesicopustular lesions of hands, feet, perineal area and face, with oesophagitis, diarrhoea and thymic atrophy. There may be impairment of phagocyte chemotaxis (9) and also of cell mediated immunity (10). Symptoms of Acrodermatitis Enteropathica only develop after weaning, and it is therefore of great interest that a zinc binding ligand has recently been demonstrated in breast milk which may augment zinc absorption (11, 12). This syndrome also develops in infants on zinc free parenteral nutrition (13, 14, 15) but has not been reported in orally fed infants. HAMBIDGE et al. (1972) (16) on the basis of low hair zinc concentrations and response to zinc therapy have described a syndrome of mild zinc deficiency in children (4–16 yr) characterised by poor growth and diminished taste sensation. In adolescents chronic mild zinc deficiency results in a syndrome of small stature, anaemia and delay in sexual maturation (17).

Copper

Copper is a component of numerous metalloenzymes including cytochrome C oxidase, tyrosinase, lysyl oxidase and dopamine β hydroxylase (18), and many of the features of copper deficiency can be attributed to the failure of specific enzymes. Copper deficiency has only rarely been reported in the survivors of premature birth (19, 20, 21). The cases presented between 3 and 6 months of age, with hypotonia, developmental delay, and pallor attributable in part to poor pigmentation. They had anaemia and neutropenia, and bone changes reminiscent of scurvey were evident on X-ray (23). Bone marrow examination showed red cell precursers with vacuolated cytoplasm and an abundance of sideroblasts. The granulolytes showed maturation arrest. Plasma, copper and caeruloplasmin levels were invariably very low. This syndrome has also been reported in infants receiving parenteral nutrition (21, 22, 23). Treatment with copper sulphate results in a prompt reticulocytosis and the haematological abnormalities revert to normal within 3 weeks.

FOETAL GROWTH AS A REFERENCE STANDARD

In the studies reported below foetal growth has been used as a reference standard in the interpretation of the results of metabolic balance studies. This is not meant to imply that the preterm infant should grow exactly the same as the foetus does in utero, or that he has exactly the same needs. If the preterm infant grew exactly like the foetus we would certainly be reassured – but it may prove not to be possible, and it may not even be necessary. The comparison is useful because it shows us how the chemical growth of the preterm infant differs from that of the foetus in utero and thus draws our attention to substances that may be growth limiting, by virtue of malabsorption, poor renal conservation or inadequate provision in the diet.

ESTIMATES OF INTRAUTERINE WEIGHT GAIN

Examination of the mean values for birth weight of infants born at different periods of gestation published by LUBCHENKO et al. (1963) (24) and by KLOOSTERMAN (1970) (25) shows them to be almost identical (26). The increase in weight of the foetus between 24 and 36 weeks gestation is exponential and occurs at a rate of 14.4 gm/kg day for an infant growing along the 50th centile. (It would be 15.6 gm/kg day for an infant growing along the 10th centile of Lubchenko and 12.2 g/kg day for an infant growing along the 90th centile.)

Comparison of postnatal weight gain with mean values for intrauterine weight gain, has shown that the smallest preterm infants seldom equal intrauterine weight gain (26) and as a result are generally below their expected weight for gestation on discharge home. If this difference in weight were due just to a reduction in body fat, it might not matter very much; however, if it were due to a more complex change in growth affecting all the components of the body then it might lead to undesirable alterations in the functions of the tissues. In order to see how the chemical growth of the preterm infant differs from that of the foetus, one must be able to compare the daily rate at which preterm infants absorb and retain different substances in their bodies, with the rate at which these same substances are laid down each day by the foetus in utero.

INTRAUTERINE ACCUMULATION RATES

Estimates of the rates of accumulation of different substances by the
foetus in utero have been made from the results of analyses of foetal
bodies given in the literature (27, 28). The exponential regression line
$(Y = Y_0 \cdot e^{kt})$ was calculated for the total amount of each substance in
the foetus expressed as a function of gestation (see fig. 1). The daily
increment of each substance was calculated using the fractional rate
constant k (Increment $- Y_t \cdot k^{days^{-1}}$). These values (26) have been used
for the comparisons in this paper.

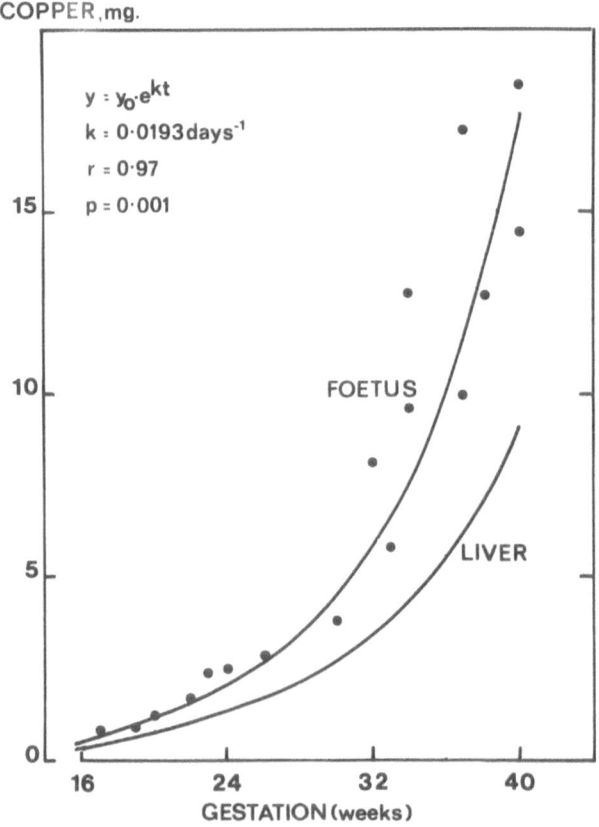

Fig. 1. Copper content of foetal bodies (27). The copper increases exponentially with
gestation and at term half the copper in the foetal body is in the liver (36).

METABOLIC BALANCE METHODS

Because of inevitable losses of milk and stool, balance techniques tend systematically to overestimate retention and in addition, during trace metal balances, contamination is always a hazard which tends to introduce more random fluctuations into the data. The methods used in these studies have been developed to reduce errors to a minimum. The milk was prepared by the laboratory staff in acid washed glass ware and frozen until required. The milk was given by syringe, and the amount given determined by weighing the bottles and syringes at the beginning and end of each day. The stools were marked with carmine and were collected onto 11.0 cm ashless filter papers which were held in place by chemically clean polythene tie pants. The infants were cleaned with a filter paper softened in a little distilled water. No ointments were used during the balance period. Urine was collected in home made polythene urine bags held in place by silicone adhesive. The urine was continuously aspirated into a chilled flask using a small diaphragm pump.

Portions of the diet, the stools and filter papers were dried and ashed, and acid extracts of the ash were analysed by atomic absorption spectrophotometry. Blank values for the filter papers were substracted from the results. The balance results given below come from a study of 6 preterm infants of mean gestation 29 weeks and mean birth weight 1191 grams. All the infants were fed pasteurised human breast milk (29, 30).

MAGNESIUM

Figure 2 gives contrasting examples of magnesium balances in two infants. The first balance commenced on day 10 and lasted three days. Balances were repeated on each infant every 10 days until discharge home. The infant on the left (J.C.) absorbed amounts close to those being laid down in utero but retained much less because he passed so much magnesium in his urine. The infant (H.M.) on the right by contrast absorbed very little magnesium until after the 40th day of life and passed correspondingly much less in his urine. One might speculate whether magnesium could ever be growth limiting in such a case. On average the 6 infants retained 1.63 mg/kg day about 56% of the intrauterine accumulation rate.

In order to verify more directly the results of these balances we have compared the composition of bones from normal foetuses (dying within

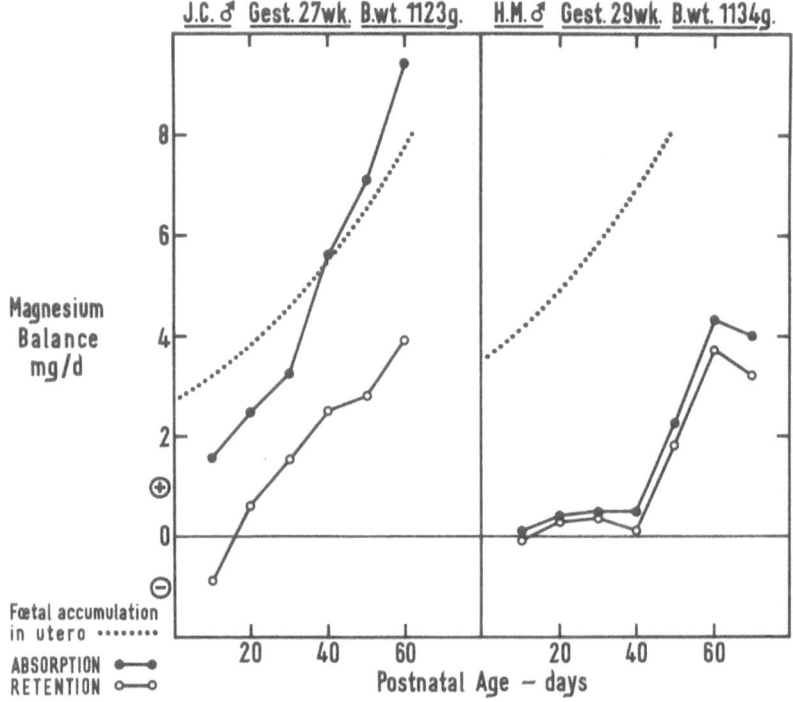

Fig. 2. Contrasting examples of magnesium balance in two infants. The difference between absorption and retention represents the amount of magnesium present in the urine. The foetal accumulation rate is given for comparison.

24 hr of birth) with the composition of bones from two groups of preterm infants dying 8–14 days after birth and > 28 days after birth. The results are shown in figure 3. The figure demonstrates the very low magnesium levels found in the femurs of preterm infants, these low levels are not just a function of reduced bone weight since the magnesium concentration (mg/100 mg dry bone weight) and magnesium: collagen ration were significantly below those of foetal bones. (p = < 0.001). These infants were, of course, very ill and these changes must therefore reflect not only the impact of premature brith but also of their fatal illnesses.

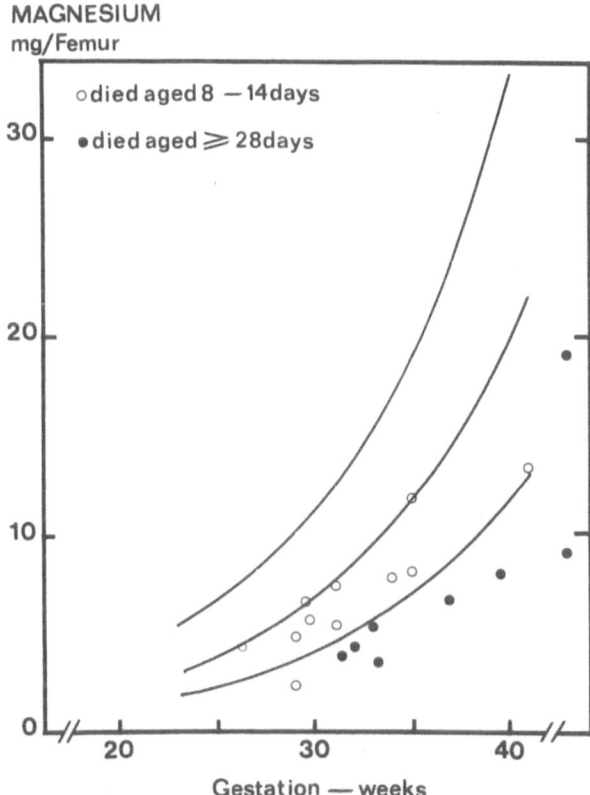

MAGNESIUM
mg/Femur

o died aged 8 — 14 days

• died aged ⩾ 28 days

Gestation — weeks

Fig. 3. Comparison of the magnesium content of the foetal femur with the magnesium content of the femurs of two groups of preterm infants dying at different times after birth. The regression line and 95% confidence limits were calculated from the results of analyses of foetal bones.

ZINC

Figure 4 gives contrasting examples of two zinc balances. These two infants and the others in the study were all in negative balance for zinc on the 10th day of life. However, whereas the infant on the left (S.R.) went steadily into positive balance by day 50, the infant on the right (J.C.) was never observed to be in positive balance at all. These results are not entirely unexpected because CAVELL and WIDDOWSON (1964) (31) found full term infants (aged 6–8 days) to be in negative balance for zinc. However, the duration and magnitude of these balances was very sur-

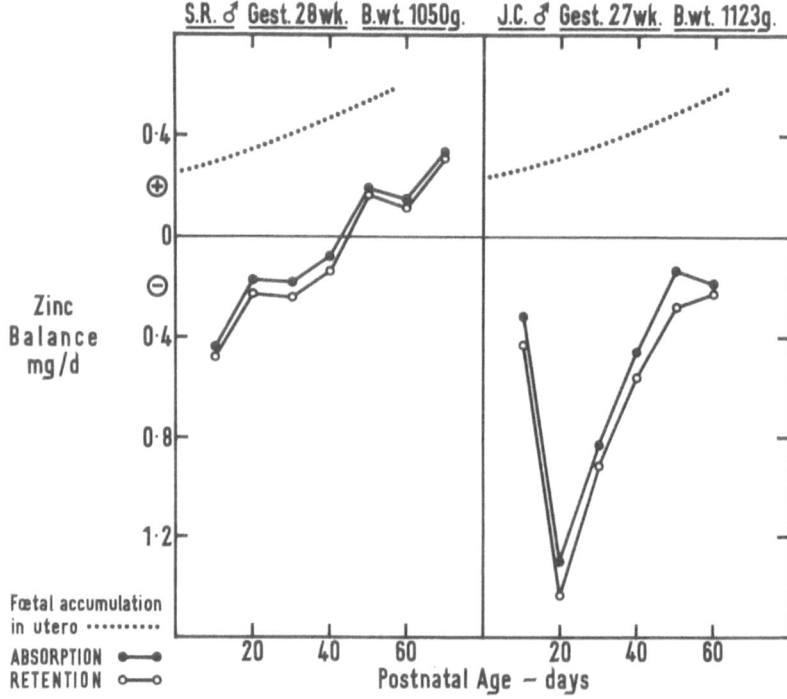

Fig. 4. Contrasting examples of zinc balances in two preterm infants. The estimated foetal accumulation rate is given for comparison.

prising because as a group they were not in positive balance on average until the 60th day of life. Figure 5 gives the results of bone analyses for zinc. Of the 18 measurements in preterm infants 15 lie below the regression line. The reduction in bone zinc is not so great as the reduction of bone magnesium, which is surprising in view of the results of the zinc balances in surviving infants. The explanation may lie in part in the fact that all these infants were seriously ill. In some cases because the introduction of oral feeding was delayed, they had to rely for varying periods on glucose infusions, and as a result, intestinal losses may have been reduced. Others received total parenteral nutrition and though no zinc was added at that time zinc was present as a contaminant in the Aminosol Solution. Figure 6 gives the results of serial measurements of plasma zinc in preterm infants. The mean values are not very different from those reported by OHTAKE (1977) (32) for healthy Japanese

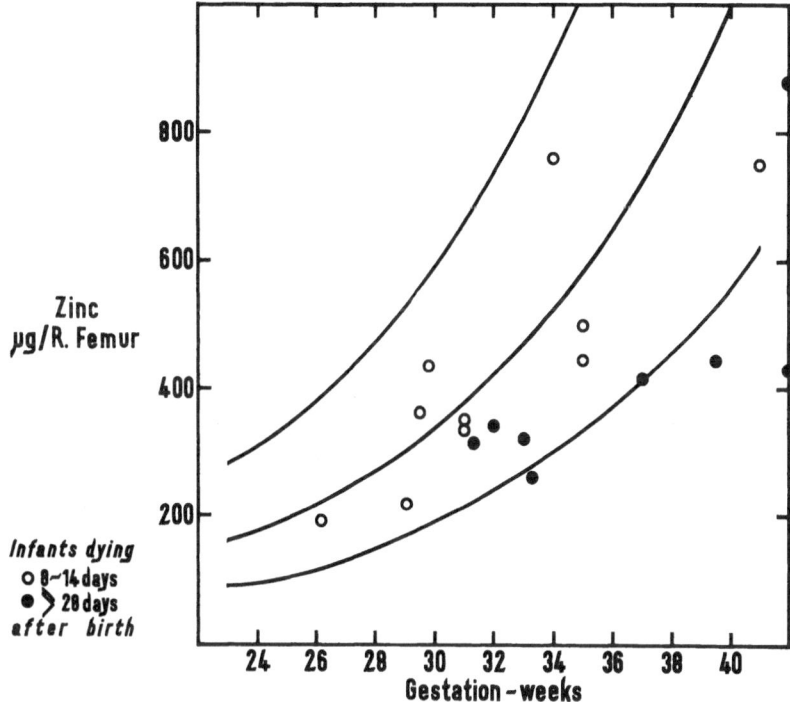

Fig. 5. Comparison of zinc content of the foetal femur with the zinc content of the femurs of two groups of preterm infants dying at different times after birth. The regression line and 95% confidence limits were calculated from the results of analyses of foetal bones.

children. What is striking is the very high incidence of low values below 50 µg/100 ml. The serial changes in a single infant (C.D.) are shown. This child had an uncomplicated clinical course and grew slowly but steadily. She exhibited no evidence of zinc deficiency though her plasma values were in the range where features resembling Acrodermatitis Enteropathica have been reported in patients receiving zinc free total parenteral nutrition (15).

It is, however, important not to equate a low plasma zinc concentration with zinc deficiency. Zinc circulates in the plasma bound to albumen, a_2 macroglobulin and transferrin (33, 34) and changes in plasma albumen produce parallel changes in plasma zinc. Until more is known about the distribution of zinc in the plasma of preterm infants the full significance of these measurements will not be known.

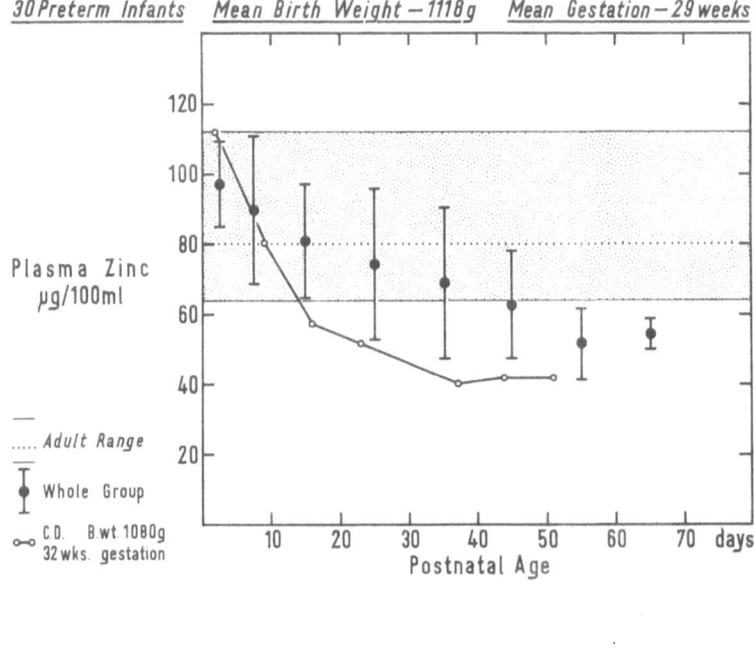

30 Preterm Infants   Mean Birth Weight — 1118g   Mean Gestation — 29 weeks

Plasma Zinc
µg/100ml

..... Adult Range

Whole Group

C.D. B.wt. 1080g
32 wks. gestation

Postnatal Age

U.C.H.M.S. 3259/279--78 V K A

Fig. 6. Changes in plasma zinc following birth in preterm infants. An example of the changes in a single infant are shown. The adult range in this figure is based on the measurements made on 42 healthy men and women.

COPPER

Figure 7 gives the results of copper balances in two preterm infants. The infant on the left (S.R.) was always in positive copper balance, and it is perhaps noteworthy that copper virtually disappeared from his urine after the 30th day. By contrast the infant on the right (H.M.) was in negative copper balance initially but went into positive balance after the 40th day of life. Neither of these infants equalled the estimated intra-uterine accumulation rates, and one must conclude that their copper stores were smaller than they might have been had they remained in utero. Measurements of copper in bone have proved to be inaccurate because of matrix interferences so at the present time we have no independent confirmation of depletion of copper in the tissues of preterm

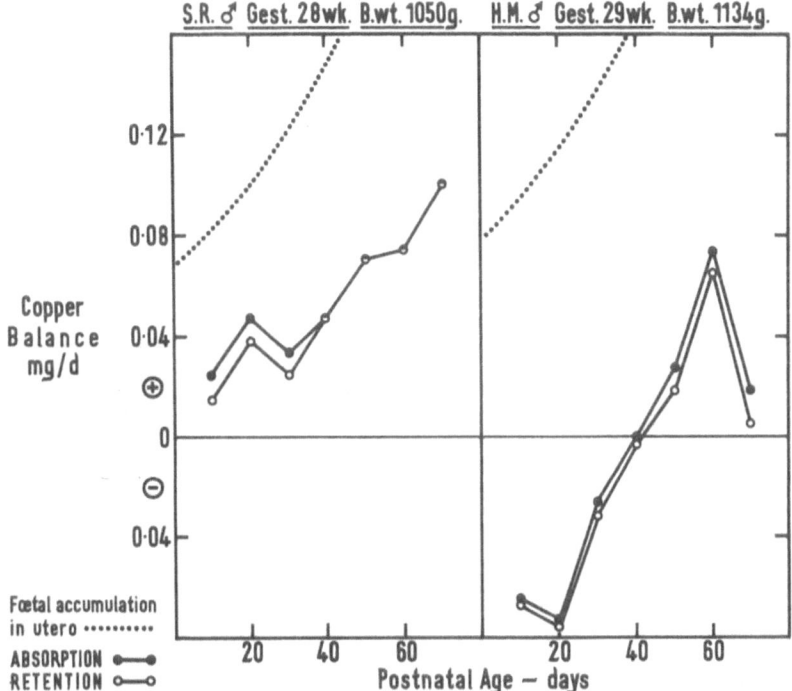

Fig. 7. Contrasting examples of copper balances in two preterm infants. The estimated foetal accumulation rate is given for comparison.

infants. Figure 1 shows that at term about half the copper is stored in the liver bound to protein that has recently been identified as a copper thionein (35). The liver is therefore the obvious place to look for depletion of copper stores.

Figure 8 shows the change in plasma copper in preterm infants following birth, and compares them with the changes that occur in full term infants (32). The plasma copper is high in the foetus and falls to very low levels with maturity. The cord blood levels of copper and caeruloplasmin are very low in full term infants and the concentrations rise very rapidly after birth as copper is released from the liver stores. By contrast the preterm infants had much higher copper levels after birth which fell quite steeply over the first 2 to 3 weeks. Thereafter, some rose to normal levels and others remained low. The serial measurements for the infant C.D. are again shown. Though her plasma copper levels fell very low, she has at present no detectable signs of copper deficiency but she is being followed up. As is to be expected the caeruloplasmin levels follow the copper levels closely.

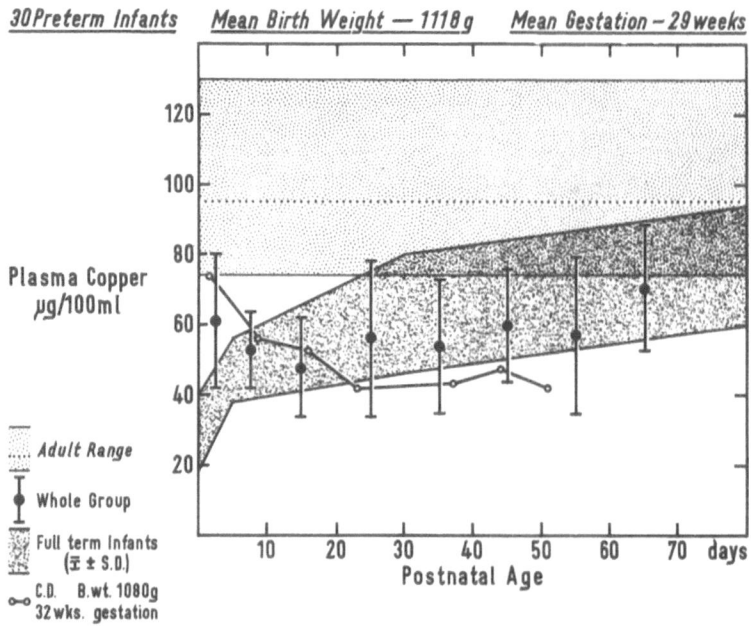

U.C.H.M.S. 3259/278-78. V.K.A.

Fig. 8. Changes in plasma copper following birth in preterm infants compared with values for full term infants (32). The adult range in this figure is based on measurements in 20 healthy adult men.

IRON

Figure 9 gives the results of an iron balance in the infant J.C. On day 10 and day 20 he was in negative iron balance. On day 30 iron supplements were given and he began to absorb amounts of iron that exceeded the intrauterine accumulation rate. Since the amount of iron absorbed also exceeded the amount required to raise his haemoglobin mass to the estimated levels iron was presumably entering his iron stores.

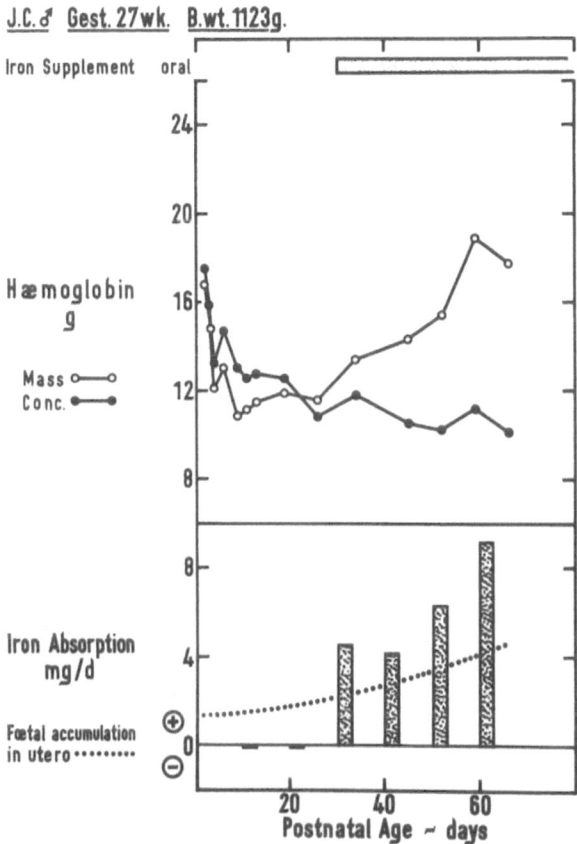

Fig. 9. Result of iron balance in one preterm infant. The haemoglobin mass was calculated from the haemoglobin concentration and the estimated blood volume (90 ml/kg).
Iron supplements (≈ 10 mg/kg day) were begun on day 30.

Figure 10 summarises all the measurements of iron absorption in
infants who received no blood transfusions. From this data it would
appear that the infants exerted no control over iron absorption, the
amount absorbed being simply a function of the concentration of iron in
the diet. Provided there are no abnormal losses of iron from vene-
puncture nor abnormal gains from blood transfusion one might tentatively conclude that an intake in the region of 5 mg/kg day would result
in iron absorption close to the foetal accumulation rate, and an intake of
rather less would probably meet their needs for haemoglobin synthesis.

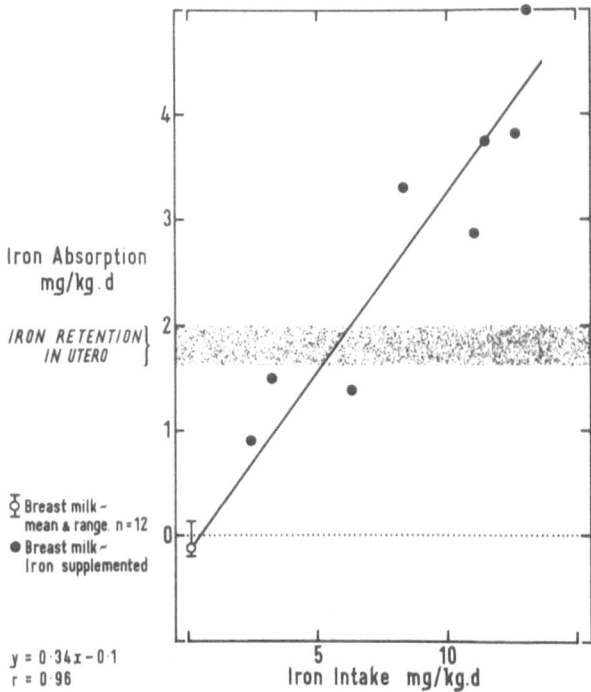

Fig. 10. Iron absorption as a function of iron intake in 6 preterm infants given different intakes of oral iron. None of these measurements were in infants who had received blood transfusion.

Figure 11 gives the results obtained in an infant who received a blood transfusion. Following the blood transfusion iron absorption became negative and did not become positive until the haemoglobin concentration fell below about 11 g/100 ml. This, and other similar results (30) suggest that a mechanism may exist for the control of iron absorption in preterm infants which cannot operate at the low levels of haemoglobin that exist in these infants.

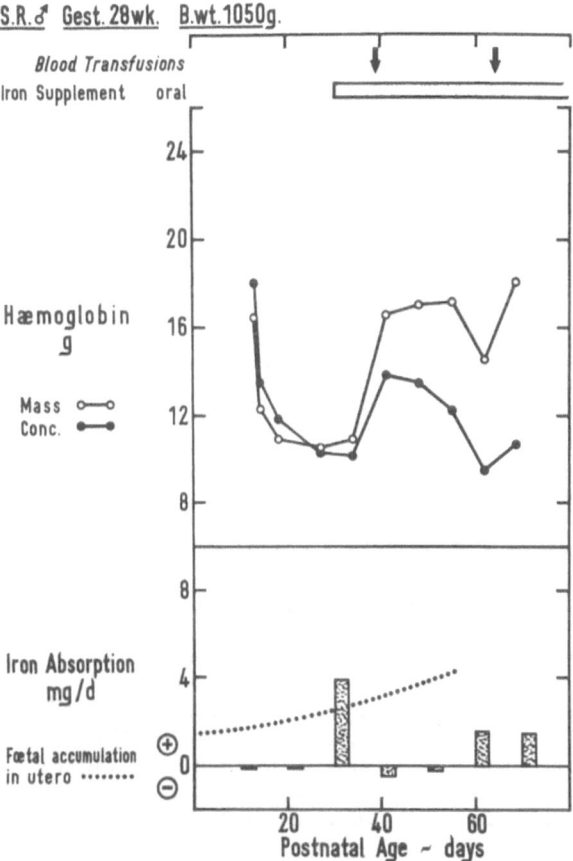

Fig. 11. Result of iron balance in an infant who received a blood transfusion on day 39, and day 65. Blood transfusion appeared to switch off iron absorption.

CONCLUSIONS

Iron and copper deficiency are known sequels of premature birth. Metabolic balance studies, together with the results of plasma measurements suggest that late copper and zinc deficiency may be more prevalent than has been supposed. Magnesium deficiency may also occur in some infants. The results of iron balances suggest that the control of iron absorption is inadequate in preterm infants, and lead to the conclusion that they are not only at risk of iron deficiency if given too little iron, but may be at risk from iron overload, if given too much.

REFERENCES

1. WACKER, W.E.C. and A.F. PARISI. (1968) New Eng. J. Med. 278:658.
2. AIKAWA, J.K. (1976) In: Trace Elements in Human Health and Disease vol. 2, Prasad, A.S. and D. Oberleas eds., Academic Press, New York, p. 47.
3. WONG, H.B. and Y.F. TEH. (1968) Lancet 2:18.
4. VALLEE, B.L. (1977) In: Biotechnological Applications of Proteins and Enzymes, Bohak, Z. and N. Sharon eds., Academic Press, New York, p. 223.
5. HURLEY, L.S. (1969) Am. J. Clin. Nutr. 22:1332.
6. HAMBIDGE, K.M., K.H. NELDNER and P.A. WALRAVENS. (1975) Lancet 2:577.
7. MOYNAHAN, E.J. (1974) Lancet 2:399.
8. MOYNAHAN, E.J. (1975) Lancet 2:710.
9. WESTON, W.L. (1977) Arch. Dermatol. 113:422.
10. GOLDEN, M.H.N., B. GOLDEN, P.S.E.G. HARLAND and A.A. JACKSON. (1978) Lancet 1:1226.
11. ECKHERT, C.D., M.V. SLOAN, J.R. DUNCAN and L.S. HURLEY. (1977) Science 195:789.
12. EVANS, G.W. and P.E. JOHNSON. (1976) Lancet 2:1310.
13. ARAKAWA, J., T. TAMURA, Y. IGARASHI, H. SUZUKI and H.H. SANDSTEAD. (1976) Acta. Chir. Scand. (Suppl.) 466:167.
14. SIVASUBRAMANIAN, K.N. (1978) Lancet 1:508.
15. SUITA, S., K. KEDA, A. NAGASAKI and Y. HAYASHIDA. (1978) J. Paediatr. Surg. 13:5.
16. HAMBIDGE, K.M., C. HAMBIDGE, M. JACOBS and J.D. BAUM. (1972) Pediatr. Res. 6:868.
17. PRASAD, A.S. (1976) In: Trace Elements in Human Health and Disease, vol. 1, Prasad, A.S. and D. Oberleas eds., Academic Press, New York, p. 1.
18. O'DELL, B.L. (1976) In: Trace Elements in Human Health and Disease, vol. 1, Prasad, A.S. and D. Oberleas eds., Academic Press, New York, p. 391.
19. AL-RASHID, R.A. and J. SPANGLER. (1971) New. Eng. J. Med. 285:841.
20. SEELY, J.R., G.B. HUMPHREY and J.B. MATLER. (1972) New. Eng. J. Med. 286:109.
21. ASHKENAZI, A., S. LEVIN, M. DJALDETTI, E. FISHEL and D. BENVENISTI. (1973) Pediatrics 52:525.
22. KARPEL, J.T. and V.H. PEDEN. (1972) J. Pediatr. 80:32.
23. HELLER, R.M., S.G. KIRCHNER, J.A. O'NEILL, JR., A.J. HOUGH, JR., L. HOWARD, S.S. KRAMER and H.L. GREEN. (1978) J. Pediatr. 92:947.
24. LUBCHENKO, L.O., C. HANSMAN, M. DRESSLER and E. BOYD. (1963) Pediatrics 32:793.
25. KLOOSTERMAN, G.J. (1970) Int. J. Gynaecol. Obstet. 8:895.
26. SHAW, J.C.L. (1973) Ped. Clin. N. Am. 20:333.
27. WIDDOWSON, E.M. and J.W.T. DICKERSON (1961) In: Mineral Metabolism, vol. II, part A, Comar, C.L. and F. Bronner eds., Academic Press, New York, chap. 17, p. 1.
28. KELLEY, H.J., R.E. SLOAN, W. HOFFMAN and C. SAUNDERS. (1950) Human Biology 2:61.
29. DAUNCEY, M.J., J.C.L. SHAW and J. URMAN. (1977) Pediatr. Res. 11:991.
30. DAUNCEY, M.J., C.G. DAVIES, J.C.L. SHAW and J. URMAN. (1978) Pediatr. Res. 12:899.
31. CAVELL, P.A. and E.M. WIDDOWSON. (1964) Arch. Dis. Childh. 39:496.
32. OHTAKE, M. (1977) Tohuku. J. Exp. Med. 123:265.
33. DOYELL, J. and J.F. SULLIVAN. (1970) Metabolism 19.148.
34. ADHAM, N.F., M.K. SONG, and M. RINDERKNECHT. (1977) Biochim. Biophys. Acta 495:212.
35. RYDEN, L. and H.F. DEUTSCH. (1978) J. Biol. Chem. 253:519.
36. WIDDOWSON, E.M., H. CHAN, G.E. HARRISON and R.D.G. MILNER. (1972) Biol. Neonate 20:360.

NITROGEN BALANCES AND PROTEIN
REQUIREMENTS OF PRETERM INFANTS

J. SENTERRE*

INTRODUCTION

Because of their rapid rate of anabolic processes, no patient faces a more critical need for protein than the low birth weight infant in the first weeks of life. However, the optimal intake of protein for these infants is still a matter of discussion.

There is some evidence for assuming that the preterm infant should continue to gain weight in a manner that is quantitatively and qualitatively similar to that occuring in utero. From the results of analyses of fetal bodies, SHAW (1) calculated that the rate of weight gain and of nitrogen retention is respectively about 15 g and 340 mg/kg body weight/day between 28 and 36 weeks of gestation.

In practice, human milk with its low protein content was widely used and is still regarded as the feeding of choice for the preterm infant (2). However, it has been shown that premature infants gain weight more rapidly (3, 4) and retain more nitrogen (5, 6) when fed cow's milk formulas of high protein content. Recently, specially adapted formulas with higher protein content than usual infant formula have been introduced on the market for feeding of low birth weight infants. However, high protein intakes may raise blood urea nitrogen, promote hyperaminoacidemia, and increase renal solute and acid load in the preterm infant (7). Therefore, there is again a tendence toward a moderate protein intake for these infants (2, 7, 8, 9).

In a previous Nutricia symposium, SNYDERMAN (10) discussed the protein requirements of preterm infants from the results of nitrogen balance studies carried out with two extremes of protein intake (2 and 9 g/kg/day). The present study reports our results of metabolic balances performed in preterm infants who received a more usual protein intake; in the range of 2.5 to 5 g/kg body weight/day.

* Maître de Recherche du Fonds National Belge de La Recherche Scientifique, Department of Pediatrics, State University of Liège, Hôpital de Bavière, B-4020 Liège, Belgium.

H.K.A. Visser (ed.), Nutrition and Metabolism of the Fetus and Infant, 195-212. All rights reserved.
Copyright © 1979 Martinus Nijhoff Publishers b.v., The Hague/Boston/London.

SUBJECTS AND FEEDINGS

The present study reports the results of 143 three-day metabolic balances
carried out in 75 healthy male preterm infants with a mean birth weight
of 1860 g (range: 1480–2180 g) and a mean gestational age of 33.4 weeks
(range: 30–36 weeks). These infants were fed pooled human milk (20
balances), human milk supplemented with 0.6% of cow's milk proteins
(9 balances), various adapted formulas (whey/casein: 60/40) with a
protein content ranging from 1.3 to 2.3 g/100 ml (87 balances), an
adapted formula with medium chain triglycerides (50% of fat) and a
protein content of 2 g/100ml (13 balances), and a half skimmed cow's
milk formula providing 2.5 g proteins/100 ml (14 balances). Each infant
was given only a single milk from birth to the end of the study. The
balances were performed between 9 and 28 days of age (mean age: 18
days). Fluid and calorie intakes were about 200 ml and 130 kcal/kg/day.

FECAL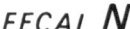

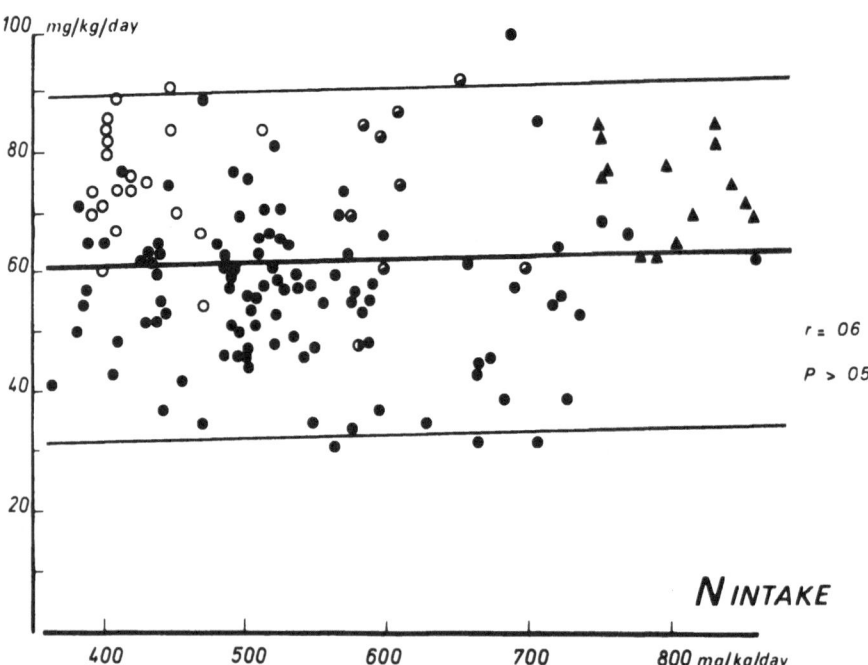

Fig. 1. Relationship between fecal excretion of nitrogen and the nitrogen intake in
preterm infants fed human milk (O), human milk enriched in proteins (◑), various
adapted formulas (●) or half skimmed cow's milk (▲).

The infants were nursed in incubators under temperature conditions complying with Hᴇʏ and Kᴀᴛᴢ's thermal neutrality (11). The metabolic balances were performed with a hammock shaped metabolic bed as previously described (12). Carmin markers were added to the first and after the last feedings. From aliquots of prepared milk, fecal homogenate and urine, total nitrogen was measured in duplicate using the classical method of Kjeldahl. Data concerning fat and mineral balances were published elsewere (13).

FECAL EXCRETION OF NITROGEN AND NET ABSORPTION OF PROTEINS

As shown in figure 1, fecal loss of nitrogen did not increase with nitrogen intake. Consequently, net absorption of proteins (N intake – fecal N/N intake) increased with nitrogen intake (fig. 2). However, fecal excretion

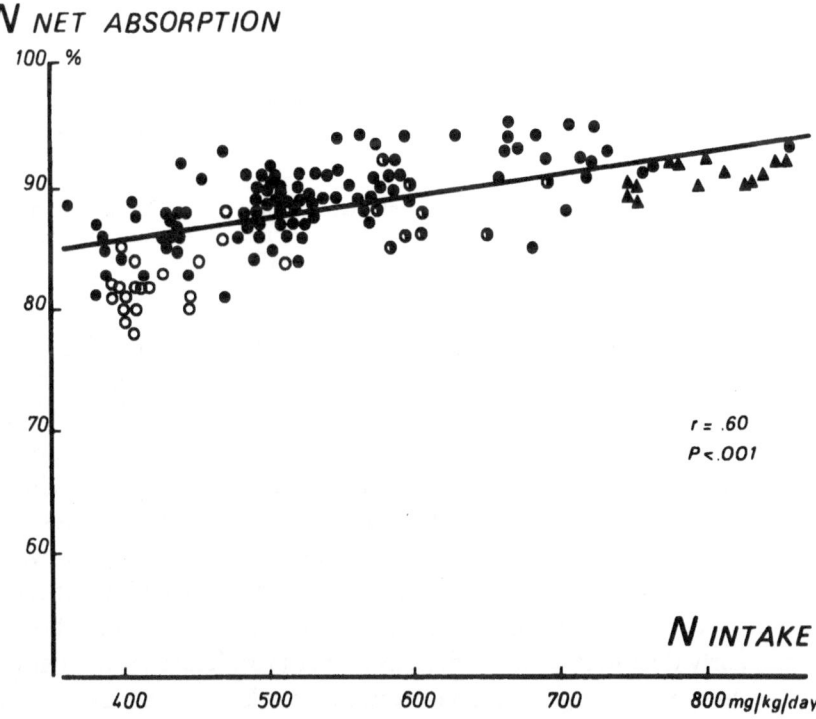

Fig. 2. Relationship between net absorption of proteins (N intake – fecal N/N intake) and the nitrogen intake in preterm infants fed human milk (O), human milk enriched in proteins (◑), various adapted formulas (●) or half skimmed cow's milk (▲).

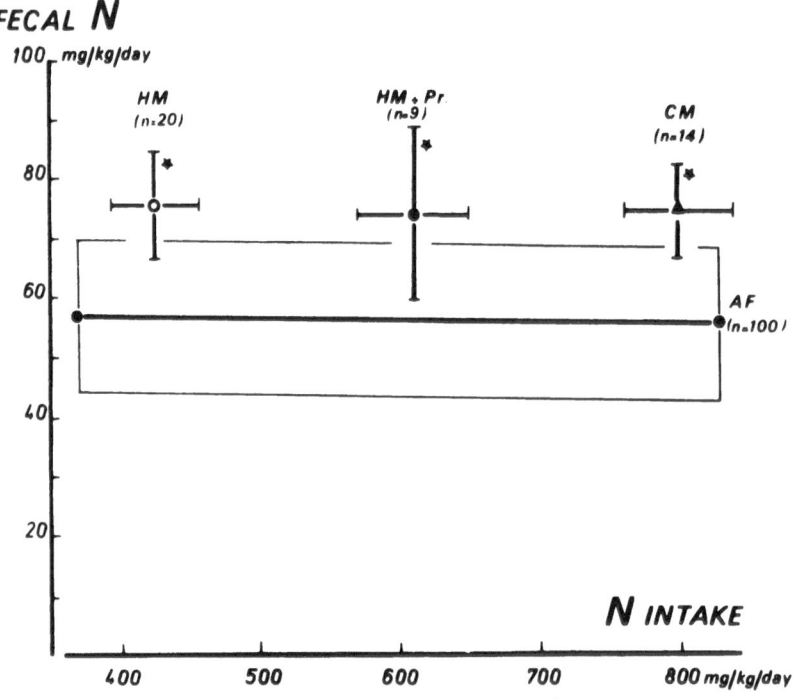

Fig. 3. Fecal excretion of nitrogen in preterm infants fed human milk (HM), human milk enriched in proteins (HM + Pr.) or half skimmed cow's milk (CM) compared to the regression line observed in infants fed adapted formulas (AF).

of nitrogen was significantly higher in the infants fed human milk or half skimmed cow's milk than in those fed adapted formulas (fig. 3). As a result, protein digestibility tended to be lower from human milk and half skimmed cow's milk than from adapted formulas. The lower apparent digestibility of proteins from human milk would seem surprising since about 25% of total nitrogen content is non protein nitrogen mainly constituted of urea, small peptides and free amino acids (14). However, human milk proteins are also caracterized by a relatively high concentration of secretory IgA immunoglobulins (15) which have been shown to be poorly degradated in the digestive tract (16). The slightly higher fecal excretion of nitrogen with half skimmed cow's milk is probably due to the high casein intake. Nevertheless, it is apparent that net absorption of proteins is very satisfactory (82 to 94% according to protein intake) in the preterm infant. True digestibility of proteins from the diet is still higher since fecal nitrogen is partly of endogenous origin (desquamation of mucosal cells, digestive secretions and bacterial debris). As shown by several studies, even prematurely born infants with very low birth weight produce proteolytic enzymes in sufficient quantity (17) to digest protein normally (18, 19). Therefore in practice, there is no indication to feed preterm infants protein hydrolysates or free amino acids which increase tonicity of the diet and are less well absorbed than oligopeptides (20).

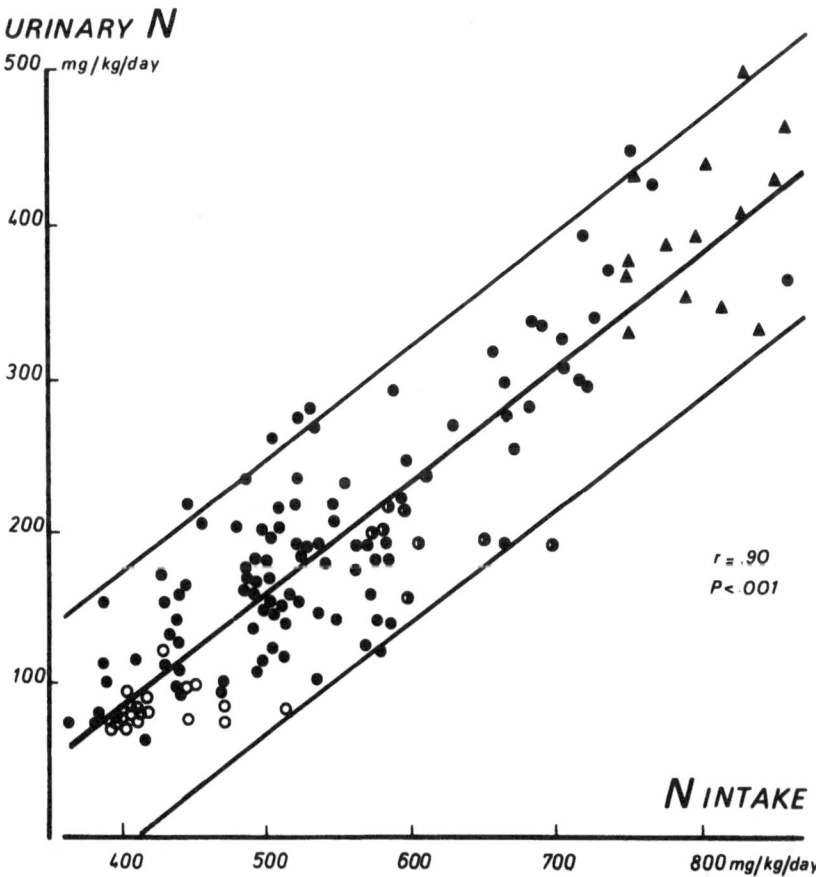

Fig. 4. Relationship between urinary excretion of nitrogen and the nitrogen intake in preterm infants fed human milk (O), human milk enriched in proteins (◑), various adapted formulas (●) or half skimmed cow's milk (▲).

URINARY EXCRETION OF NITROGEN

There was a highly significant positive linear relationship between urinary excretion of total nitrogen and nitrogen intake (fig. 4). Urinary nitrogen excretion was below 100 mg/kg/day in most infants fed 2.5 g of proteins but increased 4-fold when protein intake was doubled. The lowest values are probably close to the urinary obligatory loss of nitrogen which has been estimated to be 1.4 mg/basal calorie/day (21). By contrast, the high values indicate that when protein intake increases in isocaloric regimen, an increasing percentage of proteins are utilized for energy production.

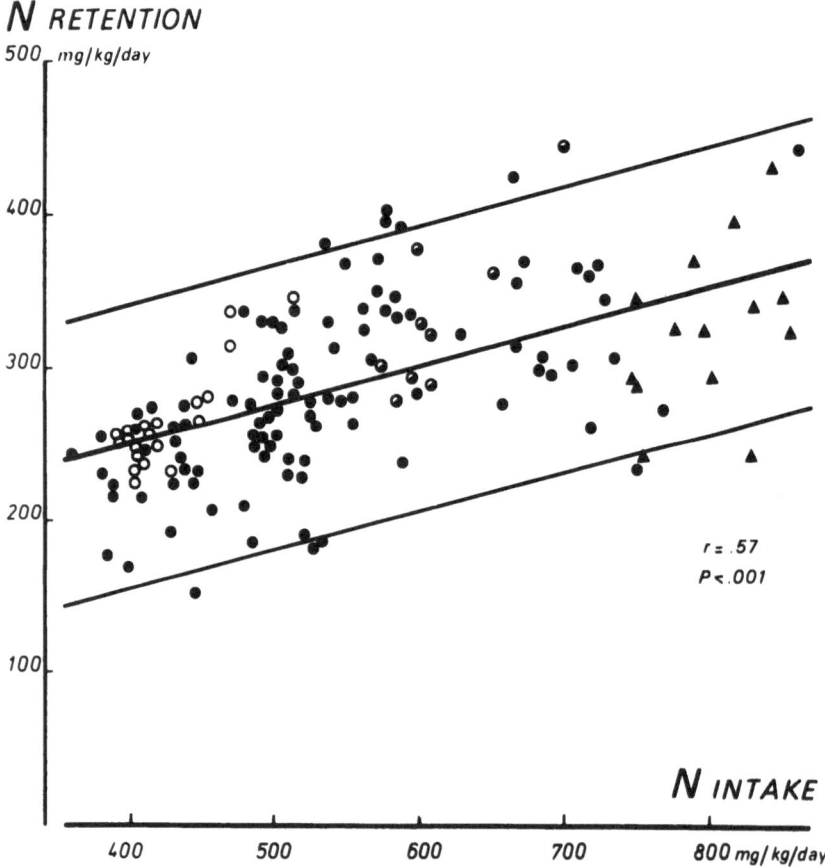

Fig. 5. Relationship between nitrogen retention and the nitrogen intake in preterm infants fed human milk (O), human milk enriched in proteins (◑), various adapted formulas (●) or half skimmed cow's milk (▲).

NITROGEN RETENTION AND NET PROTEIN UTILIZATION

In the studied range of protein intake (2.5 to 5 g/kg/day), there was a positive linear relationship between the amount of retained nitrogen and nitrogen intake (fig. 5). Mean nitrogen retention was about 250 mg/kg/day when nitrogen intake was approximatly 400 mg/kg/day, but only reached 350 mg/kg/day when nitrogen intake was doubled. As a result, net protein utilization (retained nitrogen/nitrogen intake) was inversely related to protein intake (fig. 6). These observations comply with studies performed in young animals. Indeed, when a wide range of protein intake is provided in isocaloric conditions, the response to protein supply is directly related to the logarithm of the intake; if nitrogen intake increases excessively, the improvement in nitrogen retention tends to be very small (22).

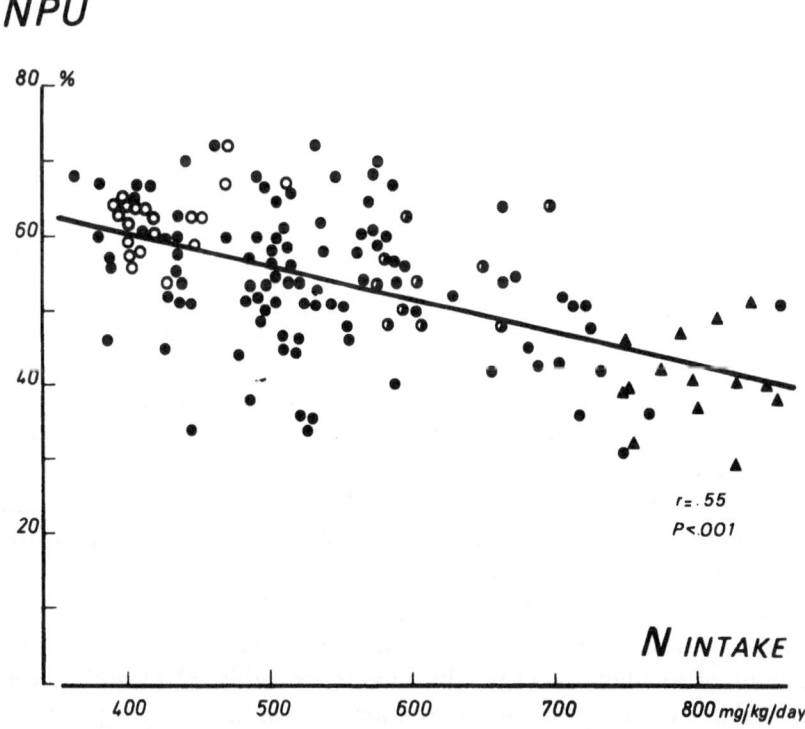

Fig. 6. Relationship between net protein utilization (NPU) and the nitrogen intake in preterm infants fed human milk (O), human milk enriched in proteins (◐), various adapted formulas (●) or half skimmed cow's milk (▲).

For a similar nitrogen intake, net protein utilization tended to be higher in the infants fed human milk (62 ± 4%) than in those fed low protein formula (59 ± 7%), but the difference was not statistically significant (table 1). However calculation of the biological value – an index of retained nitrogen related to absorbed nitrogen – showed a significant difference (76 ± 4 versus 68 ± 8%) in favour of human milk (table 1).

Table 1. *Nitrogen balance parameters (mean ± 1 SD) in preterm infants fed human milk (HM) or an adapted formula (AF) providing a similar nitrogen intake.*

	HM (n = 20)	AF (n = 21)
N intake (mg/kg/day)	424 ± 32	415 ± 26
N feces (mg/kg/day)	76 ± 9	57* ± 10
N urine (mg/kg/day)	84 ± 12	115* ± 34
N retention (mg/kg/day)	264 ± 33	243** ± 30
NPU (%)	62 ± 4	59 ± 7
BV (%)	76 ± 4	68* ± 8

*P < 0.001
**P = 0.038

NITROGEN BALANCE AND AVAILABLE ENERGY

The sensitivity of nitrogen balance to the addition or removal of energy from the diet has been clearly demonstrated in adults (23). In low birth weight infants, several studies indicate that correction of steatorrhea (18, 24) or increase of calorie intake (25, 26) may improve nitrogen retention. In the present study, mean calorie intake was similar in each diet group. However, the amount of available energy varied sometimes considerably according to the degree of fat malabsorption. For instance, mean fecal loss of fat reached 3.2 ± 1 g/kg/day in infants fed adapted formula with a high calcium content, whereas it was only 0.5 ± 0.3 g/kg/day in those fed the formula with medium chain triglycerides. To investigate in what measure nitrogen balances were influenced by such differences in the amount of available energy, the infants fed adapted formulas were divided in two groups according to their protein intake (3.0 ± 0.3 and 4.3 ± 0.3 g of proteins/kg/day). Effective calorie supply was calculated as the difference between calorie intake and fecal loss of fat. As shown in figure 7, there was a positive linear relationship between nitrogen

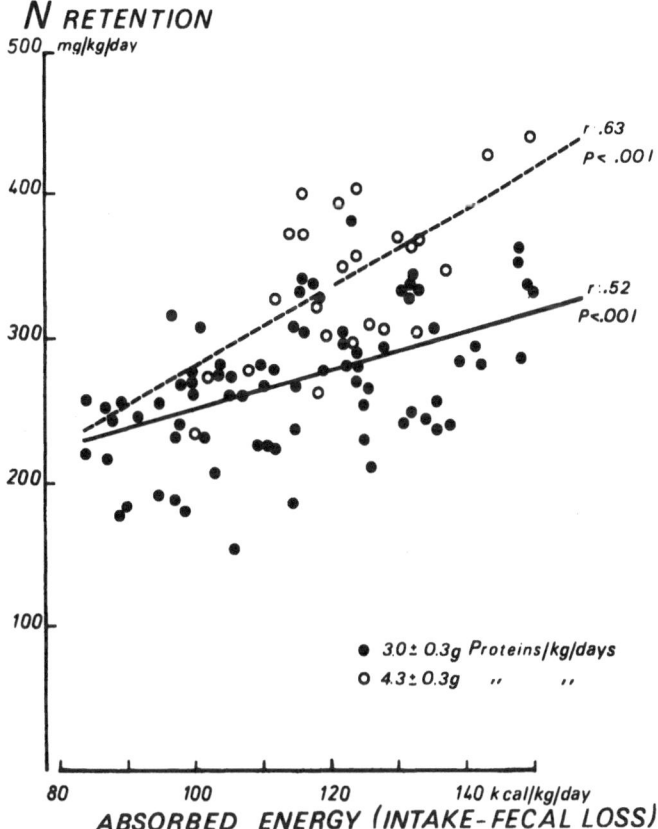

Fig. 7. Relationship between nitrogen retention and the amount of absorbed energy (caloric intake–fecal loss of calories) in preterm infants fed adapted formulas providing 3 ± 0.3 g or 4.3 ± 0.3 g proteins/kilo body weight/ day.

retention and the effective amount of absorbed energy in both groups. However, the slope of the regression line was sharper in the group fed high protein formulas. Below 100 kcal/kg/day, nitrogen retention tended to be low in both groups, when this value was exceeded the improvement in nitrogen retention was more pronounced in the high protein group. That means that, whatever protein intake, low calorie supply limits nitrogen retention whereas, for high calorie supplies, nitrogen retention is conditioned by protein intake.

BLOOD UREA NITROGEN AND SERUM AMINO ACID
CONCENTRATIONS

It is well demonstrated that high protein intake may lead to hazardous
accumulation of nitrogen metabolites in preterm infants because of the
immaturity of several enzymatic pathways and a low glomerular filtration rate (2, 7, 9).

A positive relationship between blood urea nitrogen and protein intake has been reported by numerous investigators (3, 7, 27). Such a
relationship also existed in the present study. However, the coefficient of
correlation was improved and the regression line passed through zero

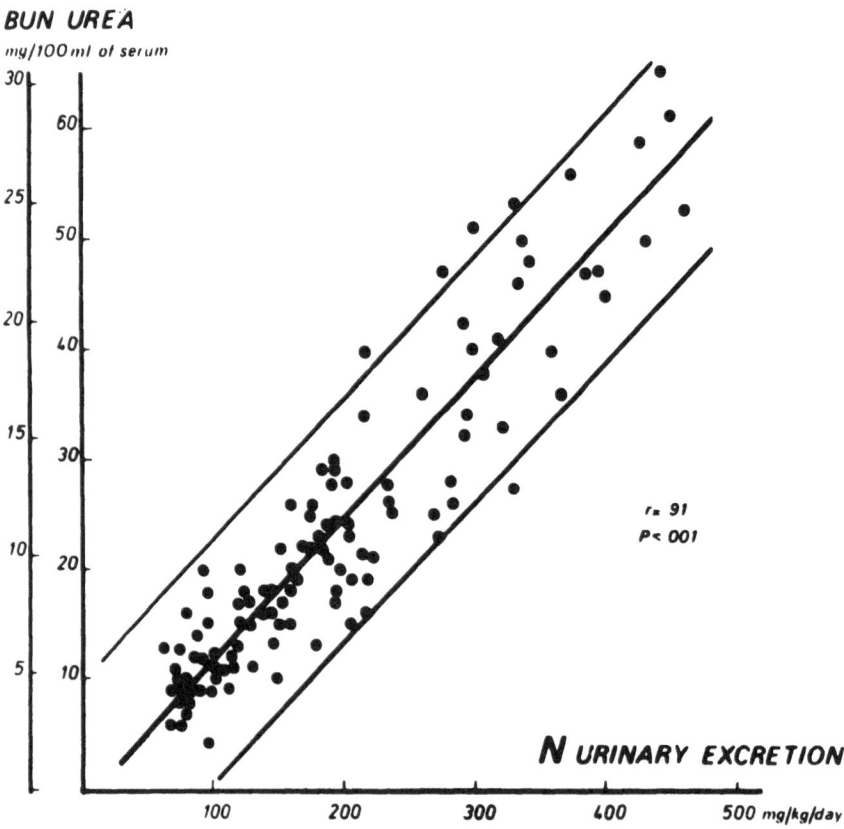

Fig. 8. Relationship between blood urea nitrogen and urinary excretion of total nitrogen
in preterm infants.

when blood urea nitrogen was related to urinary excretion of total nitrogen (fig. 8). Thus blood urea nitrogen is more largly the result of quantity of proteins utilized for energy production than of protein intake itself. Therefore, provided caloric supply is adequate, blood urea nitrogen does not necessarily increase with protein intake.

In preterm infants, high protein intake has been demonstrated to be invariably accompagnied by significant elevations of plasma levels of a number of amino acids (5, 28, 29, 30, 31, 32). Low levels are generally observed in preterm infants fed human milk (28, 29, 30). Therefore, in order to avoid distorsion of the aminoacidogram and possible toxic effects, several authors recommand feeding preterm infants with low protein diets (2, 9, 28, 29). However, the physiological supply of amino acids in these infants is by transplacental exchange. Therefore the concentrations of free amino acids in cord blood might be a more reliable

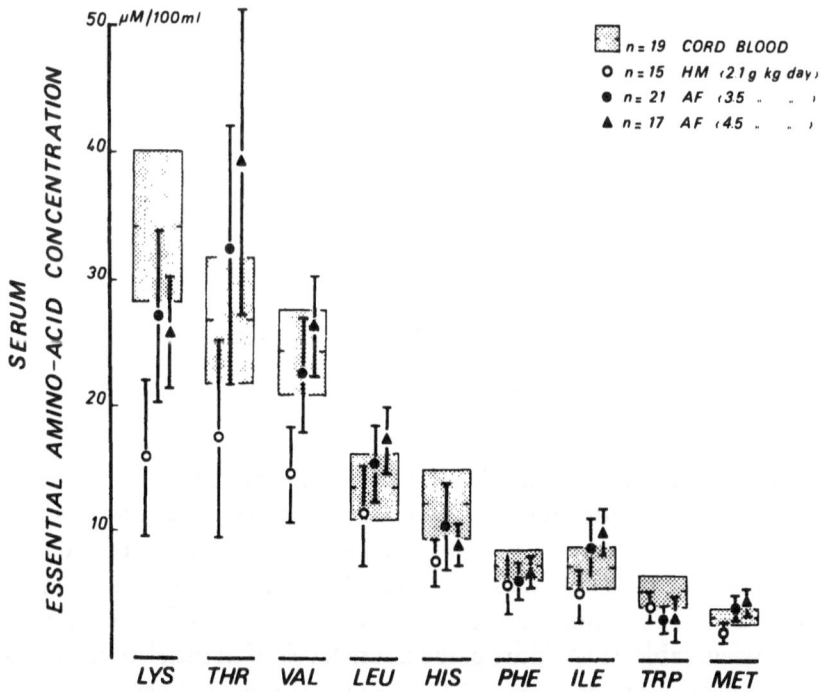

Fig. 9. Serum essential amino acid concentrations (mean ± 1 SD) in preterm infants fed human milk (HM) or adapted formulas (AF) providing either 3.5 g or 4.5 g proteins/kg/day compared to cord blood values determined in term newborn infants.

Table 2. *Serum amino acid concentrations in μ M/l (mean ± 1 SD) in cord blood of term newborn infants and in preterm infants fed human milk (HM) or adapted formulas providing 3.5 g (AF1) or 4.5 g (AF2) proteins/kg/day.*

Amino acids	HM (n = 15)	AF1 (n = 21)	AF2 n = 17)	Cord blood (n = 19)
n	(n = 15)	(n = 21)	n = 17)	(n = 19)
Age (day)	19 ± 9	16 ± 11	17 ± 7	0
Gest. (week)	33 ± 3	33 ± 3	33 ± 2	40 ± 1
TAU	244 ± 80	184 ± 56*	197 ± 39*	247 ± 63
ASP	38 ± 18*	34 ± 12*	42 ± 15*	21 ± 7
HYP	67 ± 13*	63 ± 10*	68 ± 13*	33 ± 6
THR	174 ± 78*	324 ± 97*	395 ± 135*	268 ± 51
SER	194 ± 50	233 ± 46*	219 ± 39*	179 ± 17
ASN	56 ± 21*	86 ± 19*	88 ± 25*	41 ± 6
GLU	171 ± 78	223 ± 70	196 ± 50	186 ± 61
GLN	527 ± 190	588 ± 134	661 ± 141	527 ± 147
PRO	178 ± 49	254 ± 61*	273 ± 51*	177 ± 36
GLY	240 ± 62	378 ± 69*	270 ± 52	269 ± 33
ALA	287 ± 83*	437 ± 91	413 ± 77	438 ± 75
CIT	23 ± 11	34 ± 11	35 ± 11	–
VAL	145 ± 38*	225 ± 45	264 ± 40	243 ± 34
CYS	44 ± 7	47 ± 8	60 ± 14*	45 ± 6
MET	21 ± 9*	41 ± 10*	46 ± 10*	35 ± 7
ILE	50 ± 20*	88 ± 21*	100 ± 18*	72 ± 17
LEU	113 ± 39	154 ± 31*	175 ± 25*	135 ± 25
TYR	102 ± 28*	99 ± 30*	122 ± 30*	63 ± 13
PHE	50 ± 12*	62 ± 15*	68 ± 9	74 ± 12
TRP	42 ± 11*	32 ± 10*	33 ± 18*	55 ± 12
ETH	27 ± 20	–	–	32 ± 21
ORN	145 ± 41*	152 ± 49*	174 ± 33*	104 ± 28
LYS	158 ± 62*	272 ± 69*	258 ± 43*	342 ± 60
HIS	77 ± 18*	105 ± 36	90 ± 15*	122 ± 28
ARG	103 ± 35*	125 ± 38*	114 ± 29*	81 ± 16

*$P < 0.05$ compared to cord blood value

index of optimal levels than those observed in infants fed human milk. In collaboration with RIGO (33), we determined the amino acid concentrations in cord blood in 20 term infants and in 3 groups of preterm infants during their first month of life. These infants were fed human milk or adapted formulas providing either 3.5 or 4.5 g of proteins/kg/day. As shown in table 2 and figure 9, the serum levels of essentiel amino acids in the group of infants fed 3.5 g of proteins corresponded best with cord blood values. In the infants fed human milk, most values were depressed, whereas in the group with a high protein intake they tended to be too high. The most striking difference between cord blood and postnatal values was in the level of lysine. Low lysine concentration even in the high protein group suggests that the lysine requirement of preterm infants is very high; or, that the lysine content of formulas was not entirely available because of the formation of a lysine-carbohydrate complex during heat processing. Another aspect of the amino acid requirement of the preterm infant is the possibility that certain amino acids which are not regarded as essential for more mature infants are required because of enzymatic immaturities. As other authors (2, 34, 35), we have thus far obtained evidence that cystine and taurine are in this category (30, 33).

RENAL SOLUTE AND ACID LOAD

The renal capacities to concentrate urine (36) and to excrete hydrogen ion (37) are known to be limited in preterm infants during the first postnatal weeks.

High renal solute load originates chiefly from high protein intake which is generally accompagnied by an increased mineral intake. In our study, urine concentration and renal solute load were almost twice as high in the infants fed high protein formulas as compared to those fed human milk or low protein formulas (table 3). However, even if we take into account that renal concentrating ability may be impaired in preterm infants, it is apparent that urine output was greatly in excess of obligatory water loss in all groups. Therefore, the greater margin of safety provided by low protein feedings is of little significance under usual circumstances.

Table 3. *Renal solute load (mean $\pm$ 1 SD) in preterm infants fed human milk (HM) or adapted formulas (AF) with various protein content.*

	HM (n = 20)	AF1 (n = 21)	AF2 (n = 38)	AF3 (n = 11)
N intake (mg/kg/day)	424 ± 32	415 ± 26	528 ± 38	716 ± 68
Urine output (ml/kg/day)	144 ± 11	145 ± 10	140 ± 7	135 ± 13
Urine osmolatity (mosmol/1)	103 ± 18	106 ± 24	149 ± 19	193 ± 28
Renal solute load (mosmol/kg/day)	15 ± 3	15 ± 4	21 ± 3	26 ± 4

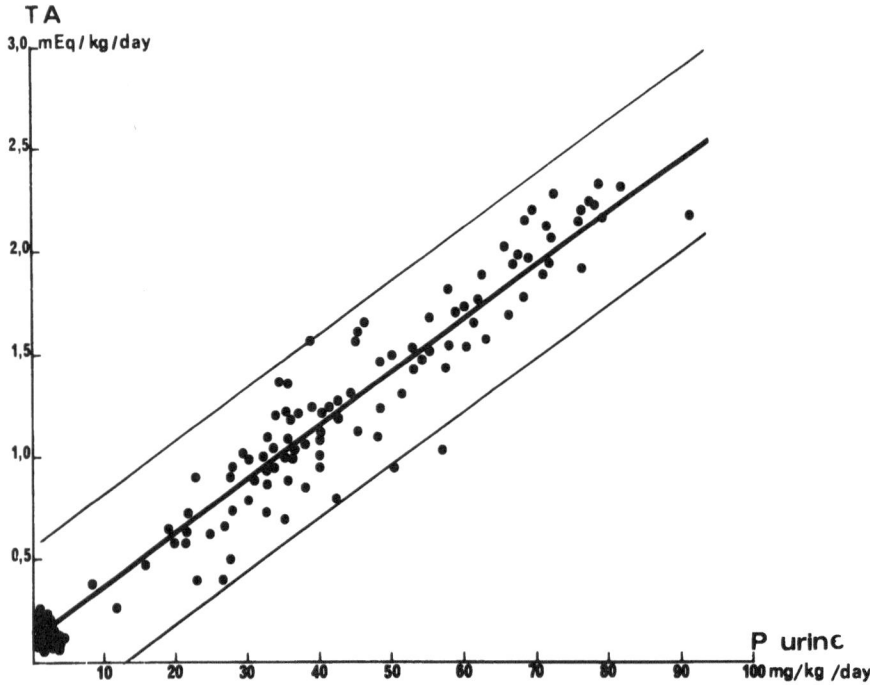

Fig. 10. Relationship between titratable acidity (TA) and urinary excretion of phosphorus in preterm infants.

The limited renal capacities to excrete hydrogen ion are more crucial. Indeed, despite a 4-fold increase of net renal acid excretion (NAE) (table 4), some preterm infants fed high protein formula presented a certain degree of metabolic acidosis (table 5). By comparing NAE values in infants fed human milk and in those fed low protein formula, it appears

Table 4. *Renal nitrogen, phosphorus and net acid excretions (mean ± 1 SD) in preterm infants fed human milk (HM) or adapted formulas providing 2.6 g (AF1), 3.3 g (AF2) or 4.5 g (AF3) proteins/kilo/day.*

	HM (n 20)	AF1 (n = 21)	AF2 (n = 38)	AF3 (n = 11)
N (mg/kg/day)	84 ± 12	115 ± 34	192 ± 41	338 ± 66
P (mg/kg/day)	1 ± 1	27 ± 9	39 ± 7	50 ± 9
TA (mEq/kg/day)	0.2 ± .1	0.8 ± .2	1.1 ± .2	1.4 ± .3
NH_4^+ (mEq/kg/day)	0.6 ± .2	1.1 ± .2	1.4 ± .3	1.6 ± .4
NAE (mEq/kg/day)	0.8 ± .3	1.9 ± .4	2.5 ± .5	3.0 ± .6

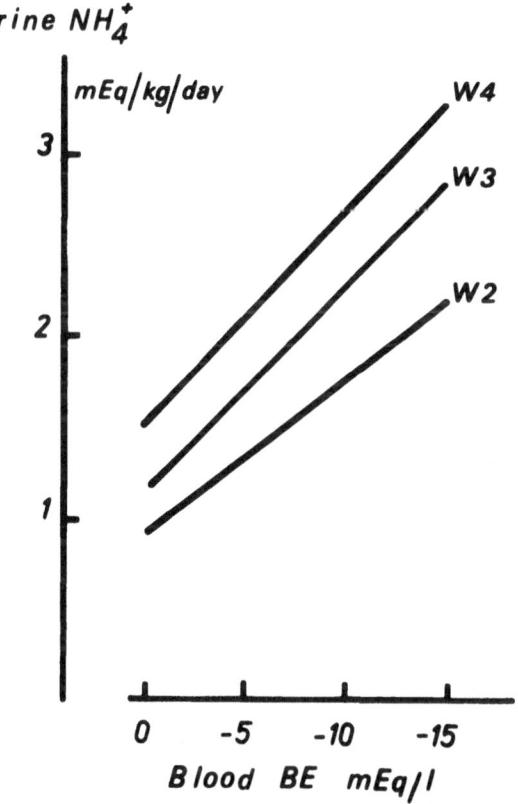

Fig. 11. Relationship between urinary excretion of ammonia and the blood base excess values in preterm infants during the 2nd, 3rd or 4th week of postnatal age.

that protein intake is not the single factor in acid load. Indeed, although nitrogen intake was similar, NAE was twice as high in infants fed low protein formula than in those fed human milk (table 4). As previously reported (13, 38, 39), differences in phosphorus load may explain that discrepancy. Indeed, in preterm infants fed human milk, phosphorus

Table 5. *Blood acid base status (mean ± 1 SD) of preterm infants fed human milk (HM) or adapted formulas (AF) with various protein content.*

	HM (n = 20)	AF1 (n = 21)	AF2 (n = 38)	AF3 (n = 11)
N intake (mg/kg/day)	424 ± 32	415 ± 26	528 ± 38	716 ± 68
pH	7.38 ± .03	7.37 ± .04	7.36 ± .06	7.35 ± .05
PCO_2 (mmHg)	43 ± 6	41 ± 7	40 ± 8	38 ± 7
BE (mEq/l)	+0.1 ± 1.6	−1.3 ± 2.3	−2.7 ± 3.8	−3.9 ± 3.1

intake is insufficient to fulfill both cellular growth and bone minerali-
zation requirements. As a result, urinary excretion of phosphorus is
practically zero wheras calciuria is high (13). On the contrary, phosphorus content of adapted formulas is generally two or three times higher
than in human milk, and the amount of absorbed phosphorus is higher
than the phosphorus retention (13). Consequently, urinary excretion of
phosphorus no longer becomes negligeable (table 4). As shown in figure
10, there was a positive linear relationship between titratable acidity
and renal excretion of phosphorus. Acidification of urine is thus satisfactory in preterm infants. Bij contrast, production of ammonia was
limited during the first postnatal weeks (fig. 11). Therefore, the buf-
fering of increased phosphorus load in addition to sulfate from protein
catabolism may lead to metabolic acidosis.

CONCLUSION

Although short metabolic balances cannot be regarded as a very precise
tools, data presented herein may lead us to several conclusions.

Protein digestibility is quite satisfactory in the preterm infants. Fecal
excretion of nitrogen does not change with nitrogen intake. Consequently, net absorption increases with protein intake. The slightly higher
fecal excretion of nitrogen observed in infants fed human milk is very
likely related to its poorly degradated secretory IgA immunoglobulins.

Nitrogen retention increases from about 250 mg/kg/day for 2.5 g
protein to 350 mg/kg/day for 5 g protein intake/kg/day. However, for a
given nitrogen intake, nitrogen retention and net protein utilization
appear to be greatly influenced by the amount of energy which is effectively available for growth.

In regard to nitrogen accumulation in utero and free amino acid
concentration in cord blood, there is some indications that 3.5 to 4 g
proteins/kg/day is the optimum intake for orally fed preterm infants.
Provided caloric supply and mineral intake are adequate, such a protein
intake will keep solute and acid loads below the renal capacities of
excretion.

Independant of the protein requirement there are, of course, immunological reasons for feeding preterm infants with breast milk, such as the
presence of defense factors or the risk of allergy to cow's milk. However,
to improve nitrogen retention and to avoid hypercalciuria, human milk
should be supplemented with proteins, preferably whey hydrolysate, and

with phosphorus. When human milk is not available, specially adapted formulas providing about 2.8 g protein/100 kcal, easily absorbed fats, and a low phosphorus load might be the best substitute.

REFERENCES

1. SHAW, J.C.L. (1973) Ped. Clin. N. Amer. 20:333.
2. GAULL, G.E. (1978) Acta Paediatr. Belg. 31:3.
3. DAVIDSON, M., S.Z. LEVINE, C.H. BAUER and M. DANN. (1961) J. Pediatr. 59:951.
4. DAVIES, D.P. (1977) Arch. Dis. Childh. 52:296.
5. GORDON, H.H., S.Z. LEVINE and H. McNAMARA. (1947) Am. J. Dis. Child. 73:442.
6. SNYDERMAN, S.E., A. BOYER, M.D. KOGUT and L.E. HOLT. (1969) J. Pediatr. 74:872.
7. RÄIHÄ, N.C.R., K. HEINONEN, D.K. RASSIN and G.E. GAULL. (1976) Pediatrics 57:659.
8. FOMON, S., E ZIEGLER and H. VAZQUEZ. (1977) Am. J. Dis. Child. 131:463.
9. Committee on Nutrition. (1977) Pediatrics 60:519.
10. SNYDERMAN, S.E. (1971) In: Metabolic Processes in the Fetus and Newborn Infant, Jonxis, J.H.P., H.K.A Visser and J.A. Troelstra eds., Stenfert Kroese, Leiden, Holland, p. 128.
11. HEY, E.N. and G.KATZ. (1970) Arch. Dis. Childh. 45:328.
12. SENTERRE, J., F. SODOYEZ-GOFFAUX and A. LAMBRECHTS. (1971) Acta Paediatr. Belg. 25:133.
13. SENTERRE, J. (1978) In: Intensive Care in the Newborn II, Stern, L. ed., Masson, U.S.A., p. 205.
14. HAMBRAEUS, L., B. LÖNNERDAL, E. FORSUM and M. GEBRE-MEHDIN. (1978) Acta Paediatr. Scand. 67:561.
15. Mc CLELLAND, D.B.L., J. Mc GRATH and R.R. SAMSON. (1978) Acta Paediatr. Scand. suppl. 271:1.
16. OGRA, S.S., D. WEINTRAUB and P.L. OGRA. (1977) J. Immunol. 119:245.
17. BORGSTRÖM, B., B. LINDQUIST and H.G. LUND. (1960) Am. J. Dis. Child. 99:338.
18. ROY, C.C., M. STE-MARIE, L. CHARTRAND, A. WEBER, H. BARD and B. DORAY (1975) J. Pediatr. 86:446.
19. WILLIAMSON, S., E. FINUCANE, H. ELLIS and H.R. GAMSU. (1978) Arch. Dis. Childh. 53:555.
20. ABIDI, S.A. (1976) Am. J. Clin. Nutr. 29:205.
21. HEGSTED, D.M. (1973) In: Therapeutic Aspects of Nutrition, Jonxis, J.H.P., H.K.A. Visser and J.A. Troelstra eds., Stenfert Kroese, Leiden, Holland, p. 65.
22. HEGSTED, D.M. (1964) In: Mammalian Protein Metabolism, Munro, H.N. and J.B. Allison eds., Academic Press, New York, Vol. 2, p. 135.
23. GARZA, G., N.S. SCRIMSHAW and V.R. YOUNG. (1976) Am. J. Clin. Nutr. 29:280.
24. TANTIBHEDHYANGKUL, P. and S.A. HASHIM. (1975) Pediatrics 55:359.
25. SATO, T. (1965) Acta Paediatr. Jap. 7:36.
26. VALMAN, H.B., R. AIKENS, Z. DAVID-REED and J.S. GARROW. (1974) Brit. Med. J. 3:319.
27. OMANS, W.B., L.A. BARNESS, C.S. ROSE and P. GYÖRGY. (1961) J. Pediatr. 59:951.
28. GAULL, B.E., D.K. RASSIN, N.C. RÄIHÄ and K. HEINONEN. (1977) J. Pediatr. 90:348.

29. RASSIN, D.K., G.E. GAULL, N.C. RÄIHÄ and K. HEINONEN. (1977) J. Pediatr. 90:356.
30. RIGO, J. and J. SENTERRE. (1977) Biol. Neonate 32:73.
31. FILER, L.J., L.D. STEGINK and B. CHANDRAMOULI. (1977) Am. J. Clin. Nutr. 30:1036.
32. ANDERSON, G.H., H. BRYAN, K.N. JEEJEEBHOY and P. CORES. (1977) Am. J. Clin. Nutr. 30:1110.
33. RIGO J. and J. SENTERRE. (1979) Manuscript in preparation.
34. STURMAN, J.A., G.E. GAULL and N.C. RÄIHÄ. (1970) Science 169:74.
35. STURMAN, J.A., D.K. RASSIN and G.E. GAULL. (1977) Pediatr. Res. 11:28.
36. EDELMAN, C.M. and A. SPITZER. (1969) J. Pediatr. 75:509.
37. SVENNINGSEN, N.W. and B. LINDQUIST. (1974) Acta Paediatr. Scand. 63:721.
38. SENTERRE, J. and A. LAMBRECHTS. (1972) Biol. Neonate 20:107.
39. SENTERRE, J. and F. BONNET. (1971) Proc. 2nd Europ. Congr. Perinatal Medecine, London, 1970, Karger, Basel, p. 264.

TAURINE IN INFANT NUTRITION

GERALD E. GAULL* and DAVID K. RASSIN**

Taurine (fig. 1) is one of the most abundant amino acids in the body (1), with the largest pool present in muscle. In mammals, taurine and inorganic sulfate are the major end products of methionine metabolism (fig. 2). Despite the fact that taurine is both ubiquitous and abundant, it takes part in few known biochemical reactions. Considerable taurine is conjugated with bile acids in liver (1), but other biochemical reactions take place to a very limited extent, if at all (2). Although there are numerous proposals for alternative pathways for the biosynthesis of taurine (cf. 2), the enzyme immediately responsible for its synthesis in physiologically significant amounts is cysteinesulfinic acid decarboxylase. There are large differences amongst species in the in vitro activity of this enzyme, as there are in the concentration of taurine itself (1). For example, the activity of cysteinesulfinic acid decarboxylase, as measured

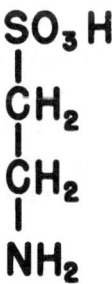

$$SO_3H$$
$$|$$
$$CH_2$$
$$|$$
$$CH_2$$
$$|$$
$$NH_2$$

Fig. 1. Structure of taurine.

*Department of Human Development and Nutrition, New York State Institute for Basic Research in Mental Retardation, Staten Island, N.Y. 10314. Departments of Pediatrics and Pharmacology, Mount Sinai School of Medicine of the City University of New York, N.Y., U.S.A.
** Department of Human Development and Nutrition, New York State Institute for Basic Research in Mental Retardation, Staten Island, N.Y. 10314. Department of Pharmacology, Mount Sinai School of Medicine of the City University of New York, N.Y., U.S.A.

H.K.A. Visser (ed.), Nutrition and Metabolism of the Fetus and Infant, 213-224. All rights reserved.
Copyright © 1979 Martinus Nijhoff Publishers b.v., The Hague/Boston/London.

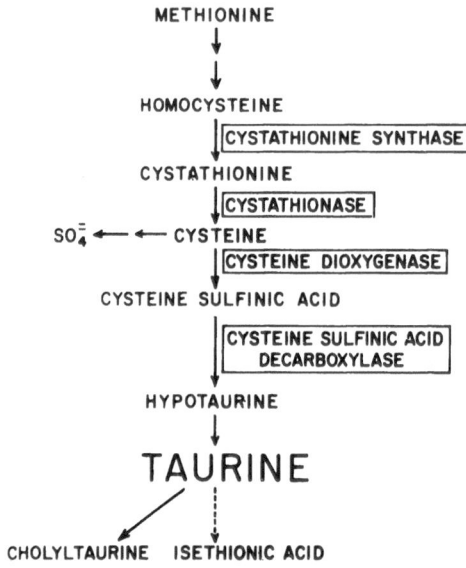

Fig. 2. Pathway of metabolism of methionine.

in our laboratory, is 1000-fold higher in adult rat liver than in adult human liver (table 1).

Interest in taurine has increased in the last decade as a result of accumulating evidence that it is involved in central nervous system function (3). A number of studies of the biochemistry, electrophysiology, and subcellular distribution of taurine have led to the belief that it is an inhibitory neurotransmitter in brain and retina. It has been shown to be transported axonally in the goldfish visual system (4, 5).

In the brain of most species at birth, taurine is the ninhydrin-positive compound present in the greatest concentration (table 2). Even in ma-

Table 1. *Hepatic cysteinesulfinic acid decarboxylase activity*

	Adult	Fetus
Man	0.32 ± 0.08 (4)	0.26 ± 0.04 (7)
Rhesus Monkey	4.97 ± 1.07 (6)	3,54 ± 0.08 (4)
Cat	4.46 ± 0.23 (6)	N.M.
Rat	468 ± 20 (5)	N.M.

Data are mean ± SEM for enzymatic activity in units of nmol/mg protein/h.
N.M. = not measured. Number of determinations are in parentheses (cf. 6).

Table 2. *Taurine concentration in brain*

Species	Neonate	Adult
Mouse	15.3	8.6
Rat	16.5	4.3
Gerbil	21.2	6.5
Guinea Pig	2.0	1.0
Rabbit	5.1	1.2
Dog	6.8	1.3
Cat	9.2	2.3
Chicken	8.9	2.3
Monkey[1]	6.9	2.0
Man[1]	3.3	1.4

Data are in μmol of taurine per gram of wet weight of whole brain.
[1] Occipital Cortex.
(Adapted from references 7, 8).

ture brain it is exceeded in concentration by glutamic acid only (1, 7, 8). In man, taurine is the free amino acid present in highest concentration during the second trimester of pregnancy (9). During this period of gestation the taurine concentration of brain is decreasing, and this decrease correlates with the increasing crown-rump length of the fetus (fig. 3). The third trimester of human gestation is unavailable for systematic study. We turned to the monkey, therefore, because sulfur metabolism in the monkey is close to that of man in many ways (10–14). The concentration of taurine in occipital lobe of rhesus monkey brain also is much higher in all fetuses studied than it is in adults (fig. 4) (9). There is no correlation between the brain taurine concentration and the gestational age of the monkeys; however, later stages of gestation in the monkey were examined than were for man. The concentration of taurine in occipital lobe decreases steadily after birth, reaching concentrations found in the occipital lobe of adult monkeys at about 7 to 9 months after birth. The concentration of taurine in fetal monkey liver is higher in every case than it is in mature monkey liver (fig. 5). The same is true in human liver. There is no significant correlation between concentration of taurine in fetal monkey liver and gestational age. After birth, however, the taurine concentration in liver decreases rapidly. Concentrations of taurine similar to those found in adult monkey liver are reached by 1–2 weeks of age (9).

When the taurine concentrations of monkey brain as well as those of

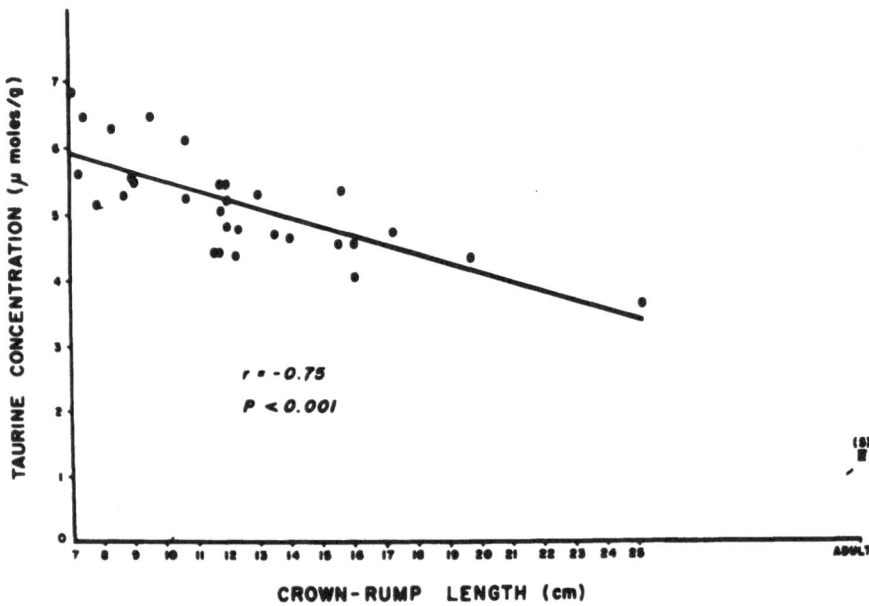

Fig. 3. Taurine concentration in human fetal occipital lobe as a function of crown-rump length. (Reference 9.)

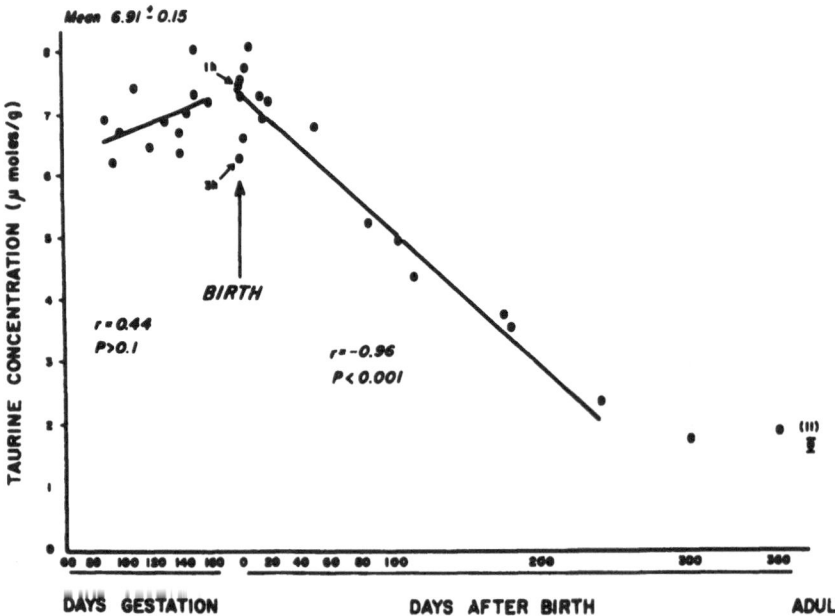

Fig. 4. Taurine concentration in rhesus monkey occipital lobe as a function of age. (Reference 9.)

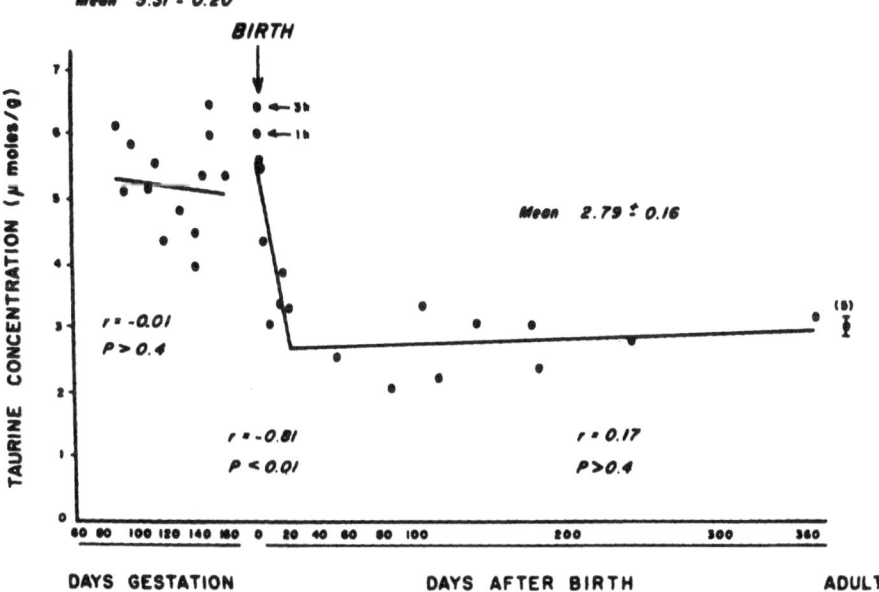

Fig. 5. Taurine concentration in rhesus monkey liver as a function of age. (Reference 9.)

neonatal rats and of neonatal rabbits are plotted as a function of weaning time (fig. 6), they decrease in a linear fashion to reach concentrations at the time of weaning equal to those found in the adult (9). The high concentration in fetal and newborn brain and its slow decrease post-natally suggest that taurine may have a role in brain development, per se, in addition to any functional role it may have in mature brain.

The origin of the very high concentration of taurine in developing brain is uncertain. The activity of cysteinesulfinic acid decarboxylase is low early in the development of rat brain (15), and it is increasing at a time when the concentration of taurine in brain is decreasing. Therefore, biosynthesis of taurine seems unlikely to account for the large concentrations found in newborn brain.

Efficient and highly selective transport systems for attaining and maintaining high intracellular concentrations of taurine in brain during development have been suggested, and such a mechanism might account for the large concentrations in newborn brain (cf. 3 and 9).

Another source for the high concentration of taurine in brain is the diet. We have reported recently that the concentration of taurine in plasma and urine of human preterm infants fed synthetic formulas de-

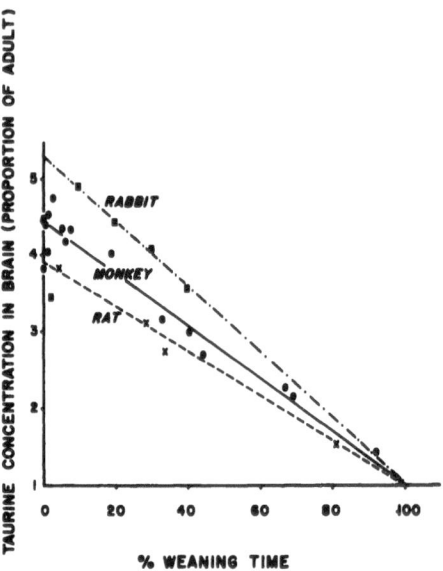

Fig. 6. Taurine concentration in brain of neonatal monkey (●), rabbits (■), and rats (×) as a proportion of the concentration in brain of the relevant adult as a function of the weaning time of each species. (Reference 9.)

rived from bovine milk decreased progressively throughout the study (fig. 7A and B) (6). Preterm human infants fed pooled human milk, in contrast, did not have such decreases. Human milk, unlike bovine milk and artificial formulas derived from it, contains a considerable amount of taurine (6). Taurine was unique among the free amino acids in this respect: most of the other amino acids were present in larger concentrations in plasma and urine of infants fed the commercial formulas than they were in plasma and urine of infants fed pooled human milk (6, 16, 17). The small concentrations of taurine in plasma of human preterm infants fed artificial formulas has been documented by others, but not commented on (18). A greater excretion of taurine by full-term human infants fed human milk than by those fed bovine milk also has been documented but not commented on (19, 20, 21).

Taurine is a major constituent of the free amino acid pool of milk from most species (table 3): In rhesus monkey, dog, cat and gerbil milk, taurine is the free amino acid present in the greatest concentration; in chimp, baboon and java monkey milk, taurine is exceeded in concentration by glutamate only; in sheep milk taurine is exceeded by glycine only

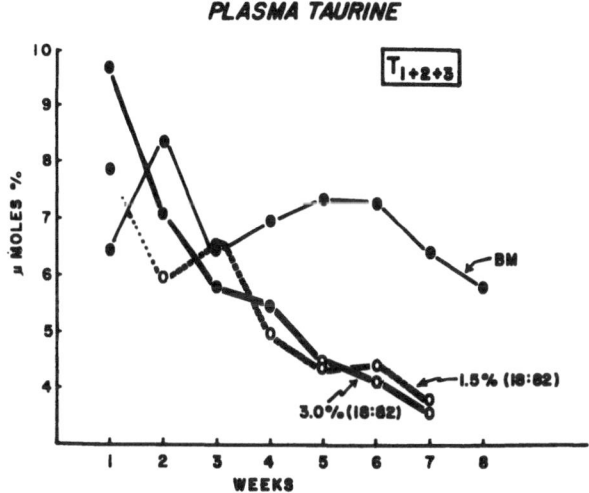

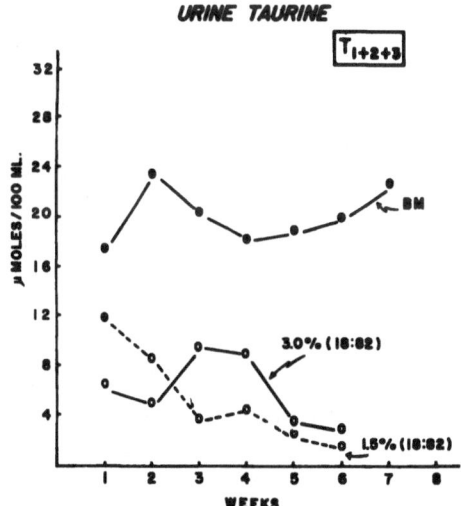

Fig. 7A+B. Effect of low taurine diet on mean plasma and mean urine concentration of taurine in preterm infants as a function of age. BM = pooled, banked human milk; 1.5% (18:82) = 1.5 g % protein made up of 18 parts bovine whey proteins and 82 parts bovine casein proteins; 3.0% (18:82) 3.0 g % protein preparation of the same formula. (Adapted from reference 6.)

Table 3. *Taurine content of milk from various species*

Species	More than 5 days after birth	Less than 5 days after birth
Gerbil	595	
Cat	287	
Beagle Dog	191	264
Mouse (C57 B1/6J)	75	
Rhesus Monkey	56	61
Baboon	38	
Man	34	41
Chimpanzee	26	71
Guinea-pig	17	
Rat	15	63
Java Monkey	14	
Rabbit	14	
Sheep	14	68
Horse	3	
Cow	1	31

Data are in μmol of taurine per 100 ml of milk. Samples were not available for all species before 5 days after birth. (Adapted from reference 22).

and in rat milk by ethanolamine only (22). The concentration of taurine in milk of man, chimp, rhesus monkey, dog, cow, sheep and rat is highest in the first few days of lactation (table 3).

The finding of a dietary requirement for taurine in the human infant is consistent with the negligible activity of cysteinesulfinic acid decarboxylase present both in fetal and in mature human liver (table 1). In order to study the transfer of taurine from mother to infant via the milk, we turned to the lactating rat. This model would provide only a minimal estimate because of the very high activity of cysteinesulfinic acid decarboxylase present in rat liver (table 1). Radioactive taurine injected intraperitoneally into lactating rats a few hours after birth is secreted in the milk and this taurine is transferred to the rat pups (fig. 8) (23). Approximately 4 μmoles of taurine is transferred via the milk to the brain of each pup in the first 5 days after birth and is still there 10 days later, providing a further illustration of the slow turnover of taurine in perinatal rat brain (23). Thus, even in the developing rat, which has a greater enzymatic capacity for taurine synthesis than most other species, dietary taurine is a significant source of tissue taurine, especially for brain.

It seems likely, therefore, that there is a dietary requirement for taurine in the rapidly growing human infant. To date, no adverse clini-

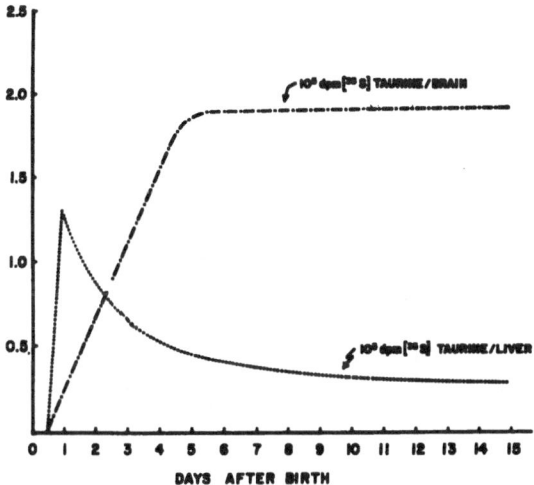

Fig. 8. Amount of [³⁵S] taurine observed in brain and liver of rat pups received via the milk of the lactating maternal rat. (Reference 23.)

cal signs attributable to taurine deficiency have been identified in human infants fed commercial formulas, although no systematic investigation has yet been made. However, cats and kittens fed a synthetic diet containing patially-purified casein as the source of protein become taurine-deficient and develop retinal degeneration. This degeneration, which eventually results in blindness, can be prevented or reversed by feeding taurine, but not by feeding methionine, cysteine, or inorganic sulfate (24, 25). Retina is especially dependent on taurine and actively resists taurine depletion. Thus, when the taurine concentration in most organs has decreased 10-fold, that in retina has decreased less than 50%; retinal degeneration appears to begin when the taurine concentration has been reduced by more than 50%. In addition, the retina of taurine-deficient kittens takes up labelled taurine more avidly than retina from control kittens (fig. 9) (26). Taken together these findings suggest that taurine has a role in the structural integrity of the retina, especially in the photoreceptor cells, in addition to its role as a neurotransmitter or neuro-modulator. It is likely also that the retina would be even more susceptible to a deficiency of taurine during early development (prior to weaning) rather than at maturity when the large pool of taurine has already been attained.

It is likely that the effects of feeding a taurine-deficient diet to the

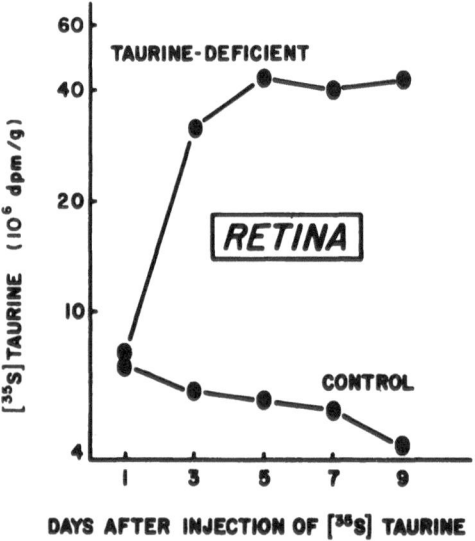

Fig. 9. [³⁵S] Taurine in retina of taurine-deficient and control kittens after the intravenous injection of 2 mCi [³⁵S] taurine. (Reference 26.)

human infant may be considerably more moderate than those observed in the kitten, for a number of reasons: The human infant conjugates bile acids solely with taurine at birth, but later develops the ability to conjugate with glycine (27–30). BRUETON et al. (31) have demonstrated that infants fed human milk remain predominantly taurine conjugators of bile acids, whereas those fed taurine-deficient formulas become predominantly glycine conjugators of bile acids. The cat conjugates bile acids with taurine only (32). It seems possible that the ability alternatively to conjugate bile acids with glycine serves to spare taurine in man. Even those human infants fed the currently available synthetic formulas usually have taurine-containing foods added to the diet within a few weeks or months of birth. The concentrations of taurine in retina of most species, although high, are not as great as in retina of the cat, and this may render it especially vulnerable. However, we should not ignore the possibility that some organs in the human infant may be adversely affected by taurine deficiency even when these organs are unaffected in the kitten. For example, taurine has been demonstrated to be involved in cardiac function in a number of species (33), and a deficiency of taurine in heart might be expected to produce abnormality of function in some individuals. In the taurine-deficient kitten, the concentration of taurine in heart is 10-fold less than in heart of control kittens. The possibility that a deficiency of taurine may be involved in the etiology of some forms of the sudden infant death syndrome, perhaps by causing cardiac arrhythmia or failure of some autonomic transmitter function, should be investigated. Finally, it should be said that the findings of BRUETON et al. (31), i.e. that the formula-fed infant tends to become a predominantly glycine conjugator rather than a predominantly taurine conjugator of bile acids, suggests that the deficiency of taurine may not be in the best interests of the infant. This is because taurine conjugated bile acids are more efficient bile acids than those conjugated with glycine (cf. 34). Furthermore, the recent work of NERVI and DIETSCHY (35) clearly establishes the importance of bile acid conjugates, specifically taurocholate pool size, in the control of hepatic cholesterol synthesis and, therefore, of total body cholesterol pool size. This whole area clearly demands thorough and systematic investigation.

It is of interest to note also that the cholesterol concentration of human milk is considerably higher than that of infant formulas curently produced. Cholesterol is a precursor in the synthesis of the bile acids which are conjugated with taurine. In collaboration with Dr. Niels Räihä in Helsinki, we have started a systematic study of the metabolic effects of taurine and cholesterol supplementation of infant formulas. It is possible that the lower absorption of lipids by infants fed some formulas is a result, at least in part, of the failure of these formulas to provide enough of these two precursors of bile acids, which are important in the absorption of fats. One cannot help but wonder also whether or not the supplementation of formulas with taurine would improve the absorption of fat soluble vitamins, such as vitamin E, and of calcium, since there then could be less soap formation between the fatty acids and the calcium.

In conclusion, there is considerable biochemical evidence for the importance of taurine during early postnatal development. Dramatic pathological findings have not been associated with a lack of taurine in the human infant but possible detrimental effects of a deficiency of taurine may emerge as more sophisticated analytical techniques are applied. In particular, studies of the interrelationships between taurine, bile salts, and cholesterol may help in understanding the function and nutritional importance of taurine in man.

REFERENCES

1. Jacobsen, J.G. and L.H. Smith, Jr. (1968) Physiol. Rev. 48:424.
2. Huxtable, R. and A. Barbeau (eds.). (1976) Taurine, Raven Press, New York.
3. Barbeau, A. and R. Huxtable (eds.). (1978) Taurine and Neurological Disorders, Raven Press, New York.
4. Ingoglia, N.A., J.A. Sturman, T.D. Lindquist and G.E. Gaull. (1976) Brain Res. 115:535.
5. Ingoglia, N.A., J.A. Sturman, D.K. Rassin and T.D. Lindquist. (1978) J. Neurochem. 31:161.
6. Gaull, G.E., D.K. Rassin, N.C.R. Räihä and K. Heinonen. (1977) J. Pediat. 90:348.
7. Sturman, J.A., D.K. Rassin and G.E. Gaull. (1977) Life Sci 21:1.
8. Sturman, J.A., D.K. Rassin and G.E. Gaull. (1978) In: Taurine in Neurological Disease, Huxtable, R. and A. Barbeau eds., Raven Press, New York p. 49.
9. Sturman, J.A. and G.E. Gaull. (1975) J. Neurochem. 25:831.
10. Sturman, J.A., D.K. Rassin and G.E. Gaull. (1970) J. Neurochem. 17:1117.
11. Gaull, G.E., J.A. Sturman and N.C.R. Räihä. (1972) Pediat. Res. 6:538.
12. Gaull, G.E., W. von Berg, N.C.R. Räihä and J.A. Sturman. (1973) Pediat. Res. 7:527.
13. Sturman, J.A., G.E. Gaull and W.H. Niemann. (1976) J. Neurochem. 26:457.
14. Sturman, J.A., G.E. Gaull and W.H. Niemann. (1976) J. Neurochem. 27:425.
15. Agrawal, H.C., A.N. Davison and L.K. Kaczmarek. (1971) Biochem. J. 122:759.
16. Rassin, D.K., G.E. Gaull, K. Heinonen and N.C.R. Räihä. (1977) Pediatrics 59:407.
17. Rassin, D.K., G.E. Gaull, N.C.R. Räihä and K. Heinonen. (1977) J. Pediat. 90:356.
18. Dickinson, J.C., H. Rosenblum and P.B. Hamilton. (1970) Pediatrics 45:606.
19. Jagenburg, O.R. (1959) Scand. J. Clin. Lab. Invest. 11:3.
20. Jonxis, J.H.P. (1951) Arch. Dis. Childh. 26:272.
21. Souchon, F. (1952) Z. Ges. Exp. Med. 118:219.
22. Rassin, D.K., J.A. Sturman and G.E. Gaull. (1978) Early Hum. Develop. 2:1.
23. Sturman, J.A., D.K. Rassin and G.E. Gaull (1977) Pediat. Res. 11:28.
24. Berson, E.L., K.C. Hayes, A.R. Rabin, S.Y. Schmidt and G. Watson. (1976) Invest. Ophthalmol. 15:52.
25. Knopf, K., J.A. Sturman, M. Armstrong and K.C. Hayes. (1978) J. Nutr. 108:773.
26. Sturman, J.A., D.K. Rassin, K.C. Hayes and G.E. Gaull. (1978) J. Nutr. 108:1462.
27. Encrantz, J.C. and J. Sjovall. (1959) Clin. Chim. Acta 4:793.
28. Sjovall, J. (1960) Clin. Chim. Acta 5:33.
29. Poley, J.R., J.C. Dower, C.A. Owen and G.B. Stickler. (1964) J. Lab. Clin. Med. 63:838.
30. Challacombe, D.N., S. Edkins and G.A. Brown. (1975) Arch. Dis. Childh. 50:837.
31. Brueton, M.J., H.M. Berger, G.A. Brown, L. Ablitt, N. Iyangkaran and B.A. Wharton. (1978) Gut 19:95.
32. Rabin, B., R.J. Nicolosi and K.C. Hayes. (1976) J. Nutr. 106:1241.
33. Grosso, D.S. and R. Bressler. (1976) Biochem. Pharmacol. 25:2227.
34. Schroten, T. (1970) In: Metabolic Conjugation and Metabolic Hydrolysis, Fishman, W.H. ed., Academic Press, New York, vol. 2, p. 75.
35. Nervi, F.O. and J.M. Dietschy. (1978) J. Clin. Invest. 61:895.

DISCUSSION

(Chairman: A. Ballabriga)

PAPER BY E.M. WIDDOWSON

J.C.L. Shaw: I was very interested to see the results of the glycine analyses of the fetal body, because we arrived in our department at a rather similar conclusion using different methods. Last summer, Dr. Alan Jackson from Jamaica was working with me for six weeks and we did some stable isotope measurements of protein turnover using ^{15}N-glycine. The results of only one infant are ready at the moment and in this infant during the first balance on the tenth day of life, glycine appeared in the urine and we were able to obtain plateau levels and calculate turnover. But, in the subsequent balances, when the baby was growing rapidly, there was no ^{15}N enrichment in the urine at all, indicating that glycine was not being converted into urea, and that therefore all the glycine administered in the diet was in fact being incorporated into body protein. We then looked at the amount of glycine in breast milk – and found of course there was very little – and we considered the possibility that in such an infant, glycine might be growth limiting.

M. Young: The free glycine concentration is also always high in fetal intra- and extra-cellular fluids, including the placenta, and is probably synthesised from essential amino acids. There are also high concentrations of arginine synthetase in animal tissues and Westall (WESTALL, R.G. (1960) Biochem. J. 77:135.) suggested some time ago that they were there in order to produce the large amount of arginine which is needed by the growing animal.

E.M. Widdowson: Of course, if the baby has not got a placenta, then maybe we should help it along.

F.C. Battaglia: I would like to congratulate you on this mammoth study.

It is a very important contribution. I think we'll all end up using these data in many, many ways.

Chemically, there are a couple of problems and I wondered how you got around them. First of all, the problem of glutamine and whether or not you have a high glutamate in part by a break-down of glutamine in the homogenate and during the chemical analyses. Secondly, I wonder, were these milks analyzed at a particular time during lactation in terms of the total aminoacid composition, in comparing the increments added to the carcass versus the milk. The only comment that I have relates to the approach you are making to compare increments acquired in the carcass for each amino acid versus the potential uptake into the umbilical stream. When we made that comparison in the lamb, that was of actual amino acid uptake, so it was flow times whole blood A-V difference. I think in tomorrow's session we'll get into the discussion of how you can get an estimate in man where you only have the A-V difference, and hopefully the A-V difference of whole blood. I am not surprised that when you look at plasma A-V differences alone versus the increment in the carcass, a pattern doesn't emerge. The other thing is, I'd be cautious, coming back to Dr. Shaw's comment, to interpret the absence of ^{15}N appearing in urea and singling out an amino acid that's limiting for growth. That's quite an assumption. In veterinary medicine, of course, there have been a whole variety of ways used to sort out which are the limiting amino acids in rapid growth.

E.M. Widdowson: Dr. Battaglia, I knew you'd ask me about glutamine and I can't tell you anything I'm afraid. So far as milk is concerned, this was mature milk collected between 4 and 8 weeks lactation. We took this stage because it is when milk is likely to be collected for milk banks and so it is the milk you would probably be feeding to your babies.

B.S. Lindblad: We gave 20 infants an alimentation of 0.10 g protein and 4 kcal/kg/hour and measured the increase of the plasma amino acids during the infusion and the decrease after we stopped the infusion. (LINDBLAD, B.S., G. SETTERGREN, H. FEYCHTING and B. PERSSON. (1977) Acta Paediatr. Scand. 66:409.) There was one amino acid that differed from the normal plasma levels and that was glutamic acid. When one sees these high figures of glutamic acid in milk and in the body composition, it should be pointed out that this is an artefact during the analysis: that we cause a decomposition of glutamine into glutamic acid.

In milk, for example, half the glutamic acid is in the form of glutamine. My question is, do you have data for taurine?

E.M. Widdowson: I was afraid Dr. Gaull would be asking me about taurine. I have no figures for it. It is a free amino acid, while most of the amino acids in the body are bound as protein.

PAPER BY J.C.L. SHAW

R.D.G. Milner: Can I ask you to go one step further and tell us your thoughts about the arguments for and against trace metal supplementation either perorally or parenterally.

J.C.L. Shaw: Unless you are going to do intravenous nutrition for only a short time, copper and zinc must be included. This is particularly important in surgical cases where losses from gastric aspiration or from fistulas are high. When to start and how much to give must still be a matter of debate. The obvious manifestations of zinc and copper deficiency are comparatively late changes, and one could guess that the body feels the deficiency before the physician is aware of it. On general grounds there seems no purpose in withholding essential nutrients. Oral supplements are more difficult. No cases of zinc deficiency have been documented yet in premature babies, and copper deficiency only rarely. These copper deficiencies resembled the late iron deficiency of prematurity in that they come on late, so we are planning to follow the babies during the first year to see what happens. We may find that we have to give premature babies copper and zinc supplements just as we give them iron supplements.

R. Zetterström: The blood copper levels in your preterm infants were very reliable. How were those babies fed? The reason why I'm asking you is that the supply of copper may vary enormously according to the food they are given. If they are formula fed, then if the powder is diluted with water, the copper content in that water may vary extremely. If you have a copper pipeline for instance, in the first tap in the morning you may have ten times as high a concentration of copper as compared with later in the day.

J.C.L. Shaw: They were all fed with breast milk and I hope that the breast milk was not diluted with water with a high copper content!

But in the balance studies we analyzed all the diets, so that we know in fact that the copper concentration was 40 μg/100 ml, which is what it should be, from other analyses.

M. Orzalesi: Dr. Shaw, did I get it right that on your last slide you were talking about iron absorption not iron retention.

J.C.L. Shaw: Well, iron absorption and iron retention are to all intents and purposes the same thing. Iron does not get out of the body.

M. Orzalesi: You postulated that the mechanism of iron absorption or retention depends on the hemoglobin level: I would like to suggest that perhaps what switches on the absorption or switches it off is not so much the hemoglobin concentration per se, but is the hemoglobin oxygen-delivering capacity – which of course depends not only on the hemo-globin concentration, but also on what kind of hemoglobin you have and if you have transfused adult blood which is capable of giving more oxygen, and the amount of 2, 3 DPG and other organic phosphates that you have in the red cells.

There is good evidence – and this is also apparent in the studies of Riegel and Versmold and Papadopoulos and Oski – that the switch in hemoglobin synthesis in reticulocytes and iron absorption depends on the oxygen-delivering capacity.

J.C.L. Shaw: You may be right. Certainly changes in hemoglobin con-centration may result in changes of oxygen delivery though changes in cardiac output can to some extent compensate for changes in oxygen content of the blood. No one knows what the messenger is that controls iron absorption at mucosal level. I think that the question of the dissocia-tion curve may not be so important, because after birth in non-acidotic infants, the normal rise in red cell 2, 3 DPG causes the dissociation curve to shift to the right with a corresponding rise in the P_{50} to a value close to that of adult haemoglobin. (WIMBERLEY, P.D., M.D. WHITEHEAD and E.R. HUEHNS. (1977) Inserm. 70:295). The consequences of giving adult blood on oxygen delivery are therefore not at all clear.

F.C. Battaglia: I'm still puzzling over the best way to present data where you're looking at increments in a newborn infant or a preterm baby. In your graphs, you present for instance for zinc or copper the accretion rate expected in fetal life and then the milligrams per day that the infant accumulated in the nursery on a particular diet. My trouble with that way of expressing is that, if a baby for example – to take an extreme – did not grow, everything in the baby would not approach the fetal accretion rate and it hasn't told us very much about a selective problem in any part of the body. Would it make more sense to present it as the accretion rate for zinc, for example, per gram of new weight gained that day? You attempted that when you mentioned that in bone you began to look at ratios to collagen.

J.C.L. Shaw: You have raised an important point; I have tried to present too much in too short a time. The magnesium retention by the preterm infants was on average 14.5 mg/100 g weight gain as against 25 mg/100g weight gain of the fetus. When we look at bone magnesium of infants dying $\geqslant 28$ days after birth magnesium is significantly reduced ($p < 0.001$) when expressed, as mg/100 g dry defatted weight; mg/100 mg N_2 or mg/100 mg of collagen.

As a group, net retention of copper by the infants was about 10% of the intrauterine accumulation, and as a group they experienced a net loss of zinc over the period studied. I think the significance of this is not obvious because we don't know how much of each element is needed for growth and how much is body reserve. All we can conclude is that the concentrations of magnesium, zinc and copper in the body appear to fall. This must result in a reduction in reserves and may lead to deficiency at some time.

PAPER BY J. SENTERRE

G.E. Gaull: Whenever we don't really know what to do, in medicine, there are two schools of thought. Dr. Senterre has admirably represented what has been referred to as the "premature-as-fetus" school and this is best seen in the slide in which the various amino acid concentrations are compared with the concentrations found in cord blood. I submit to you that the premature human infant is a new biological entity. We don't really know what the appropriate normal values are. I don't really know exactly how feed these infants. I think that one of the measurements that would be of interest in making a recommendation of any amount of protein is some measure of linear growth. In the study that we reported, the measure of linear growth was not different with pooled human milk as compared with higher protein intakes. (RAIHA, N.C.R., K. HEINONEN, D.K. RASSIN and G.E. GAULL. (1976) Pediatrics 57:659; GAULL, G.E., D.K. RASSIN and N.C.R. RÄIHÄ (1977) J. Pediat. 90:507.)

I do have a couple of questions, in addition to my philosophical comments. I notice that your base excess was only minus three or four; for the same amount of protein ours was considerably lower – about minus ten. And I'm wondering whether you think that had to do with the mineral load. Did you mention anything about protein quality? What kind of protein you were feeding as you were going up the protein scale? Finally, did you actually measure glomerular filtration rate in the infants on human milk versus the infants on the high-protein formulas?

J. Senterre: First your question about the base excess value. In the slide I showed you, the mean base excess value was indeed relatively low in the group fed on an adapted formula providing 4.5 g/proteins/kg body weight/day. In that formula the casein:whey ratio was 40:60, 50% of the fats were medium chain triglycerides and the mineral content was 0.3 g/l. Under these conditions, nitrogen retention was good and the mineral supply was relatively low. I think that is the reason why we found such a low mean value for base excess. However as shown by the high standard deviation, in some infants base excess values were below minus 8 mEq/l.

Regarding the protein quality in the slides where protein intake is going up, all the formulas used has a casein:whey ratio of 40:60 (adapted formula) except for the 14 balances carried out with half-skimmed cow's milk in which the protein quality was not modified. Concerning the glomerular filtration rate, I can say nothing because I did not measure it.

J.C. Sinclair: I was interested in your observation that you obtained higher nitrogen retention in babies who received higher digestible energy intakes on the same protein intake. I would assume those babies were also growing more rapidly. Is that true?

J. Senterre: I did not try to correlate between nitrogen retention and growth because nitrogen retention represents only about 2% of weight gain and metabolic balances were only performed during 3 days. What I can say is that our preterm infants were generally growing at a rate of about 15 g/kg/day and I cannot see any difference in growth when nitrogen retention during the short time of metabolic balance was high. The only thing I observed was a poor weight gain in the few infants who had a nitrogen retention below 200 mg/kg body weight/day during the balance period. In these cases I think it is chiefly a question of a low amount of energy available for growth either because of fat malabsorption or because of high energy expenditure.

J.C. Sinclair: I want to introduce for discussion Professor McCance's concept of homeostasis through growth. We're used so often to thinking of nutrient requirements for babies in terms of grams of something per kilo per day. But we're talking here about nitrogen largely incorporated into growing tissue. Would it advance our understanding of this problem to think of nitrogen requirements in terms of rate of weight gain of the baby during the feeding period?

J. Senterre: As calculated by Shaw, the weight gain in utero between 28 and 36 weeks of gestation is about 15 g/kg/day and the nitrogen retention about 340 mg/kg/day. It is relatively easy to get a weight gain in preterm infants similar to that observed in utero. Under these conditions I assume that it is best to get a nitrogen retention which is also close to the one calculated in the fetus. I may be wrong but with a weight gain of 15 g/kg/day I prefer to have a nitrogen retention of 340 mg/kg/day instead of a nitrogen retention of 215 mg/kg/day. But we can have a lot of discussions about it. I don't think such a nitrogen retention will accelerate the body maturation as Snyderman observed when she gave 9 g/proteins/kg/day. Under these conditions there was a nitrogen retention much higher than in utero. I don't think we derive any advantages from doing that.

E.M. Widdowson: I was interested in your observation that the fecal excretion of nitrogen was constant – more or less – whatever the nitrogen intake. This reminds me of a study we made many years ago on adults when we observed exactly the same thing. (McCANCE, R.A. and E.M. WIDDOWSON. (1947) J. Hygiene 45:59.) We did this by using bread made from Canadian wheat and English wheat, because Canadian wheat contains twice as much protein as English wheat. Most of our diet consisted of bread with the same amounts of other foods in both studies. We found just what you did: that the nitrogen in the feces was the same although the intake was twice as much on one occasion as on the other. We concluded that virtually all of the food nitrogen is absorbed and what one finds in the feces comes from bacteria, desquamation and perhaps digestive juices.

J. Senterre: I completely agree with you. My interpretation is also that fecal nitrogen is chiefly endogenous nitrogen. I can't prove it but it is very likely that true digestibility of proteins from milk is higher than the coefficient of net absorption we calculated. However, in infants on human milk net absorption of proteins is lower because a part of fecal nitrogen is probably coming from immunoglobulins.

B.S. Lindblad: You mentioned Dr. Selma Snyderman's work on the effect on the homeostasis of the different amino acids in blood during protein overload – 9 g/kg. (SNYDERMAN, S.E., L.E. HOLT, JR., P.M. NORTON, E. ROITMAN and S.V. PHANSALKAR. (1968) Pediatr. Res. 2:131.) The most typical change was a great rise of valine levels. In my paper I compare your valine levels in babies on human milk, and on the three different protein intakes, with those of Dr. Gaull and Räihä, and compare them also with our estimations in the full-term on *ad libitum* human milk. It is quite evident that we have the same levels during intake of human milk in premature and full-term babies. If you take these levels as reference of normal blood homeostasis, rather than to look at cord blood, then the levels that you see during those high protein intakes are an indication of a protein overload. I would like to have your comment on that.

J. Senterre: During the general discussion my co-worker Dr. Rigo will give some data about the increase of the plasma concentrations of some amino acids in relation to the protein intake. I can say now that there is for instance a large increase of valine in relation to protein intake.

In the table you see that concentration of valine (in micromoles per liter) is indeed higher in infants on adapted formula providing 3.5 or 4.5 g/proteins/kg/day than in those on human milk. However our impression is that the value on human milk is a bit low. On the other hand one cannot say that 225 μM/l, the value observed with a protein intake

	Valine concentration in plasma
Human milk	145 μM/l
Adapted formula	
protein intake 3.5 g/kg/day	225 μM/l
protein intake 4.5 g/kg/day	264 μM/l
Cord blood	243 μM/l

of 3.5 g/kg/day is too high when we compare with the cord blood value. The problem is that if we want to get a nitrogen retention as in utero, plasma amino acid concentrations become similar to cord blood values whereas the values observed in preterm infants fed pooled human milk look more like in protein deficiency.

B. Friis Hansen: You presented a very impressive amount of data. I was only surprised that the human milk came out so poorly – with an NPU of 60% and a biological value of only 76. So I wonder how the human milk was treated – was it heat-treated, or can you give any other explanation of these results?

J. Senterre: It was human milk from a milk-bank and it was heat-treated. It was heated at 56 °C during half an hour twice. We performed a lot of balances in preterm infants on human milk and we always found an "apparent" net protein utilization (N retention/N intake) of about 65% and an "apparent" biological value (N retention/N absorbed) of about 75%. This can be explained by the relatively high fecal loss of nitrogen (75 mg/kg/day) probably related to undigested immunoglobulins and an urinary loss of nitrogen of about 80 mg/kg/day.

E. Eggermont: Dr. Senterre, do you see any variation of protein digestibility with the age of the infants. The reason I'm asking this is that we found that the stool chymotrypsin activity decreases from birth until the age of four weeks. (Acta Paediatr. Belg., in press, 1979.)

J. Senterre: There is a small decrease in fecal excretion of nitrogen in the fourth week compared to the second week but the difference is very small (about 5 to 8 mg/kg/day). In any case protein digestibility is always very satisfactory even though there is a tendency toward a decrease in fecal excretion of nitrogen at the end of the first month.

A.G.L. Whitelaw: A brief comment. One of my colleagues in Toronto, Stephanie Atkinson, has recently compared the nitrogen content of premature milk with mature breast milk and she found that the milk produced by mothers of 28, 29, 30 week gestation babies had a nitrogen content approximately 30% higher than breast milk of mothers with at term born babies. (ATKINSON, S.A., M.H. BRYAN and G.H. ANDERSON. (1978) J. Pediat. 93:67.) She postulated that this was very fortunate, because nature seemed to be providing – or attempting to provide – some of the increased nitrogen requirements of these preterm babies. It is the normal practise in Toronto to feed the mother's own milk to her own baby and not to use pooled mature human breast milk. I wonder if you have any comments on that.

J. Senterre: I am quite sure you are right, but in practice it is difficult to realize. The milk we use comes partly from the maternity hospital. As you saw, it has a rather high nitrogen content: the net protein content, i.e. nitrogen $\times$ 6.25, is 1.3 g/100 ml. It is in fact a mixture of colostrum and mature human milk. In Strasbourg, Schneegans performed some nitrogen balances in premature infants fed on colostrum and he found a high nitrogen retention (Med. et Hyg. 35:641, 1977). I think indeed that it is better to feed a preterm infant on his mother's owns milk or on colostrum than on a mature human milk supplemented with cow's milk protein. The problem is to get it.

PAPER BY G. E. GAULL

K. Adriaensens: Is there a relationship between taurine and retrolental fibroplasia?

G.E. Gaull: I can't answer that question. It has been asked a number of times. I don't know.

C.A. Canosa: Will you recommend taurine supplementation to the milk of very low birth weight infants?

G.E. Gaull: I suppose I do. If you're a believer in Mother Nature, it's hard to resist trying to simulate human milk as closely as possible. Clearly, you change the taurine-glycine ratio of bile acids. The evidence is that taurine-conjugated bile acids are more efficient bile acids than glycine-conjugates. They make fewer entero-hepatic circulations, and they maintain the critical mycellar concentration further down the gut.

I remember when I was at medical school, we learned about Vitamin E. Everyone debated about whether Vitamin E really had a function in man. And now, we have this whole story with Vitamin E, unsaturated fatty acids, iron supplementation and hemolytic anemia in the preterm infant. There seems very little doubt, now, that we know what the function of Vitamin E is: that you really ought to supplement formulas with Vitamin E. This is true especially if you're giving vegetable fatty acids. We don't know precisely what the biological function of taurine is. I suggest to you that the circumstantial evidence is that it's very important, but what *the* function is is something that we don't know.

J.C. Sinclair: Can you tell us anything yet about the role of taurine in respect of fat absorption in premature babies fed artificial formulas?

G.E. Gaull: No.

J.C. Sinclair: Because you're not looking at this, or it's too early?

G.E. Gaull: It's too early. We don't have enough results analyzed.

H.M. Berger: Dr. Gaull, do you have any data on the effect of heat treatment, for storage of human milk, on the taurine levels?

G.E. Gaull: Taurine is an extraordinarily stable substance. It's in its fully oxydized state; there is almost nothing you can do to destroy it. I'm sure everything else in the milk would go before the taurine.

H.M. Berger: One further question. In the Birmingham study we found that when giving human milk, the taurine-glycine ratio decreased. In absolute figures, however, the amount of glycine decreased, rather than the amount of taurine increased. Have you any comment?

G.E. Gaull: I think it may have to do with the fact that you were comparing two different facts. You see, the real comparison is the so-called adapted formula with and without taurine. In your experiments, what you did was compare the taurine-glycine ratio with two variables.

There is evidence now that fat itself can alter bile acid synthesis and conjugation.

F.C. Battaglia: Just one comment and a question. The comment I have concerns grouping amino acids in terms of their concentrations in the free form in milk. I think that's perfectly valid for taurine, since it represents the total amount in the milk, but it's a meaningless comparison with the other amino acids, where the bulk of them is represented in protein. So I think a more meaningful way to compare taurine intake versus other amino acid intake is to measure the other amino acids after hydrolysis on the milk.

G.E. Gaull: We've done both.

F.C. Battaglia: In your tables, I assume you presented it as all free amino acids. That's the way I understood the tables.

G.E. Gaull: In those tables I presented the free amino acids and the only message I wanted to leave you with, was that in some animals taurine is the free amino acid present in highest concentration and in others it is second only to glutamate and in still others there doesn't seem to be any at all. I drew no further conclusions. In the protein analyses that we did, we hydrolyzed the protein. You are correct – compared with most amino acids, taurine is present in small amounts.

F.C. Battaglia: The question I had is – looking at this not in terms of infant nutrition, but in terms of fetal growth –: Do you have estimates of the total amount of taurine there is in the term infant? Let's say a 3.5 kg infant, where you don't have excretion of taurine in bile, that's representing an irreversible loss, but it's really accumulation of taurine in the nervous sytem and in other tissues. What would that come to in millimoles of taurine in the body?

G.E. Gaull: I've never really done the calculation. I know that after birth, there is a fairly striking outpouring of taurine in the urine. I was remiss in not letting this audience know that in 1951, in Archives of Disease in Childhood, the observation that infants fed human milk excreted more taurine than infants fed cow-milk formulas was made by Professor Jonxis seven years before Moore and Stein described the first automatic amino acid analyzer.

J. Senterre: Dr. Gaull, you estimated the taurine concentration in human milk as 34 μmole/100 ml. We have observed a taurine concentration of 50 μmole per 100 ml. But our human milkbank contains partly colostrum and transitional milk. Is the concentration of taurine in colostrum higher?

G.E. Gaull: Yes, it's higher. There is a systematic review of the concentration in human milk as it appears in mothers corn-fed in Iowa. (RASSIN, D.K., J.A. STURMAN and G.E. GAULL. (1978) Early Hum. Develop. 2:1.)

GENERAL DISCUSSION

R. Zetterström: Discussing the nutritional needs of preterm infants, the subject of the need of the main electrolytes has been rather much neglected. Not very much is being said about the need of sodium or potassium, for instance. With the permission of the chairman, I will present some very recent data we have obtained.

I think it's now about twenty years ago since Professor McCance and Dr. Widdowson demonstrated that the newly born has a limited capacity to eliminate sodium. (McCANCE, R.A. and E.M. WIDDOWSON. (1957) Acta Paediatr. Scand. 46:337.) Since it was considered that human milk contains a very low concentration of sodium, baby food manufacturers, in their efforts to produce an adapted formula, reduced the sodium content in their formulas.

Together with Dr. Aperia, Dr. Broberger and Dr. Herin, we have studied the pattern of sodium excretion in relation to the intake, in full-term and preterm babies. It was shown by McCance and Widdowson that the full-term baby has reduced capacity to eliminate sodium, so that when the intake is very low, the excretion goes down. In the preterm infant, there is the same inability, so to say, to excrete a load but on the other hand the preterm baby – and that stands for babies of 32 to 34 weeks of gestation – is unable to retain sodium. So, there is not a very good capacity to vary the sodium excretion in the preterm compared to the full-term baby. We have followed the excretion of sodium during the first days of life.

You can see that in the full-term baby (Fig. 1) as well as in the preterm – 32 to 34 weeks of gestation (Fig. 2), there is a peak excretion of sodium

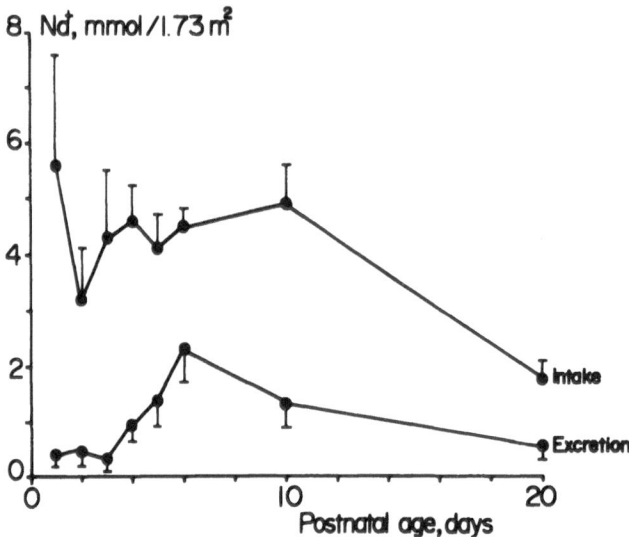

Fig. 1. Average hourly urinary sodium excretion and sodium intake in full-term infants aged 1–21 days fed breast milk from their mothers. Each filled circle represents the average of 5–7 observations. The bars represent SEM.

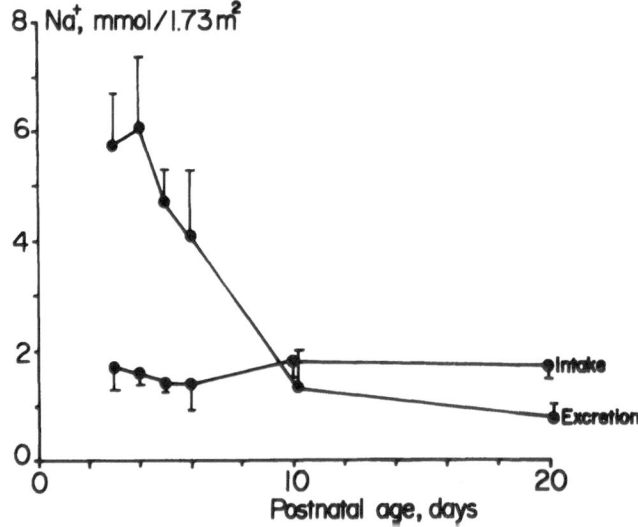

Fig. 2. Average hourly sodium intake and urinary sodium excretion in preterm infants aged 3–21 days fed pooled mature breast milk. Each filled circle represents the average of 4–9 observations.

during the fifth, sixth day after birth, and that the peak excretion is much higher in the preterm baby than in the full-term baby. When considering what the reason is for those peak excretions under normal conditions, we have of course to look for the sodium intake.

The full-term babies were fed with breast milk from their mothers and we had to find out how much sodium they were getting. The preterm infants received pooled breast milk from mothers in a later stage of lactation.

You can see that the sodium content in breast milk is not, in the early period of lactation, as low as it is considered to be in the textbooks (Fig. 3). The textbooks give values of 7–8 mmole/l, but in the early days of lactation, it's much higher and then it gradually falls. The sodium concentration is about the same in breast milk from mothers who are delivered during the 32nd–34th gestational week as in those who are delivered at term (Fig. 4). During the first period of life, breast-fed infants fed with mother's milk are thus receiving much more sodium than we thought.

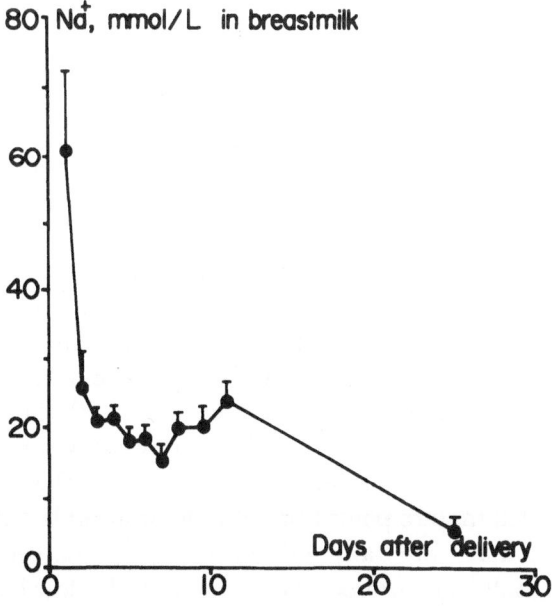

Fig. 3. Sodium concentration in breast milk from mothers who are delivered at term. The data represent mean values and the bar 1 SE.

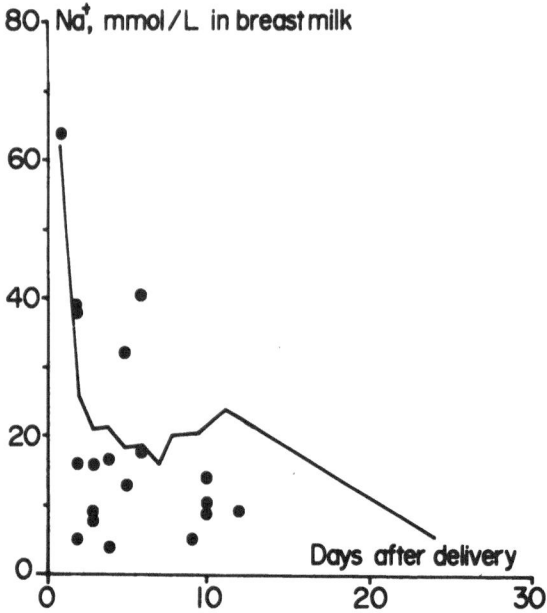

Fig. 4. Sodium concentration in breast milk from mothers who are delivered during the 32nd–34th gestation week (●). The line represents the average values observed in breast milk from mothers who have been delivered at term.

Considering the balance excretion-intake we, as illustrated in Figure 1, find in breast-fed full-term babies in the age group up to 15–20 days after birth a marked retention of sodium. Of course, this retention is somewhat over-emphasized, since the sodium losses in the sweat and in stools have not been taken into account. The reason why there is sodium retention immediately after birth remains, we think, unknown.

If we then look at the situation for preterm babies who receive breast milk from their mothers, the daily intake of sodium is about 3 to 4 mmole/1.73 m² body surface area during the first 2 weeks after birth. The intake then falls. If you compare the urinary excretion with the intake, you will find that in the very first days of life there is a slight negative balance which is corrected rather soon afterwards. On the other hand, if preterm babies are fed mature pooled breast milk or formula-fed – so-called adapted formula – the daily sodium intake will be very low: between 1 and 2 mmole/1.73 m² body surface area. If this low intake is compared to the urinary excretion, it is quite obvious that there will be a highly negative sodium balance during the first weeks of life, which will be corrected very slowly (Fig. 2). A marked deficit might remain for 2 or 3 months if the food is not supplemented with extra sodium.

There may also in full-term infants be a risk of negative sodium balance during the first weeks of life if they are fed adapted formula with low sodium concentration or mature breast milk. Of course, we do not know the significance of such a negative sodium balance during the first weeks after birth, nor do we really know why the newborn baby retains sodium under – we would say – normal conditions.

The results of these studies will be reported in detail. (APERIA, A., O. BROBERGER, P. HERIN, and R. ZETTERSTRÖM: Salt content in human breast milk during the three first weeks after delivery. Acta Paediatr. Scand., in press; and APERIA, A., O. BROBERGER, P. HERIN and R. ZETTERSTRÖM: Sodium excretion in relation to sodium intake and aldosterone excretion in newborn pre-term and full-term infants. Acta Paediatr. Scand., in press.)

K. van Acker: Professor Zetterström, did you try to correlate your sodium balances with the aldosterone levels and plasma renin activity? As far as I know there is no good explanation for the high levels in the newborn.

R. Zetterström: We have studied the urinary excretion of aldosterone and it is in the newborn infant extremely high. This is rather paradoxical when you have that peak excretion during the fifth, sixth day after birth and at that time you also have a very high aldosterone excretion. You also have a very high potassium to sodium ratio up to 3 or 4.

J. Rigo: Dr. Gaull, did you determine the taurine concentration in cord blood? I am asking this, because there are some differences in the reported values in cord blood as well as in serum of infants fed human milk.

G.E. Gaull: I have not. But you can tell from my remarks a propos of Dr. Senterre's paper, that it is not a measurement I consider highly valuable.

B.S. Lindblad: The mother's blood contains taurine and I thought that the fact that human milk contains taurine was a spill-over from the maternal blood. What about cow's blood? Why is cow's milk free of taurine?

G.E. Gaull: I don't know the answer. I really don't know why cow's milk has virtually no taurine. It's very difficult to measure. But the concentration – at least in pooled human milk – is higher than the concentration found in the mother's blood. One cannot consider it just a spill-over diffusion.

C. T. Jones: Of all the studies on taurine, the one on axonal transport is perhaps the most fascinating. Just one comment and two questions. First of all, like most of these inhibitors, cycloheximide is not specifically an inhibitor of protein synthesis and has been shown to uncouple oxidative phosphorylation.

The two questions are: Is the axonal transport of other amino acids similar to that of taurine? But the more fundamental one is: Where does the taurine go to? Does it go into cell membranes? Does it go into particular sub-cellular constituents in the optic tectum?

G.E. Gaull: I didn't make myself clear. If you inject an amino acid that is incorporated into protein into the eye of the goldfish, it will be rapidly axonally transported to the contralateral tectum after incorporation into the protein, that is, the counts come down with the TCA precipitable material. If you put cystine in, for instance, you can account for all of the radioactivity in the tectum, in the TCA precipitable material and it is cystine in protein and not taurine. Anything which is in the free amino acid pool, then, is the taurine. Taurine is exceptional among free amino acids in being transported by rapid axonal flow. That's one question.

The other question is: What is it incorporated into? It is not incorporated into anything, as far as we can tell. But there is evidence in the rat that it is bound to the synaptisomal protein. That is evidence from David Rassin in our group. (RASSIN, D.K., J.A. STURMAN and G.E. GAULL. (1977) J. Neurochem. 28:41) Certainly, there are in the synaptisomes high capacity, low KM systems for uptake of taurine.

Your comment about cycloheximide is of course correct, but other protein inhibitors will do the same thing, they also inhibit the axonal flow of taurine.

M. Young: I just wondered if you had compared its rate of transport up the axon with a non-metabolizable amino acid, such as AIB or any of the others.

G.E. Gaull: Yes. Even AIB is not rapidly axonally transported.

A.H. Markum: What is the concentration of taurine in human milk of the mothers with preterm babies compared to those with full-term babies?

G.E. Gaull: I can't answer that question. We are going to be able to give you an answer, because we are aware of the work done in Toronto on the higher concentration of nitrogen in the milk of mothers with preterm born babies. We now have the milks collected from a number of the mothers that we're presently studying and we will do both true protein and analyze the non-protein nitrogen fraction. I think that this will be a very interesting thing to do, but I don't know how it's going to come out.

A. Ballabriga: At the recent meeting of the International Pediatric Association, Dr. Kobayashi and his group presented data on the analysis of human milk at different periods after birth and they showed that during the first 3 weeks of life there was an increase of the level of taurine. My question is, when did you take your samples for the measurement of the concentration of taurine in the brain, because in different animals there are differences in the degree of brain development.

G.E. Gaull: In every animal the taurine concentration in the milk is highest, when the animal is born and then it falls of gradually, so that it is related to birth and not so much to brain development at birth. We don't know what the function of taurine in brain is. There is certainly a lot of evidence that taurine is probably an inhibitory neuro-transmitter or neuro-modulator. However, there is much more taurine in brain than one needs to account for some sort of neuro-transmitter substance. We think – and this is pure speculation – that taurine probably is related to membranes or to cyto-skeletal structure. What you see when you grind up the cell is that it's in the cytosol and it's not attached to anything. But its charges are such that it might well have a loose association in phospholipid membranes.

A. Ballabriga: I have asked this question because if taurine plays a role as neuro-transmitter, we know that the amount of taurine in human breast milk is increasing after birth. Would it not be logical that in guinea-pig milk or in monkey milk the concentration of taurine will go down because the degree of brain development in these animals at birth was different?

G.E. Gaull: The only thing we can say right now is that, in the five or six species that we have checked, the concentration of taurine in milk is always highest early and falls.

H.L. Greene: You have presented some data on the retina and have implied at least that what's going on in the retina may be in fact something similar to what may be going on in the brain. When cats have become taurine deficient and develop their blindness, is there a morphologic change and, if so, is this reversible by giving taurine?

G.E. Gaull: Yes, there is a morphological change. There is degeneration of the photoreceptor cells and this is reversible in the early stages by the administration of taurine and not by the administration of any of the precursors of taurine. (Cf. HAYES, K.C. (1976) Nutr. Rev. 34:161.)

H.L. Greene: Is this change reversible after a period of time or is it just during the first few stages?

G.E. Gaull: After several weeks, it's not reversible. You have to have the taurine concentration in retina fall to below 50% and it takes about 6 months to do that. But before that, you get changes in the electro-retinogram which are readily identifiable in the cat. One can feed the taurine early and reverse it. I'd like to make clear that that was not work from my laboratory; that was work that had gone on long before we ever got into it.

J.D. Baum: May I ask a very short question and make a philosophical comment? The short question is: Did you measure the differences in taurine concentration between early milk and late milk from a mother at a given feed? The philosophical consequence of that is that at this time of explosion of knowledge on the refined studies on the composition of milk, should we not have some convention in defining how the samples are taken before presuming that we know what the baby eats. It is a presumption that milk expressed at a certain time in a feed reflects what the baby would have, if it were naturally feeding at the breast. Your very impressive studies on the term babies were presumably free-range living babies feeding at the mother's breast and that's very impressive. But other experiments on milk samples may depend very much on how they are collected.

G.E. Gaull: I certainly agree with you and I don't think it's a philosophical question. We have very carefully defined ours as pooled human
milk by Finnish mothers. The mothers bring the milk to collecting points.
These are known donors. The milk is then pooled and, if you look at
successive pools of milk collected in that way, you come out with answers
very close to the figure I gave. So I don't think that our data is at all
presumptive. On the contrary, I think it's very carefully defined. I think
what is interesting is why the full-term infants show more striking deficiencies in the plasma and urine concentrations than the preterm.

J. Rigo: I would like to give you some more information concerning
protein requirements of preterm infants. In our study with Dr. Senterre,
we measured the serum amino acid concentration in preterm infants and
in cord blood of full-term infants (Fig. 5). The premature infants fed
human milk have a low serum concentration of essential as well as of total
amino acids. The concentration of essential amino acids increases in
relation to the protein intake, and in infants given 3.5 to 4.5 g/proteins/
kg/day, it is similar to cord blood values, with the exception of lysine
whose concentration is decreased.

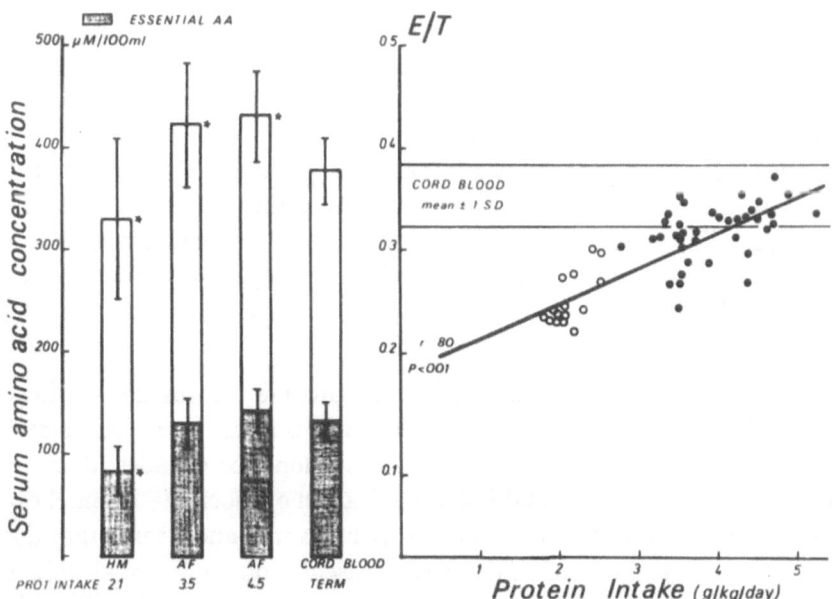

Fig. 5.

On the other hand, as reported by several investigators, the ratio of essential to total amino acids (E/T ratio) is also a useful indicator of the protein nutritional status. There is a positive linear relationship between the E/T ratio and protein intake. However, protein intake must reach 4.5 g/kg/day in order to obtain an E/T ratio similar to that in cord blood. This is because essential amino acids increase with the increase of protein intake. Thus, if we want to obtain an E/T ratio in serum similar to that in cord blood with an intake of 3.5 g/proteins/kg/day, it will be necessary to increase the E/T ratio in the protein given. Indeed, it has been reported that the E/T ratio in blood depends on the E/T ratio in the formula. The quality of the protein must be considered when discussing the optimal composition of an amino acid solution for parenteral nutrition.

A. Ballabriga: We still don't know if we have to use formulas, which give a total protein intake of about 2.7–3.0 g/proteins/kg/day, or to use formulas – as Dr. Senterre suggests in his studies – which give 3.5–4.0 g/proteins/kg/day. Generally infants that have been fed with 2.5 or 3.8 g/proteins/kg/day did clinically well; there were no differences from a clinical point of view. There was the same increase in weight and length. There was no real difference in the percentage of infants with metabolic acidosis. However, I think, we need to know more about the long-term prognosis. In my opinion the problem is not about biochemical differences, we need long-term observations, up to 8 years, as late neurological effects can become evident after 6 or 7 years.

Dr. Gaull, it has been shown in animal experiments that amino acid concentrations in blood cannot be related to amino acid concentrations in tissue. This means that we don't know about the concentrations of branched chain amino acids in the brain when we know the concentrations in blood.

G.E. Gaull: I think that the nutritional outcome is a function of how carefully we look at some things. If all you do is measure the length and weight of the infant, as pediatricians have done for decades, than an infant who grows bigger and faster – at least in our society – is somehow better. But I don't think that necessarily holds true and I think that the later neurological outcome, the cardio-vascular outcome are all things that have to be taken into account, or our weight gain is a Pyrrhic victory. As to your second remark, again I agree with you.

J. Senterre: It all depends what you are looking for. You may have a good growth in length, but at the same time you may have not enough calcium or magnesium in the bones, not enough zinc in the body. When you give infants a low protein intake, you will have a lower nitrogen retention. We try in these infants to have postnatal retention of calcium, magnesium and zinc as close as possible to the retention in utero. I try to give enough nitrogen to have a good retention of nitrogen, without reaching toxic amino acid concentrations in blood. Now, we cannot say that cord blood levels are optimal levels, but at the same time we can be sure that these levels are not toxic levels.

B.S. Lindblad: I agree that your cord blood levels are high. I think it's important to sample all the time from the same compartment. The peripheral venous plasma level before the first feed, on the first day of life, *not* the level of cord blood, may represent the normal level and should be compared to the subsequent levels. This might be important, as the branch-chained amino acid levels are correlated to insulin levels. (FELIG, P., O.E. OWEN, J. WAHREN and F.G. CAHILL JR. (1969) J. Clin. Invest. 48:584). A high level could result in greater insulin release and we do not know what that would mean.

J. Senterre: Our data are term cord blood values and if you take cord blood values at preterm delivery, at 32 weeks of gestational age, you have still higher cord blood values. I think these are not really high values for a preterm infant. In utero, they do have such high values.

J.C. Sinclair: I'd like to comment on the design of clinical experiments to look at the question of the impact of neonatal feeding policy on long-term mental development. If we're going to pursue this suggestion seriously, it will affect the way one designs feeding studies in the future. It would be desirable to insure that one enrolled groups that were comparable with respect to prognosis for mental development in such feeding studies. Whatever is measured by this thing called social class, or any other indicators that one could have in hand at the time of birth, should preferably be documented and used prospectively as a basis for forming groups anticipated to be comparable with respect to mental development. One would also want to hold under tight control any co-interventions which are known to affect mental development. It's a formidable problem to do that over a long period of time, until the final outcomes are measured. Although it's right to say that long-term follow-up is needed, a serious pursuit of that goal will demand that feeding studies be organized in a somewhat different way from the way feeding studies have been planned in the past.

D. Hull: Dr. Shaw, in your careful balance studies on the very immature babies, have you got any measurements on how much of the metals is lost or might be lost through the skin? I am curious to know from Professor Zetterström how much sodium and water relatively is lost through the skin of the premature babies, because I think this is going to influence the balance a little. Have measurements been made?

J.C.L. Shaw: There are estimates of iron losses and they come out at about 0.1 of a mg/kg/day. But that's a very crude estimate taken from estimates in adults and cutting them down on a meter square basis. As far as zinc and copper are concerned, there are measurements in sweat. But I have absolutely no idea how much is lost by a premature baby each day. One has to do this by keeping them in plastic and then dipping them in baths, rinsing them off in distilled water, collecting it all and drying it and analyzing it. I've not done that.

R. Zetterström: In regard to the losses of sodium in sweat I think that will only increase the negative balance. We were more interested in those factors related to a negative balance than those retaining sodium.

J. Senterre: Dr. Shaw, you showed data about a premature infant on human milk with a good magnesium absorption, but a high urinary excretion of magnesium. Did you measure simultaneously urinary excretion of calcium and phosphorus? If you put a little phosphorus in the milk perhaps you will depress urinary excretion of magnesium.

J.C.L. Shaw: We did phosphorus and calcium balances on this baby and I can't remember the results, so I can't exactly tell you. As is well known, the phosphorus content of urine of babies on breast milk is very low indeed and it's quite possible that increasing the phosphorus content in the diet one might influence magnesium balance.

A. Ballabriga: Dr. Shaw, do you think that we have to supplement the formulas for premature babies with copper and zinc?

J.C.L. Shaw: Certainly, the artifical formulas should be supplemented up to the level of breast milk and I think most of them are. There was a copper deficiency case reported in a preterm infant fed a non-supplemented formula. (SEELY et al. (1972) New Eng. J. Med. 286:109.) I don't think that it should be increased substantially at the moment, until we have more evidence on the effect of augmenting copper intake on the copper absorption and until we know whether in fact babies are getting copper deficiency in any numbers.

HUMAN MILK

COMPOSITION OF HUMAN MILK

LEIF HAMBRAEUS*, MD

The neonatal period represents one of the most, if not *the* most critical and vulnerable period in mammalian life, particularly with respect to nutrition. Not only is there a pronounced demand for the availability of essential nutrients to cover the requirement of the rapid growth and maturation of the tissue but furthermore, due to the immaturity of those organs involved in the regulation of the endogenous metabolism, i.e. liver and kidney, there is a reduced tolerance for deviations in the food intake.

One essential illustration of the assumption that mammalian milk is specifically adapted to fulfil the nutritional requirement of the newborn offspring seems to be the significant and obvious differences in the nutrient content which are observed when milk specimens obtained from various species of mammals are compared (table 1) (1). It is consequently logical to assume that human breast milk represents the optimal food for the human infant comprising the ideal composition with regard to the essential nutrients and perhaps also the non-essential nutrients in order to obtain optimal growth, development and maturation. Consequently the recommended dietary allowances for babies are mainly

Table 1. *Composition of milk obtained from different mammals, and the growth rate of their offspring.*

	Content of milk (%)				Days required to double birth weight
	Protein	Fat	Carbohydrate	Ash	
Man	0.9	3.8	7.0	0.2	180
Cow	3.4	3.7	4.8	0.7	47
Buffalo	3.8	7.4	4.8	0.8	
Goat	2.9	4.5	4.1	0.8	19
Sheep	5.5	7.4	4.8	1.0	10

* Institute of Nutrition, University of Uppsala, Uppsala, Sweden.

H.K.A. Visser (ed.), Nutrition and Metabolism of the Fetus and Infant, 253-262. All rights reserved.
Copyright © 1979 Martinus Nijhoff Publishers b.v., The Hague/Boston/London.

based on the analogy with breast-fed infants. (2) Nevertheless presently available data on both volume and composition of human milk are incomplete and there is a need for more modern studies (3). As seen in table 1 human breast milk already with respect to its crude composition seems to represent one extreme with a high lactose content and relatively low protein and mineral content. The table furthermore illustrates that there seems to be a direct relationship between the protein content as well as the protein-energy per cent on the one hand and the rate of growth of the offspring on the other as was suggested already in 1898 by BUNGE (4).

Although there consequently are obvious differences between the various mammalian species with respect to the crude composition of milk this refers not only to quantitative differences with respect to the major components but also to substantial qualitative differences. This is illustrated in table 2 which shows that in addition to the difference in protein content from the quantitative point of view as shown in table 1, there is

Table 2. *Casein/whey protein ratio in milk obtained from various mammals.*

Human	0.3		
Indian elephant	0.6		
Mouse	1.1	Kangaroo	1.0
Cat	1.1	Northern fur seal	1.1
Pig	1.4	Dolphin	1.3
		Lion	1.6
		Polar bear	1.9
Dog	2.5	Blue whale	2.0
Camel	2.9	Rhesus monkey	2.2
Buffalo	4.6	Hamster	2.5
Cow	4.7	Rat	3.2
Sheep	5.1	Guinea pig	4.4
Goat	6.3		

(Source: JENNESS, 1974. ref. 1)

Table 3. *Classification of milk nutrients (according to JENNESS and SLOAN (5)).*

Organ and species specific
Organ specific but not species specific
Not organ specific but species specific
Neither organ *nor* species specific

also a significant difference in the qualitative protein composition. Thus the casein/whey protein composition is remarkably different when milk from various mammals are compared, human milk once more being one extreme.

JENNESS and SLOAN (5) have divided the various constituents of milk into four major classes based on their milk specificity. This classification which is illustrated in table 3 seems to be a valid basis whenever the composition of milk and its physiological implication is to be discussed.

In this paper I will focus on some qualitative aspects on the milk and species specific components of human milk and their possible nutritional implication. I will, however, not comment upon the immunological aspects neither the immunoglobulins as they will be covered in the following paper(s).

No doubt the proteins represent some of the most essential components in milk as the availability of essential amino acids is a necessary requisite for the formation of new protein during the rapid growth after birth. It is also a well-known fact that milk contains a very heterogenous mixture of proteins some of them being both organ and species specific. The isolation and characterization of milk proteins is however complicated by the fact that there is a considerable tendency of the milk proteins to associate and form complex structures, a tendency which also differs with respect to various species. This has made the definition of the specific physiological and immunological characteristics of milk proteins difficult. As bovine milk has by far been most extensively studied, both methodology and nomenclature has been almost extensively devoted to bovine milk and not always suited for studies of human milk. Our knowledge regarding the nitrogen and protein composition of human breast milk and its variation during different physiological and pathological conditions has consequently for a long time been very limited.

There are however two major characteristics of human milk which makes it different from milk of other species. First human milk has a very high content of non-protein nitrogen, which constitutes as much as 25% of the total nitrogen. Interestingly, this was described many years ago by MACY and her collaborators (6) who performed a series of outstanding studies on the composition of human milk. However, her results have oddly enough been overlooked for many years. Thus it has wrongly been assumed that the protein content of human milk is 1.1–1.2%, an estimation which is based on the determination of total nitrogen and the use of the conversion factor 6.38 to give "crude protein". This however represents an overestimation by 20–25% (7).

Table 4 shows the composition of the non-protein nitrogen according to the literature and verified by us (6, 8, 9). It is seen in the table that 50% of the non-protein nitrogen is derived from urea; free amino acids and peptides constitute another 25% and creatinine, creatine and uric acid 15%. The nutritional significance of some of these compounds has however not been evaluated satisfactorily. It should, however, be remembered that SNYDERMAN et al. in 1962 described unessential nitrogen as a limiting factor for optimal nutritive value in the feeding of infants (10).

The other characteristic of human milk is the protein composition. It has earlier been stated that casein constitutes about 40% of the total protein in human milk versus 80% in bovine milk (1). However, recent analyses by LÖNNERDAL show that the casein percentage in human milk might be as low as 20% (11). This discrepancy might be due to the fact that a valid method for the quantitative estimation of casein is still lacking and casein is still defined as the protein fraction which precipitates at pH 4.6. However, if the nitrogen contents of the various human whey protein fractions, i.e. a-lactalbumin, lactoferrin, lysozyme, serum albumin and the immunoglobulins (secretory IgA, IgA, IgG, and IgM) are subtracted from the total nitrogen content there is only about 20% left to be constituted by casein. Our findings indicate that the earlier values of 40% are probably due to the co-precipitation with casein of other protein fractions such as the whey proteins. Of further interest is the fact that there are also significant differences in the physico-chemical characteristics of human casein resulting in another curd formation in the stomach than that of bovine casein, which might have a physiological implication.

The nutritional significance of the casein/whey protein ratio in human milk still has to be evaluated. It should, however, be observed that due to the specific amino acid composition of casein versus the whey proteins, this gives rise to certain characteristics of the amino acid composition of

Table 4. *Non-protein nitrogen content in human milk (values refer to mg $N/100$ ml)*

References	Urea-N	Creatine-N	Creatinine-N	Uric acid	a-Amino-N	% recovery
DENIS and						
MINOT (8)	12.6	1.5	2.1	0.8	7.2	73.5
MACY (6)	18.0	1.1	1.1	2.2	5.0	86.4
Own analyses	16.2	1.7	4.3	not determ	6.9	

the human milk versus cow's milk which is in agreement with the metabolic capacity of the infant and which will be further commented upon in another paper during this symposium. Thus the methionine/cystine ratio is extremely low in human milk while it is extremely high in casein (7). Furthermore, the content of the aromatic amino acids phenylalanine and tyrosine is much lower in the whey proteins than in casein. Consequently, human milk results in a much lower load of methionine and of the aromatic amino acids than cow's milk. This is in agreement with the limited capacity during the neonatal period to metabolize these amino acids.

The composition of the whey proteins is also rather specific for the human milk as illustrated in table 5, which shows the protein composition of the whey proteins in human mature milk versus that in bovine milk. It is seen that a-lactalbumin and lactoferrin are the two dominating whey proteins in human milk with secretory IgA as the third dominating protein. β-lactoglobulin, however, which is by far the dominating whey protein fraction in bovine milk, is completely lacking in human milk and the content of lactoferrin in bovine milk is almost negligible. The nutritional significance or immunological implication of these differences has still to be further elucidated.

The lactoferrin content of human milk is worth further comments. This is a milk-specific iron-binding glycoprotein, which is closely related to transferrin and that specifically binds two ferric ions with incorporation of two molecules of bicarbonate. It has earlier been assumed to be saturated with iron to about 10–40% (12). Recent analysis at our laboratory by FRANSSON and LÖNNERDAL has, however, revealed the iron

Table 5. *Whey protein composition in human milk and cow's milk (the values are given as mg protein/ml)*

Protein	Human milk	Cow's milk
a-lactalbumin	1.6	0.9
β-lactoglobulin	–	3.0
Lactoferrin	1.7	0.012
Lysozyme	0.4	0.0001
Serum albumin	0.4	0.3
Immunoglobulins		
IgA	1.4	0.03
IgG	0.01	0.6
IgM	0.01	0.03

(Source: HAMBRAEUS and LÖNNERDAL, unpublished observations.)

saturation of lactoferrin to be only 2–6% in milk from well-nourished Swedish mothers (13).

It is known that lactoferrin plays an essential role in the defence against gastrointestinal infections which has been assumed to be due to the fact that as it mainly occurs in unsaturated form in human milk, it binds iron so strongly that it makes it unavailable for the bacteria. Consequently, the growth of certain bacteria i.e. Escherichia coli, Staphylococci and Candida albicans is inhibited. Saturation of lactoferrin with iron, however, seems to reverse its bacteriostatic effect (14).

It has also been supposed that lactoferrin plays an essential role for the iron absorption on the intestines of the infant as it has been observed that the iron in human milk is absorbed to a much higher degree (50–75%) (15) than iron in infant formula (2–10%), where it is in the form of ferrum reductum or easily absorbable iron salts. However, only about 30% of the total iron content in human milk is bound in lactoferrin, whilst the remaining two thirds occur in the fat fraction and the low molecular fraction of human milk (13). Interestingly, we have observed that milk specimens obtained from Ethiopian mothers, malnourished and well nourished, had a very high lactoferrin content (16). This has been assumed to be due to the fact that the iron intake in the Ethiopian population is extremely high being about 300–500 mg/day (17).

It is consequently thought to be of interest to further study the effect of the iron status of the mother and her nutritional status on the iron saturation of lactoferrin as well as on the iron distribution in the other compounds present in human milk. This might give further information about the role of lactoferrin on the iron absorption as well as the explanation why iron is so well utilized from human milk.

It is obvious that there is a variation in the content of the various protein components with time of lactation and this is illustrated in table 6, which shows the content of total nitrogen, non protein nitrogen as well as of the two milk specific whey proteins a-lactalbumin and lactoferrin in Swedish mothers as well as in non-privileged Ethiopian mothers (18). It is seen that the content of the specific proteins decreases during lactation in a way similar to that of total nitrogen while the non-protein nitrogen is more constant. Although the non-privileged Ethiopian mothers had an intake of almost all nutrients except iron below 60% of recommended dietary allowances (17), almost no qualitative differences were observed as illustrated in the table. It is thus shown that the qualitative composition of breast milk is influenced to a remarkably low degree by the

Table 6. *Nitrogen and protein content in human milk and its variation during lactation (the values refer to mg/ml)*

	Duration of lactation (months)				
	0–0.5	0.5–1.5	1.5–3.5	3.5–6.5	> 6.5
TOTAL NITROGEN					
Swedish mothers	3.05	1.93	1.61	1.48	
Ethiopian non-privileged mothers		2.50	1.77	1.69	1.74
NON-PROTEIN NITROGEN					
Swedish mothers	0.43	0.46	0.41	0.38	
Ethiopian non-privileged mothers		0.43	0.36	0.34	0.33
LACTOFERRIN					
Swedish mothers	3.53	1.94	1.65	1.39	
Ethiopian non-privileged mothers		2.64	1.67	1.72	1.48
a-LACTALBUMIN					
Swedish mothers	3.62	3.26	2.78	2.68	
Ethiopian non-privileged mothers		3.58	2.76	2.65	2.58

(From HAMBRAEUS et al. 1978, ref. 18.)

nutritive status of the mother. It is therefore of special interest that FORSUM and LÖNNERDAL recently reported that when a low-protein diet containing about 7–8 energy per cent protein and a high protein diet containing 20–23 energy per cent protein were fed to well-nourished Swedish lactating mothers there was a significant difference in the nitrogen composition of the breast milk (19). Thus there was a significant and pronounced increase in the non-protein nitrogen content when a high protein diet was given instead of a low protein diet. This was partly due to an increase in the urea concentration but an increase in the concentration of the milk-specific proteins, i.e. a-lactalbumin and lactoferrin was also observed constituting about 12–19% increase or about 1.5 g more protein per day to the infant (table 7).

I have so far concentrated my discussion to the nitrogen and protein content of human milk mainly for two reasons, first, we have been most engaged in the study of these compounds at our laboratory and, secondly, it seems to be the components of human milk where we have gained most new data during the last few years. I also want to refer to the

Table 7. *Output of total nitrogen, non-protein nitrogen (NPN) and true protein in milk from mothers fed experimental diets for 4 days. (the values refer to g/day)*

	Total N $\bar{x}$ SD	N P N $\bar{x}$ SD	Protein $\bar{x}$ SD
Low protein diet	1.46 ± 0.07	0.32 ± 0.01	7.15 ± 0.47
High protein diet	1.88 ± 0.12	0.44 ± 0.05	8.75 ± 0.45
Level of significance	0.01 > p > 0.001	0.05 > p > 0.01	0.05 > p > 0.01

(From FORSUM and LÖNNERDAL, 1978, ref. 19.)

most interesting studies performed by GAULL, RÄIHÄ and their colla-borators (20) which give further evidence for the nutritive significance of the specific characteristics regarding the protein composition.

With respect to the energy content of human milk it is assumed that about 50% of the energy is derived from fat. The fat content shows significant diurnal variations being high in early mornings (21). Of special importance is the fact that the milk obtained at the end of a breast feeding has a higher fat content than the foremilk (21). This has been assumed to be of significance for the regulation of appetite in the breast fed baby. The variation in the breast milk composition with special reference to its fat content furthermore results in the fact that it is still very difficult to perform an accurate evaluation of the exact energy intake of the infant during breastfeeding. The realistic energy content of the breast milk is almost impossible to determine as the sampling technique will markedly influence the total fat and energy intake. It could therefore be stated that we still lack accurate data regarding the fat intake and energy intake in breast-fed babies.

Human milk fat contains a substantial amount of unsaturated fatty acids such as oleic acid and linoleic acid while the saturated fatty acid content is lower than in cow's milk. The composition of the fat is in-fluenced by the mothers diet (22). It is still open to question whether it is desirable to increase the content of polyunsaturated fatty acids in infant feeding either by manipulating the mother's diet or by altering the fatty acid composition of the infant formula.

Lactose represents the other energy source of human milk and plays a significant role as human milk is especially rich in lactose which consti-tutes about 7% or 40 energy per cent. Interestingly, there seems to be a reverse relationsship between the fat and lactose content when milks from various species are compared (23). Although not being an essential nutrient, lactose has been reported to have a beneficial effect on the absorption of minerals (23) and also for the protein utilization (24).

With respect to the mineral composition of human milk it is a well-known fact that human milk has a remarkably low mineral content, which probably is of physiological importance as it results in a lower renal solute load for the immature infant kidney. So far relatively few minerals have been sufficiently studied in order to constitute a basis for the recommendation of intake during infancy. Consequently, the essentiality of the mineral content in breast milk cannot be accurately evaluated. Furthermore it is still open to discussion whether the presence of trace minerals is essential as the infant has had an opportunity to store these in the tissues during the intrauterine life when they are derived from the mother. As milk represents a rich source of calcium and phosphorous it is however of interest to note that calcium content of human milk is about half of that of cow's milk and that the calcium/phosphorous ratio is 2:1 instead of 1,2:1 as in cow's milk.

Finally a few comments regarding the vitamin content. The human milk obtained from well-nourished women seems to furnish the infant with acceptable amounts of the water-soluble vitamins as well as of the fat soluble vitamins A and E. The vitamin D content has been intensively discussed during the last few years as WIDDOWSON and her collaborators have described the occurrence of water soluble vitamin D sulphate which should be biologically active (25). The necessity to supplement vitamin D to breast-fed infants is consequently worth further studies.

In conclusion it can be stated that human milk shows a series of characteristics with respect to the composition which probably has a significance from the nutritional and metabolic point of view for the infant. As our recommendations regarding the optimal nutrient intake during infancy are based on the assumption that breast milk composition represents the optimal nutrient intake, it is urgently needed that our knowledge regarding the human milk composition and its relation to various physiological and pathological parameters is further studied.

REFERENCES

1. JENNESS, R. (1974) In: Lactation: A Comprehensive Treatise, vol. III, Larsson, B.I.. and U.R. Smith eds., Academic Press, New York, p. 3.
2. ALFIN-SLATER, R.B. and D.B. JELLIFFE. (1977) Red. Clin. N. Amer. 24:3.
3. FOMON, S. (1974) Infant Nutrition, ed. 2, W.B. Saunders Co., Philadelphia, Pa.
4. BUNGE, G. (1898) Lehrbuch der Physiologische Chemie, ed. 4, Berlin & Leipzig.
5. JENNESS, R. and R.E. SLOAN. (1970) Abstr. Dairy Sci. 32:599.
6. MACY, J.G. (1949) Am. J. Dis. Child. 78:589.
7. HAMBRAEUS, L., E. FORSUM and B. LÖNNERDAL. (1977) In: Food and Immunology. Symposia of the Swedish Nutrition Foundation XIII, Hambraeus, L., L.Å. Hansson and H. McFarlane eds., Almqvist & Wiksell, Stockholm, p. 116.
8. DENIS, W. and A.S. MINOT. (1919) J. Biol. chem. 37:353.
9. FORSUM, E. and B. LÖNNERDAL. (1978) Unpublished observation.
10. SNYDERMAN, S.E., L.E. HOLT, Jr, J. DANCIS, E. ROITMAN, A. BOYER and M.E. BAYLIS. (1962) J. Nutr. 78:57.
11. LÖNNERDAL, B. (1978) Unpublished observation.
12. BULLEN, J.J., H.J. ROGERS and L. LEIGH (1972) Brit. Med. J. 1:69.
13. FRANSSON, G.-B. and LÖNNERDAL, B. (1978) XI Int. Congr. Nutr. Abstr. Rio de Janeiro, p. 152.
14. REITER, B. (1977) Personal communication.
15. MCMILLAN, J.A., F.A. OSKI, G. LOURIE, R.M. TOMARELLI, and S.A. LANDAU. (1977) Pediatrics 60:896.
16. LÖNNERDAL, B., E. FORSUM, M. GEBRE-MEDHIN and L. HAMBRAEUS. (1976) Am. J. Clin. Nutr. 29:1134.
17. GEBRE-MEDHIN, M. and A. GOBEZIE. (1975) Am. J. Clin. Nutr. 28:1322.
18. HAMBRAEUS, L., B. LÖNNERDAL, E. FORSUM and M. GEBRE-MEDHIN. (1978) Acta Paediatr. Scand. 67:561.
19. FORSUM, E. and B. LÖNNERDAL. (1978) XI Int. Congr. Nutr. Abstr. Rio de Janeiro, p. 151.
20. RÄIHÄ, N.C.R., K. HEINONEN, D.K. RASSIN and G.E. GAULL. (1976) Pediatrics 57:659.
21. HYTTEN, F.E. (1954) Brit. Med. J. 1:176.
22. INSULL, W., J. HIRSCH and T. JAMES. (1959) J. Clin. Invest. 38:443.
23. KRETSCHMER, N. (1972) Sci. Amer. 227:73.
24. FORSUM, E. (1975) Nutr. Rep. Int. 11:5.
25. LAKDAWALA, D.R. and E.M. WIDDOWSON. (1977) Lancet 1:167.

IMMUNE FACTORS IN HUMAN MILK

B. CARLSSON*, J.R. CRUZ**, B. GARCIA**, L.Å. HANSON*,
and J.J. URRUTIA**

During recent years much information has accrued concerning factors in human milk which may help the breast-fed infant in its defense against infections. Some of these factors, especially those with specific immune functions, will be briefly reviewed.

LEUCOCYTES IN HUMAN MILK

Large numbers of leucocytes are present in human milk during late pregnancy and the first few weeks of lactation. These cells are primarily macrophages, in some samples up to 80% of the cells. The macrophages contain IgA antibodies in the cytoplasm (1) presumably originating from the mammary gland and therefore supposedly representing the local synthesis of such antibodies. No specific function has been demonstrated for the milk macrophages, but it has been suggested that they might protect the mammary gland against infection. It cannot be excluded that the macrophages or their content of IgA can play a role in the defense against microorganisms in the infant's gut.

T-lymphocytes are also recognized in the milk (2, 3). According to PARMELY et al. (4) and OGRA and OGRA (5) the T-lymphocytes in milk show a different reactivity against mitogens and antigens than do T-lymphocytes in peripheral blood, suggesting that they represent different populations. It is possible that the milk T-lymphocytes may be part of a cell-mediated local immune response and that they provide some form of immunity to the neonate; it has been demonstrated that tuberculin positivity can be transferred to the baby by breast feeding (6, 7).

Human milk also contains B-lymphocytes which primarily produce

* Department of Immunology, Institute of Medical Microbiology and Department of Pediatrics, University of Göteborg, Göteborg, Sweden.
** Institute of Nutrition of Central America and Panama (INCAP), Guatemala City, Guatemala.

H.K.A. Visser (ed.), Nutrition and Metabolism of the Fetus and Infant, 263-271. All rights reserved.
Copyright © 1979 Martinus Nijhoff Publishers b.v., The Hague/Boston/London.

IgA antibodies (8). It is still unknown whether these cells represent the lymphoid cell population of the mammary gland or whether they reach the milk through the circulation. Observations in women with a Salmonella typhimurium infection during lactation have indicated that intestinal exposure may result in antibodies appearing in the milk (9). Experimental studies in rabbits (10) and in swine (11) have also suggested that intestinal exposure may be the initiator of milk antibodies. Intestinal colonization of women in late pregnancy with E.coli resulted in the appearance of leucocytes in milk a few days later forming plaques which could be recognized due to presence of secretory IgA antibodies against the O antigen of the colonizing strain (12). Experimental studies by Roux and coworkers (13) have strongly supported the notion that there is a homing of lymphoid cells from the gut after intestinal antigenic exposure, moving via the lymph and circulation to the mammary gland. The initiation of this homing seems to take place in the Peyer's patches in the gut and it is presumably directed by Ia-antigens on the epithelial cells of the mammary gland. Appearance of such Ia-antigens in the gland is under hormonal influence (14).

   The homing to the mammary gland of specific IgA-producing cells after they have been exposed to antigens from the intestinal content, in the Peyer's patches, is probably part of a generalized homing process of IgA producing cells to the mucous membranes of exocrine glands (fig. 1). As a result the breast-fed baby is provided in the maternal milk with antibodies of the secretory type against a number of intestinal microorganisms to which the baby may be exposed after birth.

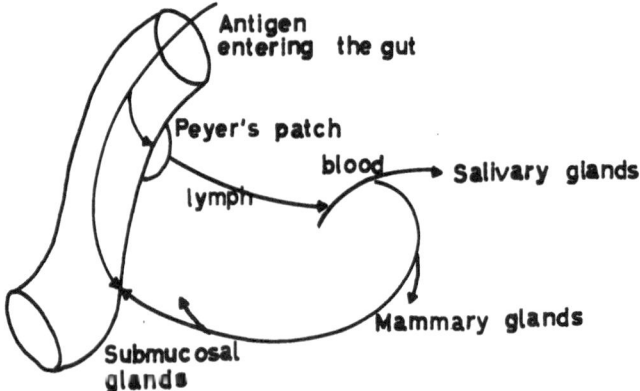

Fig. 1. Homing of IgA producing cells to exocrine glands after stimulation in the gut.

THE SECRETORY IgA ANTIBODIES OF HUMAN MILK

As a consequence of the homing mechanism, human milk contains large amounts of secretory IgA (SIgA). The SIgA is composed of two IgA monomers stabilized by two polypeptide chains, the J-chain and the secretory component. The resulting antibody molecule is resistant against enzymic degradation and pH-changes (15, 16).

Using a new technique for specific quantitation of SIgA (17) it was found that the initial values in colostrum were as high as 18.5 g/l, rapidly diminishing to slightly less than 1 g/l. It was noted that, simultaneously with the decrease, there was an increase in volume which made the total output of secretory IgA rather constant, as has been indicated in earlier studies (18, 19). We found that the concentration of SIgA is not significantly different in women from privileged and under-privileged groups in Ethiopia (20) and Guatemala (table 1) (21). This agrees with earlier

Table 1. *Levels of secretory IgA (g/l) and specific IgA antibodies (% of reference) in milk samples from rural and urban Guatemalan women.*

		Socio-economic group		
		Rural (n = 10)	Urban poor (n = 10)	Urban elite (n = 10)
SIgA/l		0.626*	0.836	1.024
SIgA/24 h		0.309	0.357	0.456
anti E.coli	a	13.9	17.3	37.1
	b	6.9	6.7	20.2
anti Salmonella A	a	8.5	10.5	12.4
	b	4.2	4.1	6.7
anti Salmonella B	a	10.0	11.2	12.6
	b	4.7	3.8	6.6
anti Salmonella C_1	a	12.0	21.3	31.5
	b	5.6	9.8	18.5
anti Salmonella C_2	a	9.2	12.9	11.8
	b	4.3	4.5	6.4
anti Salmonella D	a	8.1	9.9	12.8
	b	4.0	3.7	6.9
anti Salmonella E	a	15.9	21.6	26.8
	b	7.9	8.1	15.8
anti cow's milk	a	10.3	11.2	36.7
	b	5.5	5.1	19.6

* mean
a: antibody level/unit of volume
b: antibody level corrected for 24 h milk volume

studies on milk from Pakistani women where the levels of E.coli anti-bodies were the same as in healthy Swedish women although the Paki-stani women were severely under-nourished (22). Preliminary observa-tions in the Pakistani women suggested that their milk volumes were exceedingly low, however, diminishing their total output of secretory IgA. They were under heavy stress, with their children admitted to hospital for severe disease, so further studies are required to define whether or not lactation failure will result in decreased volumes but not lowered concentrations of milk components.

Human milk contains antibodies against a number of O and K anti-gens of E.coli. Such antigens are virulence factors of E.coli, especially the K1 antigen found on about 80% of strains causing neonatal sepsis and/or meningitis (23). This may be one reason why such infections are more common in infants which have had little breast feeding than in matched controls who get milk SIgA anti-K1 (24). In milk from exposed mothers high levels of antibodies of enteropathogenic E.coli are found (20). They also have SIgA antibodies against Shigella (25) and against E.coli and Vibrio cholerae enterotoxin (26). SIgA antibodies against Salmonella antigens are also recognized in milk (21).

In investigations of milk samples from urban elite, urban poor and rural women in Guatemala it was found that the antibody levels against E.coli enterotoxin, against E.coli O antigens and certain Salmonella O antigens were often higher in the urban elite women (table 1). The ex-planation for this is not yet obvious, but it may be related to the fact that the urban elite women use processed food which is not available to the poor women. The differences in titres can not be explained by dif-ferences in concentrations of SIgA or differences in volumes of milk which are similar in the three groups (21).

The milk also contains antibodies against viruses such as rota-virus (27) and polio-virus (28). The mode of function of the milk SIgA anti-bodies to various microbial antigens may simply be binding and neu-tralizing viruses and binding bacteria blocking their attachment to the epithelium of the gut preventing further steps of the infection process. In fact such an anti-adherence activity of milk antibodies to E.coli has been demonstrated (20, 29, 30).

INTESTINAL EXPOSURE AND VACCINATION INFLUENCING THE MAMMARY GLAND IMMUNE RESPONSE

Exposure of mucous membranes is known to induce a local secretory IgA production (16). From the above-mentioned observations of the homing process it is, however, obvious that exposure of the intestinal mucosa involving Peyer's patches will result in a transfer of the secretory IgA response also to distant exocrine glands like the mammary gland. It can therefore be expected that repeated exposure of the intestinal mucosa should result in a continuous production of milk IgA antibodies. Such repeated exposures may explain the fact that the milk contains antibodies against such a large number of different antigens from enterobacteria. It would otherwise be difficult to understand how the reportedly short lived SIgA response could be present against such an array of antigens. Still it seems unlikely that the mothers have been exposed within months to so many various antigens.

In a recent study we noticed that it was possible to boost an already existent local immune response by parenteral vaccination. Thus, Pakistani women who had been naturally exposed to V.cholerae had antibodies in the saliva as well as in the milk against the lipopolysaccharide of V.cholerae. A parenteral vaccination not only increased the serum antibodies, as expected, but also the milk and saliva antibodies with a response that was dominated by SIgA (31). In contrast, Swedish women who had no local response in the form of SIgA antibodies against the V.cholerae in the saliva or milk did not show any booster effect on SIgA of parenteral vaccination (21). It therefore seems possible to boost the milk SIgA antibody titres by parenteral vaccination if a local response already exists. In the absence of such a response the parenteral vaccination will have no effect on the SIgA levels.

More recently, it has been noted that in lactating women who already have secretory IgA antibodies in their milk against polio-virus, peroral vaccination with live polio-virus lowers these titres. This was especially evident if cholera vaccination was performed simultaneously, but peroral administration of polio vaccine alone was found to significantly diminish the titres in 6 out of 10 women as well (21). The interpretation of the finding is not yet apparent, but may be related to a local consumption of the virus SIgA antibodies, or possible induction of tolerance in the gut. Further studies will have to investigate this possibility and also determine whether or not it is possible to boost the milk antibody

response, instead by using an inactivated polio vaccine given parenterally. Anyhow, these studies indicate that it is possible to modulate the
local antibody response of the mammary gland occurring as SIgA antibodies in the milk.

FOOD ANTIBODIES IN HUMAN MILK

As a consequence of the assumption that the Peyer's patches sample
antigens from the intestinal content exposing lymphoid cells that home
to exocrine glands, it can be expected that milk contains antibodies
against food proteins also and not only against antigens from more or
less invasive microorganisms. Antibodies against cow's milk have been
demonstrated in human milk (32, 33). Significantly lower levels of SIgA
milk antibodies to cow's milk were found in groups of under-privileged
mothers from Guatemala, where cow's milk is not included in the diet,
than in an urban elite group (table 1).

The role of food antibodies in the gut is not clear, but since Walker et
al. (34) found that antibodies can diminish the uptake of native un-
degraded food proteins in the gut and increase the amount of degraded
material absorbed, it is possible that the cow's milk antibodies in the
human milk play a similar role in the infant. This was analysed in a
comparative study of infants which were directly transferred from breast
feeding to artificial feeds and infants which were kept on mixed feeding,
that is breast feeding and artificial feeds, for more than 3 weeks. It was
seen that the infants on mixed feeding had significantly lower titres of
serum antibodies against cow's milk proteins than the others (32). This
suggests that the milk SIgA antibodies may diminish the systemic exposure to potentially allergenic food components. This may be of relevance till the time when the infants' own SIgA production in the gut can
take over such an activity. On this basis it may be suggested that breast
feeding should be prolonged, and a period of mixed feeding, including
breast milk, should be inserted before weaning of infants with atopic
heredity.

NON-SPECIFIC HOST-DEFENSE FACTORS IN HUMAN MILK

The difference in pH and consistency of the stool of the breast fed baby
compared to that of the artificially fed is striking. The reason for this
difference is multifactorial. Presumably the SIgA antibodies may add to

the reduction in bacterial numbers and prevention of the attachment of the bacteria to the epithelium of the intestine. Many other components may, however, take part in this like lactoferrin which has been shown to be bacteriostatic by binding iron which is required as a growth factor for bacteria (35). Obviously, the bacteria produce chelating agents which bind iron in competition with lactoferrin. In the presence of antibodies the production and/or release of these chelating agents is interfered with and as a result lactoferrin binds the iron and the bacteriostatic effect becomes more evident than with antibodies or lactoferrin alone (36). Other components such as lysozyme and bifidus factors may add to the conditions that seem to make lactobacilli thrive in contrast to E.coli which are found in lower numbers in breast-fed infants than in non-breast-fed (37).

Taken together, human milk contains many components which may with combined efforts diminish the number of potentially pathogenic microorganisms in the infants' gut. With the lower numbers of such pathogens the chances for the SIgA antibodies to prevent attachment of the microorganisms to the epithelial membranes of the gut may be better (30). The efficiency of these various host-defense factors in human milk may be an important reason why repeated studies have indicated that breast-fed infants have less frequent infections, especially in the gastrointestinal tract, than artificially fed (38, 39, 40, 41).

CONCLUSIONS

Human milk contains in early lactation considerable numbers of macrophages as well as T- and B-lymphocytes. The biological significance of these cells has not been settled.

The dominating immunoglobulin in milk is secretory IgA which presumably is locally produced in the mammary gland. The special structure of these SIgA antibodies make them resistant against proteolysis, so they can function in the gastrointestinal tract. It seems that this local antibody response is closely connected with exposure to antigens in the intestine. As a result the human milk contains antibodies of the secretory IgA type against a large number of antigens of various microorganisms appearing in the gut, such as E.coli, V.cholerae, Shigella, Salmonella and polio- and rota-virus. These antibodies may primarily function by binding the microorganisms, hindering them from attaching to and infecting via the mucous membrane of the gut.

Recent findings have indicated that it is possible to boost an already existent mammary gland antibody response by parenteral vaccination.

Human milk also contains antibodies against food proteins which may be of importance to prevent the development of food allergy in atopic infants. Through a prolonged period of mixed feeding with human milk and artificial feeds while the infant develops its own secretory IgA system, a diminished exposure to the potential allergens of the artificial feeds may result, decreasing the risk for atopic allergic reactions.

Human milk contains several non-specific host-defense factors including lactoferrin which may aid in lowering the number of potential pathogens in the infants' gut, aiding the secretory IgA antibodies in their role as preventors of contact between microorganisms and host tissue.

ACKNOWLEDGEMENTS

This work has been supported by SAREC, the Swedish Medical Research Council (No. 215), the Wenner-Gren and Arla Foundations and Ellen, Walter and Lennart Hesselman Foundation for Scientific Research. J.R. Cruz was receiving a WHO grant.

REFERENCES

1. PITTARD, W.B., S.H. POLMAR and A.A. FANAROFF. (1977) J. Reticuloend. Soc. 22:597.
2. SMITH, C.W. and A.S. GOLDMAN. (1968) Pediat. Res. 2:103.
3. DÍAZ-JOUANEN, E.P. and R.C. WILLIAMS. (1974) Clin. Immunol. Immunopathol. 3:248.
4. PARMELY, M.J., D.B. REATH, A.E. BEER and R.E. BILLINGHAM. (1977) Transpl. Proc. 9:1477.
5. OGRA, S.S. and P.L. OGRA. (1978) J. Pediat. 92:550.
6. SCHLESINGER, J.J. and H.D. COVELLI. (1977) Lancet 2:529.
7. MOHR, J.A., R. LEU and W. MABRY. (1970) J. Surg. Onc. 2:163.
8. MURILLO, G.J. and A.S. GOLDMAN. (1970) Pediat. Res. 4:71.
9. ALLARDYCE, R.A., D.J.C. SHEARMAN, D.B.L. McCLELLAND, K. MARWICK, A.J. SIMPSON and R.B. LAIDLAW. (1974) Brit. Med. J. 3:307.
10. MONTGOMERY, P.C., B.R. ROSNER and J. COHN. (1974) Immun. Common. 3:143.
11. BOHL, E.H. and L.J. SAIF. (1975) Infect. Immun. 11:23.
12. GOLDBLUM, R.M., S. AHLSTEDT, B. CARLSSON, L.Å. HANSON, U. JODAL, G. LIDIN-JANSON and A. SOHL-ÅKERLUND. (1975) Nature 257:797.
13. ROUX, M.E., M. McWILLIAMS, J.M. PHILLIPS-QUAGLIATA, P. WEISZ-CARRINGTON and M.E. LAMM. (1978) J. Exp. Med. 147:934.
14. KLARESKOG, L., U. FORSUM and P.A. PETERSON. In manuscript.
15. TOMASI, T.D. and J.M. BIENENSTOCK. (1968) Adv. Immunol. 9:11.
16. HANSON, L.Å and P. BRANDTZAEG. (1979) In: Immunologic Disorders in Infants and Children, Stiehm, E.R. and V.A. Fulginiti eds., W.B. Saunders, Philadelphia, Pa., In press.

17. SOHL-ÅKERLUND, A., L.Å. HANSON, S. AHLSTEDT and B. CARLSSON. (1977) Scand. J. Immunol. 6:1275.
18. McCLELLAND, D.B.L., J. McGRATH and R.R. SAMSON. (1978) Acta Paediatr. Scand. suppl. 271:1.
19. SCHUBERT, J. and A. GRÜNBERG. (1949) Schweiz. Med. Wochenschr. 79:1007.
20. HANSON, L.Å., S. AHLSTEDT, B. CARLSSON, S.P. FÄLLSTRÖM, B. KAIJSER, B.S. LIND-BLAD, A. SOHL- ÅKERLUND and C. SVANBORG- EDEN. (1978) Acta Paediatr. Scand. 67.577.
21. HANSON, L.Å., B. CARLSSON, J.R. CRUZ, B. GARCIA, J. HOLMGREN, S.R. KHAN, B.S. LINDBLAD, A.-M. SVENNERHOLM, B. SVENNERHOLM and J. URRUTIA. (1978) National Institute of Child Health and Human Development Conference on the Immunology of Breast Milk. In press.
22. CARLSSON, B., S. AHLSTEDT, L.Å. HANSON, G. LININ-JANSON, B.S. LINDBLAD and R. SULTANA. (1976) Acta Paediatr. Scand. 65:216.
23. ROBBINS, J.B., G.H. McCRACKEN, E.C. GOTSCHLICH, F. ØRSKOV, I. ØRSKOV and L.Å. HANSON. (1974) New Engl. J. Med. 290:1216.
24. WINBERG, J. and G. WESSNER. (1971) Lancet 1:1091.
25. CARLSSON, B., T. MEITERT, E. GARON, L. COGULESCU and L.Å. HANSON. In manuscript.
26. HOLMGREN, J., L.A. HANSON, B. CARLSSON, B.S. LINDBLAD and J. RAHIMTOOLA. (1976) Scand. J. Immunol. 5:867.
27. SIMHON, A. and L.J. MATA. (1977) Lancet 1:39.
28. HODES, H.L., R. BERGER, E. AINBENDER, M.M. HEVIZY, H.D. ZEPP and S. KOCHWA. (1964) J. Pediat. 65:1017.
29. SVANBORG- EDEN, C. and A.-M. SVENNERHOLM. (1978) Infect. Immun. 22:790.
30. HANSON, L.Å., S. AHLSTEDT, B. CARLSSON, B. KAIJSER, P. LARSSON, I. MATTSBY BALTZER, A. SOHL-ÅKERLUND, C. SVANBORG-EDÉN and A.-M SVENNERHOLM. (1978) In: Secretory immunity and Infection, Mc Ghee J.R., J. Mestecky and J.L. Babb eds., Plenum Publishing Corporation, p. 165.
31. SVENNERHOLM, A.-M., J. HOLMGREN, L.Å. HANSON, B.S. LINDBLAD, F. QUERESHI and J. RAHIMTOOLA. (1977) Scand. J. Immunol 6:1345.
32. HANSON, L.A., S. AHLSTEDT, B. CARLSSON and S.P. FÄLLSTRÖM. (1977) Int. Arch. Allergy appl. Immunol. 54:457.
33. McCLELLAND, D.B.L. and T.T. McDONALD. (1976) Lancet 2:1251.
34. WALKER, W.A., M. WU, K.J. ISSELBACHER and K.J. BLOCH. (1975) J. Immunol 115:854.
35. BULLEN, J.J. (1976) In: Acute Diarrhea in Childhood (Ciba Foundation Symposium 42), Amsterdam, North-Holland, p. 149.
36. GRIFFITHS, E., J. HUMPHREYS, A. LEACH and L. SCANLON. (1978) Infect. Immun. 22:312.
37. HAENEL, H. (1970) Am. J. Clin. Nutr. 23:1433.
38. TASSOVATZ, B. and A. KOTSITCH. (1961) Ann. Pediat. 8:285.
39. GERRARD, J.W. (1974) Pediatrics 54:757.
40. HANSON, L.A and J. WINBERG. (1972) Arch. Dis. Childh. 47:845.
41. GOLDMAN, A.S. and C.W. SMITH. (1973) J. Pediat. 82:1082.

THE EFFECTS OF PASTEURISATION ON
IMMUNE FACTORS IN HUMAN MILK

J.D. BAUM*, MA, MSC. MD. FRCP, DCH

The recent literature on human milk emphasises the specificity of its biochemical composition which sets it apart from even the most modern humanised milk formulas. Thus there remains little doubt that for the term infant the ideal food is his own mother's fresh milk. There is less certainty, however, about the optimal food for pre-term infants.

Recently, ATKINSON et al. (1) have compared the composition of the milk from mothers of pre-term infants with milk from mothers of term infants, the milk samples being collected at comparable times after birth. This small study showed that the total nitrogen content of the milk of the mothers who delivered pre-term was significantly higher than the milk from the mothers who delivered at term. In the absence of evidence to the contrary this might be interpreted to mean that the ideal food for a pre-term infant is his own mother's fresh pre-term milk.

There has been a recent growth of knowledge relating to the antimicrobial properties of human milk. Lactoferrin for example has been shown to serve the dual purpose of an iron transport protein and a bacteriostatic agent for E. coli (2). Milk IgA has been shown to offer a wide range of specific immunity to the baby reflecting the bacterial flora of the individual mother and her baby (3). The specific function of the large number of lymphocytes and macrophages in human milk are currently under active investigation taking a lead from the report of PITT et al. (4) who showed that in newborn mice the cellular component of the species specific milk could protect against experimentally induced necrotising enterocolitis. This information in conjunction with biochemical considerations strongly supports the practice of feeding pre-term infants with their own mothers' fresh milk.

There are, however, problems in securing the supply of fresh milk from the baby's own mother for all pre-term infants in Special Care Baby

* Clinical Reader in Paediatrics, Oxford University, John Radcliffe Hospital, Headington, Oxford, England.

H.K.A. Visser (ed.), Nutrition and Metabolism of the Fetus and Infant, 273-283. All rights reserved.
Copyright © 1979 Martinus Nijhoff Publishers b.v., The Hague/Boston/London.

Units. In a recent survey at the John Radcliffe Hospital we have shown that 56% of the mothers of babies admitted to the United initially wanted to try to breast feed their infants but that of these mothers only 70% were successful in sustaining their lactation throughout the period of the baby's admission. The failure rate was particularly high among the mothers of the infants of lowest birth weight who spent the longest time in the Unit. The reasons for this low success rate in sustaining lactation are manyfold. They include the fact that mothers with social disadvantage are over-represented in the population whose babies come to the Special Care Baby Unit. These mothers are likely to be the least motivated in sustaining their lactation and beset with the greatest difficulties in maintaining constant contact with the Special Care Baby Unit. Even among the babies whose mothers do maintain lactation successfully, there are problems in securing supplies of the baby's own mother's fresh milk for each feed throughout the hospital stay.

It follows from this that if one decides on a policy of feeding all babies in the Special Care Baby Unit on human milk, one is forced into providing some system of human milk banking. In rationalising the establishment of a human milk bank one must weigh the potential advantages of using human milk in terms of nutrients, humoral immunity and possible cellular immunity against the disadvantages or hazards of such a system in terms of bacterial and viral contamination, the presence of drugs and environmental chemicals and the variation in the nutritional value of the pooled milk. In the present discussion I shall only deal with two of the variables in this exercise of rationalisation, namely the bacterial safety of the milk and the preservation of humoral immune factors in the milk.

THE PATHWAY OF DONATED MILK FROM PRODUCER TO CONSUMER

In order to clarify the magnitude of the problems of milk handling I will trace the pathway that milk follows in the Oxford human milk banking system from donor to consumer. Milk is predominantly collected from mothers in their homes who either donate expressed breast milk (expressed by hand or by milk pump) or drip breast milk, the milk that drips spontaneously from the non-feeding breast, which occurs in about 20% of breast feeding mothers (5) This milk is collected into sterile containers and kept in the home refrigerator or freezer. The problems of a bacterial contamination at this stage include faults in hand washing technique, breast cleanliness and the degree of sterility of the milk receptacle. There are also problems in relation to the temperature of the home refrigerator or freezer which will have an effect on the rate of bacterial growth. The temperature of the average refrigerator and freezer is $+4\,°C$ and $-20\,°C$, respectively, but there is wide variation depending on the quality of the individual machine and seasonal climatic variations. There are also variations in the period of time that the milk stays at home prior to collection by the milk collection volunteers. The milk is transported to the hospital in picnic-type freezer boxes, the temperature of which is not guaranteed but frequently no colder than $+5\,°C$. The time taken for the milk to travel from the home to the hospital varies from a half hour to several hours according to the distance from the hospital and the route taken.

The milk on arrival in the hospital is transferred from the picnic freezer box into the reception refrigerator at $+4\,°C$. As soon as possible after the milk has arrived in the reception refrigerator, and as soon as the milk arriving frozen has thawed, the individual donations are pooled and the pooled milk poured into bottles for pasteurisation. Following pasteurisation a sample of milk from one of the bottles is sent for bacteriology, while the rest of the milk bottles are frozen to $-20\,°C$ to await use pending the results of the post-pasteurisation bacteriology. If the milk is declared "clean" it is marked as such and remains deep frozen until it is used.

On the day prior to use the bottles are taken out of the freezer in accordance with the nursery demands and placed in the dispensing refrigerator to thaw overnight. The following day small aliquots of milk are poured from the 100 ml bottles which can then be used on the ward to deliver the small volumes of milk required by the very low birth weight babies avoiding the problem of large volumes of milk standing around in the nursery in unrefrigerated conditions.

A diagramatic representation of the temperature pathway of the milk from consumer to the baby is shown in figure 1. It can be seen that the milk leaves the mother at $37\,°C$ and, in most homes, is placed in the deep freeze at $-20\,°C$; it is then transported to the hospital reception refrigerator and allowed to thaw; it is then pasteurised, frozen, thawed and delivered to the baby at nursery room temperature. Thus the milk goes through five major changes of temperature involving four changes in physical state in its pathway from the donating mother to the baby in the nursery.

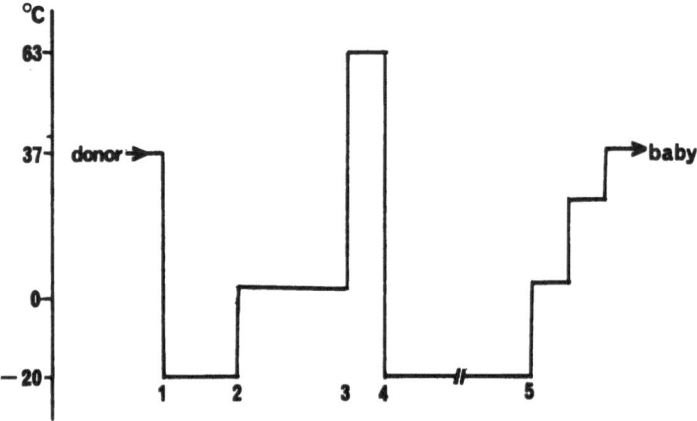

Fig. 1. The temperature profile of human milk from donor to baby.

THE BALANCE BETWEEN BACTERIAL SAFETY AND THE PRESERVATION OF THE IMMUNE FACTORS IN MILK

For each bacterial species a thermal death line can be drawn indicating the number of surviving bacteria at a given temperature against the duration of exposure to that temperature. This is illustrated in figure 2. Since the vertical scale is logarithmic the milk never, theoretically, becomes strictly sterile. Thus the time required to reach a given bacterial count in the milk will depend upon the degree of bacterial contamination of the initial milk sample. While each bacterial species has its own thermal death line it appears that for the majority of common milk organisms exposure at 62.5 °C for 30 min will greatly reduce the colony count.

The problem of achieving clean milk without destroying the immune proteins in milk is illustrated in figure 3. The dotted line represents a theoretical statement of the destruction of milk IgA in comparison with the thermal death line for E. coli. This suggests that there is a margin of discrimination which should allow bacterial destruction with immunoglobin preservation provided that the system of heat treatment is precise.

There have been a number of studies published relating to the effects of various forms of heat treatment on the destruction of immune factors in human milk (7, 8, 9, 10, 11). The major conclusions are summarised in table 1. The various authors agree that IgA is well preserved under the conditions of classical pasteurisation (that is 62.5 °C for 30 min), but that

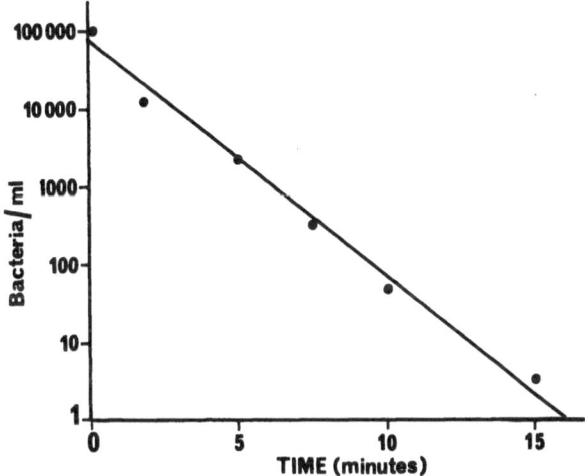

Fig. 2. The thermal death line for E. coli (redrawn from a paper given by H. Burton at a Symposium on the protective properties of human milk and the effects of processing on them (6)).

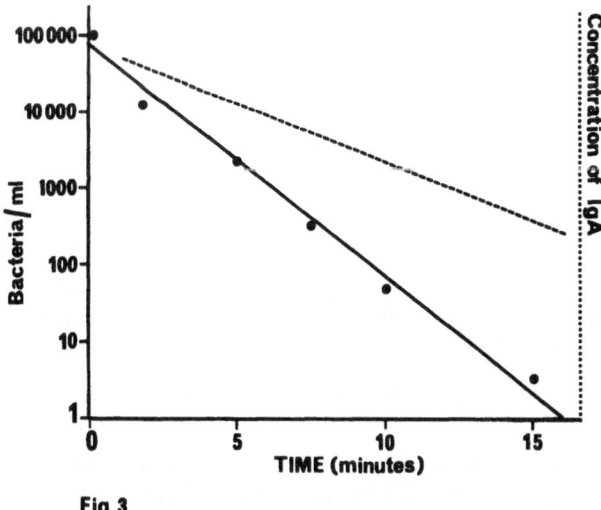

Fig 3

Fig. 3. Comparative thermal destruction of E. coli and IgA (redrawn from a paper given by R.L.J. Lyster at a Symposium on the protective properties of human milk and the effects of processing on them (6)).

Table 1. *The percentage survival of some immune factors in human milk with different heat treatments.*

	Evans et al. (ref. 7)		Ford et al. (ref. 8)			Liebhaber et al. (ref. 9)	Gibbs et al. (ref. 10)		Raptopoulou-Gigi et al. (ref. 11)	
	$62.5\,°C \times 30'$	$73\,°C \times 30'$	$62.5\,°C \times 30'$	$72\,°C \times 15'$	$100\,°C \times 15'$	$63\,°C \times 30'$	$62.5\,°C \times 30'$	$100\,°C \times 3'$	$62.5\,°C \times 30'$	$100\,°C \times 15'$
IgA	100	0	80	50	–	67	80	0	100	0
Lysozyme	76	2	100	65	0	–	64	0	–	–
Lactoferrin	43	1	40	5	–	–	–	–	100	0

it is destroyed progressively under conditions of greater time and temperature exposure. The same holds true for lysozyme. EVANS et al. (7) and FORD et al. (8) found that less than 50% of lactoferrin survived pasteurisation. However RAPTOPOULOU-GIGI (11) reported that 100% of the lactoferrin survived. This discrepancy is interesting in that EVANS et al. and FORD et al. describe the exact experimental conditions used for the milk heat treatment, employing 2 ml of milk in a test tube immersed in a precisely controlled temperature bath. RAPTOPOULOU-GIGI et al. on the other hand do not describe the experimental conditions employed and it is possible that herein lies the difference in the heat destruction of lactoferrin reported.

An additional biological test of the preservation of the bacteriostatic factors in human milk has been reported by FORD et al. (8) and GIBBS et al. (10). In these experiments milk was inoculated with E. coli and incubated for 4 hr at 37 °C. Growth of E. coli achieved was compared when the milk was raw, pasteurised and boiled. As shown in figure 4 pasteurised milk was similar to raw milk in its bacteriostatic effect in contrast to boiled milk in which the E. coli grew rapidly. This suggests that the immunologically active bacteriostatic factors in human milk were largely intact after pasteurisation.

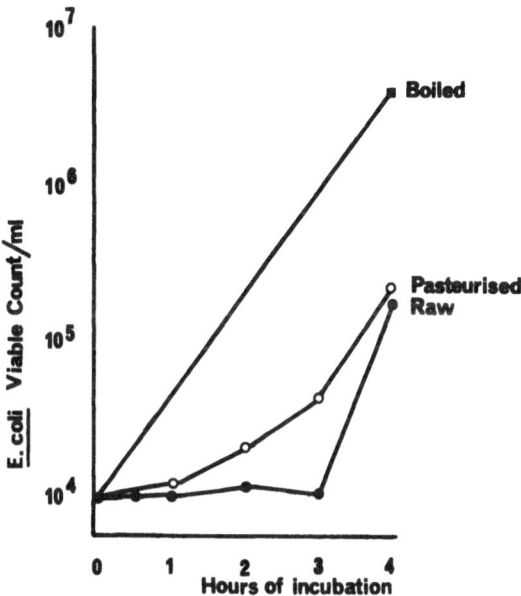

Fig. 4. Multiplication of E. coli, as viable count/ml, during incubation at 37 °C with raw, pasteurised and boiled milk (10).

PRECISION IN PASTEURISATION

It is likely that there is a relatively small difference in the time/temperature exposure of milk which will effectively remove bacteria and that which will destroy the immunologically active proteins. In order to steer this narrow course on a daily basis in a Special Care Unit human milk bank, some system of accurate and automated heat treatment is necessary. The Oxford Human Milk Pasteuriser* was designed to meet these requirements(10). It is automated so that bottled milk is accurately exposed to 62.5 °C for 30 min. The temperature profile of this pasteurisation process is shown in figure 5. However, even a simple system such as this will only subject the milk in the bottles to a reliable time/temperature exposure if there is constancy in the milk bottle design itself. Figure 6 shows the temperatures of milk exposed to pasteurisation in two alternative milk bottles, a rounded glass bottle in comparison with an elon-

*Available from Vickers Ltd., Medical Engineering, Priestley Road, Basingstoke, Hants.

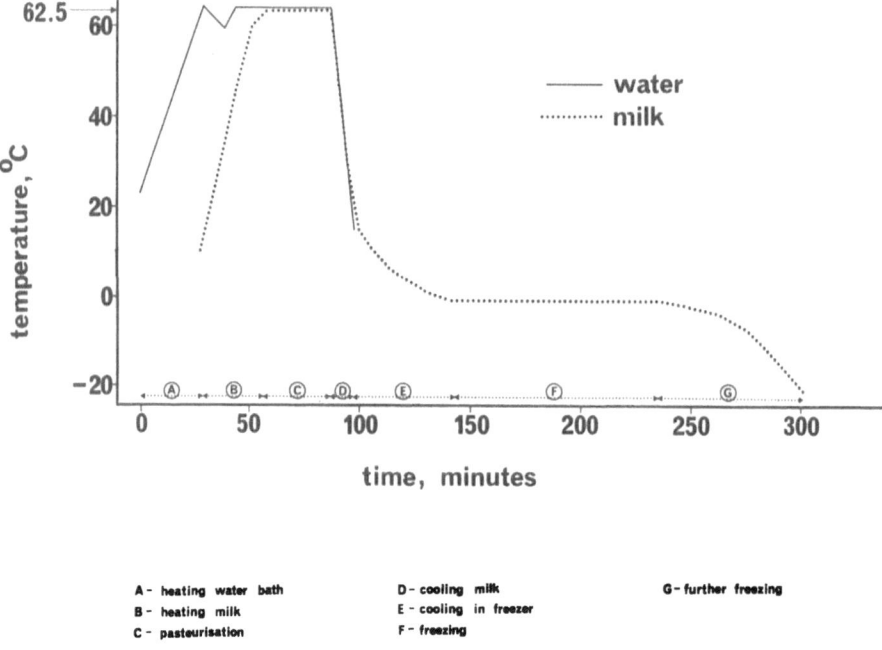

Fig. 5. The time/temperature profile during the pasteurisation of 40 × 100 ml bottles of human milk using the Oxford Human Milk Pasteuriser.

gated plastic bottle rectangular in its cross section. However, these differences are small and are only shown to illustrate the detailed considerations necessary if one is aiming to expose milk to a very precise heat treatment.

THE EFFICIENCY OF THE OXFORD PASTEURISER IN ELIMINATING BACTERIA

We have shown that provided the initial bacterial count is overall less than 10^6 colonies/ml then the Oxford Pasteuriser will effectively produce a "sterile" milk (10). More recently, LUCAS and ROBERTS (12) have shown that this is particularly true for the pathogenic organisms E. coli, staph. aureus and Group B β-haemolytic streptococci. The same study shows that in the case of organisms that are less certainly pathogenic, although the counts were greatly reduced following pasteurisation a strictly sterile "milk" was not uniformly produced.

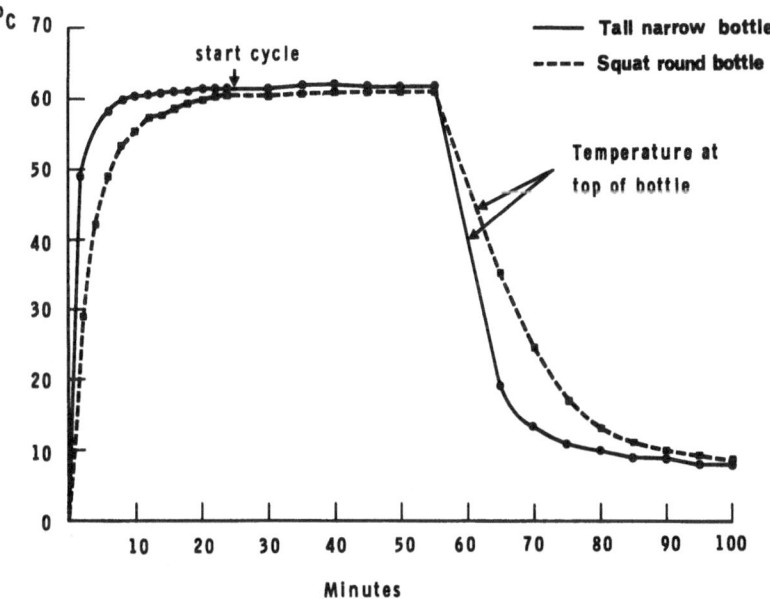

Fig. 6. A comparison of the milk temperatures during pasteurisation inside a squat cylindrical glass bottle compared with an elongated plastic bottle rectangular in its cross-section. The latter bottle design is better suited for rapid heat exchange. (This data was made available by courtesy of P. ROLFE and P. GODDARD, The Department of Bio-Engineering, Department of Paediatrics, John Radcliffe Hospital.)

The conclusion from these experiments is that provided the initial milk is relatively clean then the Oxford Pasteuriser is efficient in producing a "sterile" milk. The most important details which we have found to require attention in producing a clean milk are: strict attention to hand washing by the mother; treatment of the milk collecting utensils with a hypochlorite solution; and storage of the milk in the home freezer rather than refrigerator.

CELLULAR IMMUNITY

It seems unlikely that one can devise a simple form of human milk banking which will secure the delivery to the infant of immunologically functional human milk cells. If one refers back to the pathway that the milk must travel from the donor in the home to the infant in the Special Care Baby Unit, it appears that the amount of handling and changes in temperature and physical state, to which the milk will be subjected, make it unlikely that enough live human milk cells will survive to have any worthwhile effects. This is an important negative consideration, since there has been a move towards the use of unpasteurised pooled banked human milk on the assumption that the avoidance of heat treatment will give the baby the advantage of live human milk cells.

CONCLUSIONS

Ideally pre-term infants should receive their own mothers fresh milk for each feed. However, for the majority of infants in Special Care Baby Units this is not a practical proposition. If one believes that there are advantages in giving human milk to pre-term infants, some form of human milk banking must be used.

It is unlikely that one can usefully deliver live human milk cells from a human milk bank. This being the case there seems little purpose in using raw or untreated pooled human milk, since such a system carries with it the unknown hazard of giving certain doses of live bacteria in the milk. There is no information on which to base any criteria for acceptable doses of bacteria given to infants in this way.

Using a precise system of pasteurisation it is possible to greatly reduce or eliminate bacterial contamination from a milk pool while preserving the majority of the immunologically active proteins. In this way it seems possible that one can achieve the best compromise of bacteriological safety and immunological advantage. Such a system however in no way reduces the importance of strict attention to cleanliness and care in every stage throughout the process of the collection and handling of the donated milk.

REFERENCES

1. ATKINSON, S.A., M.H. BRYAN and G.H. ANDERSON. (1978) J. Pediat. 93:67.
2. BULLEN, J.J., H.J. ROGERS and L. LEE. (1972) Brit. Med. J. 1:69.
3. LODINOVA, R. and V. JOUJA. (1977) Acta Paediatr. Scand. 66:705.
4. PITT, J., B. BARLOW and W.C. HEIRD. (1977) Pediatr. Res. 11:906.
5. LUCAS, A., J.A.H. GIBBS and J.D. BAUM. (1978) Early Hum. Develop. 2:351.
6. Symposium Report (1978) Arch. Dis. Childh. 53:684.
7. EVANS, T.J., H.C. RILEY, L.M. NEALE, J.A. DODGE and V.M. LEWARNE. (1978) Arch. Dis. Childh. 53:239.
8. FORD, J.E., B.A. LAW, V.M.E. MARSHALL and B. REITER. (1977) J. Pediat. 90:29.

9. LIEBHABER, M., N.J. LEWISTON, M.T. ASQUITH, L. OLDS-ORROYO and P. SUNSHINE. (1977) J. Pediat. 91:897.
10. GIBBS, J.H., C. FISHER, S. BHATTACHARYA, P. GODDARD and J.D. BAUM. (1977) Early Hum. Develop. 1:227.
11. RAPTOPOULOU-GIGI, M., K. MARWICK and B.B.L. McCLELLAND. (1977) Brit. Med. J. 1:12.
12. LUCAS, A. and C.D. ROBERTS. (1978) Brit. Med. J. 1:80.

FEEDING PRE-TERM INFANTS WITH RAW
AND HEAT-STERILISED HUMAN MILK:
EFFECTS ON FAECAL FLORA

L.A. GOTHEFORS* and PAMELA A. DAVIES**

Bacterial infection, particularly that caused by enteric organisms, occurs more commonly in pre-term than in mature infants. In the last ten years the care of low birth weight babies has become increasingly technical and complex, and survival rates, especially in the smallest infants, are continuing to rise. As this intensive care becomes regionalised, certain units tend to have relatively large numbers of very small, often ill babies, in whom both the risks of infection and the use of antimicrobial drugs are increased; and illnesses such as necrotizing enterocolitis have also increased, perhaps in parallel. The scientific basis for the antimicrobial properties of human milk has now become more firmly established (1), and there has been renewed interest in the ability of such milk to augment the pre-term newborn's fragile defences against infenction. When the food is human rather than cow's milk there is also evidence that certain at least of the constituents are more effectively assimilated, and that metabolic imbalance is less (2, 3, 4). The fact of establishing and continuing lactation, too, may be of psychological help to a mother, faced as she often is with a period of separation from her baby after birth.

Since the beginning of the century the healthy mature breast-fed infant has been considered to develop an intestinal flora predominating in bifidobacteria and lactobacilli. Although there are now known to be many exceptions to this rule (H.B. LUNDEQUIST and J. WINBERG, personal communication), it is probably still true to say that the growth of Gram-negative enteric bacteria capable of causing serious infection is suppressed, a state of affairs which should be of benefit to the low birth weight infant. Previous work on the flora of ill and low birth weight infants fed a dried cow's milk has shown that they have larger numbers of

* Present address: Department of Paediatrics, University Hospital, S-90185 Umeå, Sweden.
** From the Departments of Bacteriology, Royal Postgraduate Medical School, and Paediatrics and Neonatal Medicine, Hammersmith Hospital, London.

H.K.A. Visser (ed.), Nutrition and Metabolism of the Fetus and Infant, 285-295. All rights reserved.
Copyright © 1979 Martinus Nijhoff Publishers b.v., The Hague/Boston/London.

Escherichia coli in their faeces than do mature healthy well-grown infants fed the same milk (5). Immature infants who are fed on human milk are usually unable to suck at the breast, and the expressed milk used in the past has been boiled and terminally autoclaved and given by tube. Such heating to high temperatures destroys IgA, lactoferrin and lysozyme (6), and these are all important antimicrobial proteins. The latter may, on the other hand, be largely preserved by a precise system of pasteurisation (7, 8). We have studied the faecal flora of pre-term infants fed raw (unheated) human milk, heat-sterilised (as above) human milk (pasteurised milk unfortunately not being available to us), and modified dried cow's milk to see what differences if any could be found in their faecal flora.

PATIENTS AND METHODS

Patients

The 27 infants studied were among those admitted to the neonatal intensive care units of Hammersmith Hospital and Queen Charlotte's Hospital, London, during a 9 month period between June, 1977 and February, 1978. Eighteen infants, selected because their mothers wished to breast feed, were given human milk; 7 of them were fed raw milk, and 11 heatsterilised milk. The remaining 9 infants were fed modified dried cow's milk. The mother's permission for the study was obtained in every case. Details of birth weight and gestational age are shown in table 1. The majority of the infants were ill initially and 17 of the 27 were given one or more courses of animicrobial drugs systemically (usually benzyl penicillin and gentamicin). Five of the 27 were fed to begin with via in-

Table 1. *Birth weight and gestational age in those fed raw or heated human milk, or cow's milk.*

	Number of infants	Birth weight (median and range) g.	Gestational age (median and range) w.
Fresh human milk	7	1550 (760–1920)	32 (26–37)
Heat-sterilised human milk	11	1410 (700–1860)	31 (28–35)
Modiefied cow's milk	9	1510 (965–1940)	32 (30–36)

dwelling oro- or nasojejunal silastic tubes, the remainder by indwelling oro- or nasogastric polyvinyl tubes. Intravenous dextrose or dextrose saline supplements were needed initially in some infants.

Milks

Human milk

i) *Unheated:* Milk from the infants own mother was always used unless her supply failed, but frequent supplementation was necessary from the supplies of other mothers on the lying in wards or later at home. Milk was usually expressed using an Egnell breast pump, but occasionally manually. It was stored at 4 °C for no longer than 6 hr, or for longer periods at -20 °C.

ii) *Heated:* This was collected as above, but then heated to > 100 °C for 15 min before being stored at 4 °C for 24 hr, or deep frozen until use.

An analysis of representative samples (made by D.B.L. McClelland, Edinburgh) showed that levels of IgA, lactoferrin and lysozyme were unexceptional in raw milk that had been deep frozen, but were destroyed, as expected, by the heat sterilisation.

Dried cow's milk

Two modified (low protein, partially or completely filled and demineralised) feeds of cow's milk (Cow and Gate Premium and SMA Gold Cap), commercially prepared elsewhere, were used.

Bacteriological specimens

Stool specimens were transported under oxygen free nitrogen to the laboratory and processed in an anaerobic glove box. The following media were inoculated with serial dilutions up to 10^{-8}: blood agar, neomycin blood agar, tomato juice agar, MacConkey agar, a 'Bifid medium' and Saboraud dextrose agar. After incubation (up to 5 days for the anaerobic cultures) the plates were examined and organisms forming visible colonies were subcultured and further identified with Gram stain, gas liquid chromatography and some biochemical tests. All manipulations were carried out in the anaerobic glove box. Quantitative counts were achieved by noting the number of colonies of each type on a suitable dilution plate.

RESULTS

These are shown in tables 2, 3 and 4 and figures 1 and 2. The only difference which could be ascribed to the feeding of raw (unheated) human milk was that Clostridia species, and perhaps Bacteroides species had a reduced incidence during the first week of feeding (table 2). Unlike the situation in healthy mature infants (9), the faecal flora did not become stabilised for 2 to 3 weeks after birth. Escherichia coli was a common organism and feeding with raw human milk did not reduce its incidence (tables 2 and 3). Coliforms in fact dominated in numbers

Table 2. *Incidence of some microorganisms in faecal specimens from pre-term infants, aged 3–7 days, in relation to diet.*

	Raw breast milk (12 spec)	Heated breast milk (18 spec)	Cows milk derivatives (16 spec)
Clostridium	1	4	7
Bacteroides	2	1	7
Bifidobacterium	2	1	4
Lactobacillus	1	1	2
Escherichia coli	10	2	7
Klebsiella/Enterobacter	8	4	2
Staphylococcus epidermidis	8	10	9
Candida	5	7	3

3–7 days

Table 3. *Incidence of some microorganisms in faecal specimens from pre-term infants, aged 14–35 days, in relation to diet.*

	Raw breast milk (9 spec)	Heated breast milk (13 spec)	Cows milk derivatives (17 spec)
Clostridium	4	9	10
Bacteroides	3	1	4
Bifidobacterium	3	2	3
Lactobacillus	4	1	3
Escherichia coli	7	4	11
Klebsiella/Enterobacter	7	4	8
Staphylococcus epidermidis	6	10	10
Candida	4	4	3

14–35 days

Table 4. *Clostridium species (vegetative and spore-forming) in faecal specimens from pre-term infants in relation to diet. Number of specimens* yielding organisms.*

	Raw breast milk	Heated breast milk	Cows milk derivatives	Total no.
C. perfringens	2	4	5	11
C. sporogenes	2	1	6	9
C. difficile	1	1	6	8
C. felsineum	1	2	4	7
C. putrificium		1	5	6
C. scatologenes	1	1	3	5
C. ramosum		2	2	4
C. butyricum	1		2	3
C. fallax	1	2		3
C. beijerinckii			2	2
C. cadaveris			2	2
C. paraputrificum	1	1		2
C. septicum		1	1	2
C. subterminale		1	1	2
C. tertium	1	1		2
C. aminovalericum			1	1
C. cellobioparum		1		1
C. ghoni			1	1
C. glycolicum		1		1
C. innocuum	1			1
C. novyi		1		1
C. rectum			1	1
C. sphenoides			1	1
C. species not identified	3	4	9	16

*Raw breast milk: 21 from 7 infants
Heated breast milk: 31 from 11 infants
Modified cow's milk: 33 from 9 infants.

(figures 1 and 2), in contrast to what is seen in the healthy term breast-fed infant. Bifidobacteria and lactobacilli were not found to be at all prominent although they were seen more frequently, compared with the total number of specimens, in those infants fed breast milk whether raw or heated, after the second week of life (table 3). They did not, however, dominate the flora as in the healthy infant fed at the breast (figure 3). The normal skin micro-organism Staphylococcus epidermidis was commonly found in the faeces particularly during the first week (figure 1), in high numbers.

Candida was also found commonly (tables 2 and 3) and higher numbers were present in infants fed cow's milk (figures 1 and 2).

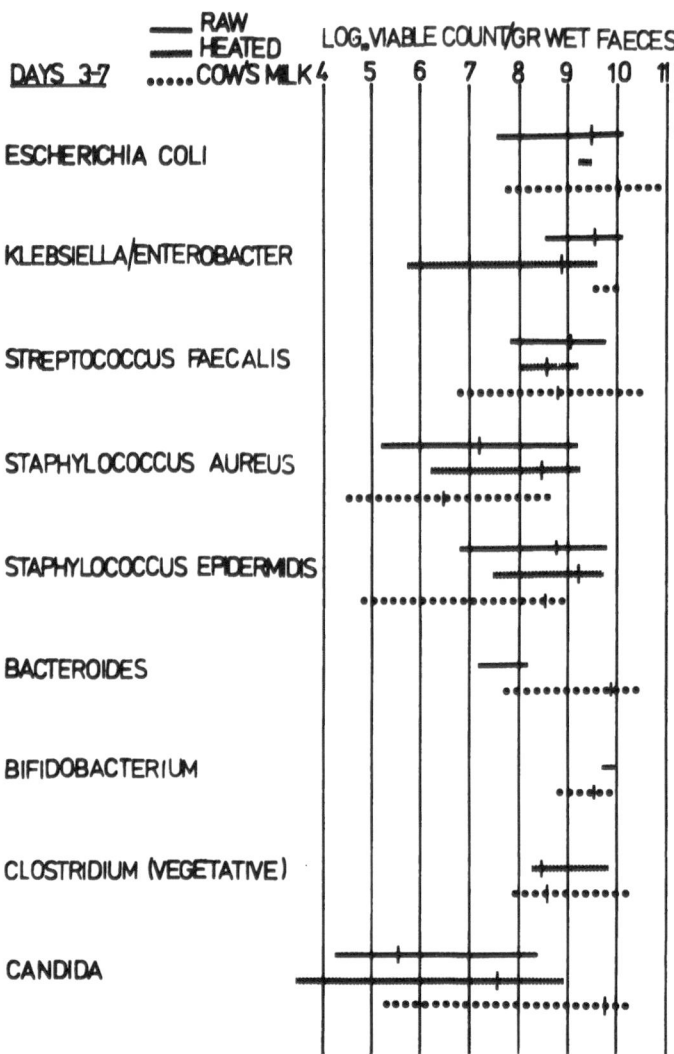

Fig. 1. Log$_{10}$ viable count/g wet faeces in pre-term infants, aged 3–7 days, in relation to diet.

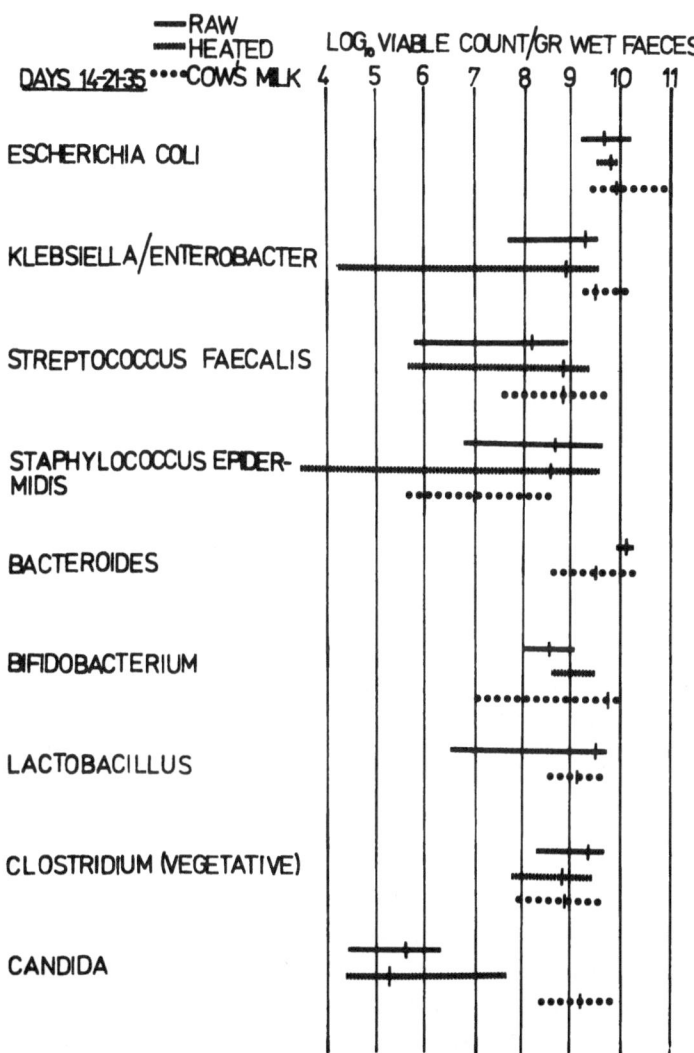

Fig. 2. Log$_{10}$ viable count/g wet faeces in pre-term infants, aged 14-35 days, in relation to diet.

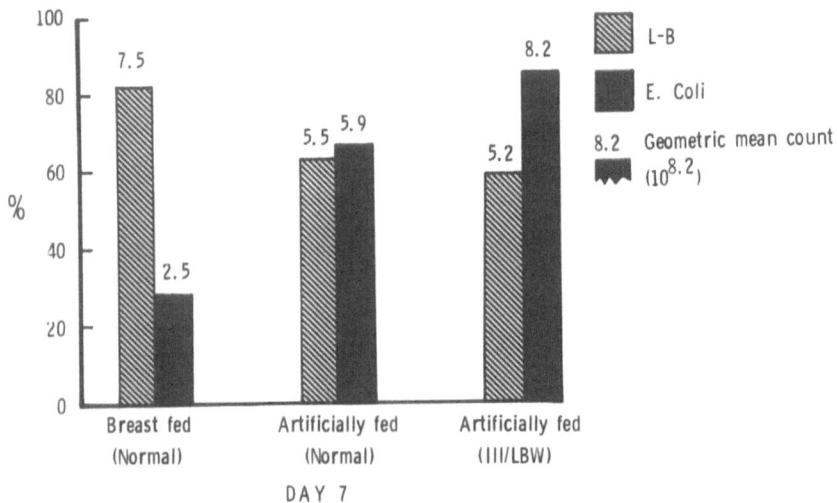

Fig. 3. Percentage colonization and nubers of Lactobacilli/bifidobacteria and Escherichia coli on day 7 in breast and artificially fed normal infants and in ill/LBW infants. (Reproduced with permission from Stern, L., Friis-Hansen, B. and Kildeberg, P. Ed's. 'Intensive Care in the Newborn'. Masson Publishing U.S.A. Inc.)

DISCUSSION

The unique antimicrobial properties of breast milk have been summarised in recent reviews (1, 10). The very immature infant, more prone to bacterial infection than the healthy mature baby, should theoretically benefit most from its anti-infective action. As he is unable to suck at the breast however, when such milk has been fed to him in the past it has traditionally first been sterilised by heating to high temperatures. Such treatment is now known to destroy some at least of the vital constituents, such as immunoglobulin, lactoferrin and lysozyme (6), which together act in the bowel to prevent invasion by pathogenic microorganisms. Whether the physico-chemical properties of milk, so essential in promoting colonization with lactobacilli and bifidobacteria are inactivated by heating is unknown. Renewed efforts are now being made to collect human milk safely for feeding in the raw or pasteurised state (8, 11, 12,

13, 14), and to assess the effects of any processing on its constituents.

As far as we are aware, detailed studies of the faecal flora of very immature infants fed raw or heat treated human milk exclusively for several weeks after birth have not been made previously, and indeed, detailed anaerobic studies of the faecal flora of infants in general are very few (5, 15). In presenting these results, we have to say that among the immature, usually ill babies studied in our referral unit and another intensive care unit, faecal flora was quite different from that of the normal breast fed infant. In a previous colonization survey at Hammersmith Hospital (5), it was found that artificially fed low birth weight and/or ill infants had higher numbers of Escherichia coli in their faeces than did healthy artificially fed babies. Thus it seemed likely that raw breast milk fed to the immature baby might not reproduce the same flora, at least quantitatively, when compared to that of the healthy mature infant fed at the breast. That there would be so little apparent difference in faecal flora of the 3 groups we studied was, however, unexpected and disappointing. A reduction in Clostridia and Bacteroides species during the first week was the only important finding in the human milk fed infants, and coliform organisms, particularly Escherichia coli dominated their flora, whether milk was fed raw or heated.

This is not to say that there is little point is using human milk for its antimicrobial properties in pre-term infants. More conclusive evidence will have to be sought in qualitative rather than quantitative changes of flora and in the small bowel as well as in the large bowel. The anti-adherence effect of IgA on Escherichia coli found with unheated breast milk may still be active in the gut lumen without necessarily changing the numbers of organisms there or in the faeces. There are reports suggesting that the use of fresh or stored human milk has played a substantial role in preventing or controlling bacterial gastroenteritis in pre-term infants (16, 17, 18), but there are no good studies to show that such babies have a lower incidence of other serious infections compared to these fed cow's milk. Colostrum and early milk are the richest in most of the antimicrobial factors (19, 20), but there are difficulties in collecting large amounts for use in neonatal intensive care units. Preliminary reports suggest that the nitrogen content of milk from women prematurely delivered is higher than that after term delivery (21), a finding which may lessen the argument that the protein content is too low for satisfactory growth. We feel that women giving birth to pre-term infants should be encouraged to lactate whenever possible.

SUMMARY

The known anti-infective properties of human milk have led to renewed interest in its use for pre-term infants who are more susceptible to infection than those born at term. As there have been no previous studies of the faecal flora of immature babies fed raw human milk exclusively, we have investigated this in a small number of infants, and compared results with a group fed sterilised human milk, in which the antimicrobial proteins sIgA, lysozyme and lactoferrin were destroyed by heating, and a group fed modified dried cow's milk. The median gestational age of the 27 infants studied in this way was 32 weeks, and median birth weight 1430 g. There were no significant differences of weight or gestation between the 3 groups. Many of the babies were ill and more than half of them received systemic antimicrobial drugs (usually benzyl penicillin and gentamicin), at some time during the first 5 weeks of life, the period of the study.

It was found that in all infants the flora did not become stabilised for several weeks after birth. The feeding of raw human milk did not reduce the incidence or numbers of Escherichia coli, and coliform organisms dominated the flora. Bifidobacteria and lactobacilli, although more often seen in the human milk fed groups after 2 weeks of age, were not present in large numbers. Both these findings are at variance with those in healthy mature breast-feeding infants. Clostridia and Bacteroides species had a reduced incidence during the first week of feeding raw human milk, and the clostridial flora was much more varied in the cow's milk fed group than in either of the other two.

We have therfore not demonstrated large quantitative differences in faecal flora between infants fed raw, or heat sterilised human milk, or modified dried cow's milk. It is still possible that advantage might lie with the raw milk fed group where qualitative changes are concerned, for the anti-adherence effect of sIgA on Escherichia coli for instance might be active in the gut lumen without necessarily changing the numbers of organisms there or in the faeces.

ACKNOWLEDGEMENTS

We are most grateful to Professor D.A. Mitchison for making the resources of his department available to us, and for his guidance. We have also had many helpful discussions with Professor Rosalinde Hurley, Dr. Naomi Datta and Dr. David Harvey. Miss Bodil Bäcklund, supported by a generous grant from Action Research for the

Crippled Child, carried out much of the technical work, and we would like to thank as well Mr. Ian Blenkharn who gave us similar help. L.G. was supported by fellowships from the Royal Society and British Council, also acknowledged with gratitude. The study would not have been possible without the generous help of the nursing staff at both hospitals.

REFERENCES

1. HANSON, L.A. and J. WINBERG, (1972) Arch. Dis. Childh. 47:845.
2. WIDDOWSON,E.M. (1965) Lancet 2:1099.
3. GAULL, G.E., D.K. RASSIN, N.C.R. RAIHA and K. HEINONEN. (1977) J. Pediat. 90:348.
4. RASSIN, D.K., G.E. GAULL, N.C.R. RAIHA and K. HEINONEN. (1977) J. Pediat. 90:356.
5. GRAHAM, J.M. (1975) Ph.D. thesis, University of London.
6. RAPTOPOULOU-GIGI, M., K. MARWICK and D.B.L. McCLELLAND. (1977) Brit. Med. J. 1:12.
7. FORD, J.E., B.A. LAW, V.M.E. MARSHALL and B. REITER. (1977) J. Pediat. 90:29.
8. GIBBS, J.H., C. FISHER, S. BHATTACHARYA, P. GODDARD and J.D. BAUM, (1977) Early Hum. Develop. 1:227.
9. HAENEL, H. (1970) Am. J. Clin. Nutr. 23:1433.
10. MATA, L.J. and R.G. WYATT. (1977) Am. J. Clin. Nutr. 24:976.
11. LIEBHABER, M., N.J. LEWISTON, M.T. ASQUITH, L. OLDS-ARROYO and P. SUNSHINE. (1977) J. Pediatr. 91:897.
12. LIEBHABER, M. N.J. LEWISTON, M.T. ASQUITH and P. SUNSHINE. (1978) J. Pediat. 92:236.
13. EVANS T.J., H.C. RYLEY, L.M. NEALE, J.A. DODGE and V.M. LEWARNE. (1978) Arch. Dis. Childh. 53:239.
14. WILLIAMSON, S., J.H. HEWITT, E. FINUCANE and H.R. GAMSU. (1978) Brit. Med. J. 1:393.
15. LONG, S.S. and R.M. SWENSON. (1977) J. Pediat. 91:298.
16. SVIRSKY-GROSS, S. (1958) Ann. Paediatr. (Basle) 190:109.
17. TASSOVATZ, B. and A. KOTSITCH. (1961) Ann. Pediatr. (Paris) 27:285.
18. LARGUIA, A.M., J. URMAN, J.M. CERIANI A. O'DONNELL, O. STOLIAR, J.C. MARTINEZ, J.C. BUSCAGLIA, S. WEILS, A. QUIROGA, and M. IRAZU. (1974) Arch. Argent. Ped. 72:109.
19. GOTHEFORS, L. (1975) Thesis, University of Umea, Sweden.
20. McCLELLAND, D.B.L., J. McGRATH and R.R. SAMSON. (1978) Acta Paediatr. Scand. Suppl. 271.
21. ATKINSON, S.A., M.H. BRYAN and G.H. ANDERSON. (1978) J. Pediatr. 93:67.

PSYCHO-SOCIAL IMPLICATIONS OF
BREAST FEEDING

M. P. M. RICHARDS*

The possible psychological advantages of breast-feeding to children have been long debated. Many people have made strong positive statements while others have claimed that these lack any supporting evidence. Despite a good deal of research on the topic (1) most of the evidence does remain inconclusive. A major reason for this is that many studies have employed inadequate methodology.

Typically, studies of this problem take two groups of children, one breast-fed, the other bottle-fed, and compare them on a single or small number of characteristics. These have included both the incidence of specific behaviour patterns such as thumb-sucking, or more global ratings such as "orality", "dependency" or learning abilities. The implicit assumption is that because the two groups are selected on one characteristic – the method of feeding – this factor will be causally related to any differences found between the two groups of infants. But this assumption is likely to be false. At least in industrialised societies, breast-feeding mothers are not a random cross-section of the population. They tend to be of upper social class (as rated by their husbands' occupations) and have received more education than mothers who choose to bottle-feed. So, the whole environment, both social and material, in which their children grow up will tend to differ from that of bottle-fed children. Any part of this may be responsible for any differences that may be found in the children.

In most European countries there have been wide variations in the incidence of breast-feeding over the past few decades. Most countries experienced very low rates in the late 1950s and 1960s but have had a considerable increase since that time. Figures as low as 10% of mothers breast-feeding when they were discharged from hospital were reported a few years ago while today, in Britain, rates at discharge may be as high as

* Medical Psychology Unit, University of Cambridge, England.

H.K.A. Visser (ed.), Nutrition and Metabolism of the Fetus and Infant, 297-304. All rights reserved.
Copyright © 1979 Martinus Nijhoff Publishers b.v., The Hague/Boston/London.

60 or even 80%. Clearly as the incidence changes, the characteristics of the breast-feeding subsample will vary and in turn this may have influences on the development of the children. When breast-feeding receives little encouragement and the incidence is low only mothers who are strongly motivated and who feel able to resist the social pressures for bottle-feeding are likely to establish lactation. In many hospitals in Britain today breast-feeding is strongly encouraged and, unless there is a medical problem that prevents lactation, mothers may find it hard not to breast-feed – at least while they are in hospital.

Given these problems, not only is a very careful matching of groups required before one can find evidence of the effects of breast-feeding *per se*, but one must not expect to find a universal answer to the question. Given that the choice of feeding method is based on social and cultural factors and that we are dealing with developmental processes which are dependent on a social world, we may expect varying answers to the question of the psychological effects of breast-feeding in differing social and cultural settings and at different historical times. In the extreme case the effects of not breast-feeding a child in the Third World may well be death from infection and malnutrition whereas in Britain the effects on infant health are minimal (2).

The final general point that must be considered is that breast- and bottle-feeding are descriptions of techniques of *feeding*. The composition of the milk given might have an influence on the psychological development of children. However, the composition of breast-milk is determined, in part, by the mother's diet and many different things can be put in a bottle. Heavy metal and pesticides, for instance, have been recorded as contaminants of breast-milk and have been shown to influence the development of the baby's central nervous system and behaviour (3, 4). These compounds have also been found as contaminants of formulas and these themselves vary widely in composition. In addition, the reconstitution of powdered formulas is another variable in the process that can have important consequences (5). However, my main concern in this paper is not the effects of milk composition itself but of the way in which the milk is given – from the breast or a bottle. Here again there tends to be an assumption that each method tends to be relatively uniform and that individual variation between mothers in each group is relatively unimportant. However, as far as effects on development are concerned the quality of the whole relationship between the parent and child is probably the key issue. Feeding is but one part of that relationship and one must therefore be cautious in discussing it in isolation.

Having mentioned some of the complications of the question, I want to consider a recent British study that suggests that the method of infant feeding does have long-term effects on cognitive development.

This study by RODGERS (6) set out to replicate an earlier one by MENKES (7) which had found that the percentage of a clinical sample of children with learning disorders who had been breast-fed was much lower than in a control group. 13.8% of those with learning disorders had been breast-fed compared with 47.2% of a group with neurological disorders other than learning difficulties. RODGERS set out to replicate this finding using data from the British National Survey of Health and Development (1946 birth cohort). This sample of 5362 people was selected from all the legitimate singleton births during one week in 1946 and have been followed to adulthood. Of these 1133 were entirely bottle-fed and 1291 were never bottle-fed. Tests of picture intelligence and mechanical word reading were completed at 8 years of age as were other tests of non-verbal ability and mathematical attainment at 15 years. Analysis showed that low scores on all tests were more likely for the bottle-fed children. Additionally the sentence completion scores for those who were part breast-fed and part bottle-fed varied with the age of transfer from breast to bottle and was intermediate between the never breast-fed and never bottle-fed groups. So there appears to be a kind of dose response curve.

As one might expect there were a number of variables which differed significantly between the breast-feeding and bottle-feeding groups. Breast-feeding was more common in families of higher social class, in families where either parent had received some secondary schooling, in families where parents showed more interest in the children's primary schooling and for children of lower birth rank (first-born children were most likely to be breast-fed). It was less common for boys than girls and for those of lower birth weight. As these factors are all likely to be correlated with intellectual performance, regression techniques were used to give "corrected" values for the 8-year and 15-year-old tests. This procedure showed that after correction, significant differences remained between the breast-fed and bottle-fed groups on all the test scores except the 8-year-old word reading test.

These results are strongly suggestive of a direct connection between feeding method and later intellectual performance. Of course, it is always possible that there are other unknown variables that influence both the incidence of breast-feeding and intellectual development and this possibility can only be ruled out by more detailed longitudinal studies. However, this study provides the most convincing evidence that is available as yet.

If we assume for the moment that there is a direct connection between feeding method and intellectual development, the question arises of what processes might be involved. Factors related to milk composition could be implicated, but here I want to discuss possible psychological processes.

For this I will use data from the Cambridge Longitudinal Study (8) of 80 low-risk cildren. As part of this study, observations of feeding sessions were made during the first 10 post-partum days and at 8 weeks. There were many differences between breast- and bottle-feeds and many of these seemed independent of background variables associated with choice of feeding method (9). In essence, for many mothers, each method of feeding seemed to represent a different kind of social situation. Breast-feeding was generally a time of close social interaction between mother and baby. Breast-feeds lasted longer and there was more kissing, rocking and affectionate touching. Mother and baby were more often alone and mothers were much less likely to talk to other adults or children during a breast-feed. On the other hand, bottle-feeding was a situation that was limited to the feeding itself. Most mothers seemed largely concerned with getting food into the baby. Behaviour patterns related to the efficiency of feeding predominated – rubbing, patting, jiggling and concern about bringing up the wind were more common. Other people were more often present and frequently were the main focus of the mother's social attention.

The idea that feeding played a rather different part in the whole of the social relationship between mother and baby for the two groups is further supported by some follow-up data (10, 11). For instance, the amount of affectionate touching seen in the first ten days in the feeding situation showed strong correlations with amounts of maternal contact and voca-lisation recorded in non-feeding interactions over the first 7 months in breast-feeding families but not in bottle-feeding ones. This might suggest that breast-feeding does form part of the whole style of social interaction which shows quite strong continuities over the first few months. Bottle-feeding couples also showed continuities in social interaction but these did not extend to the feeding situation itself.

The observational data also indicate that breast-feeding may itself be a

more truly interactive situation than bottle-feeding. During breast-feeding a mother's behaviour is more dependent on and related to what the
baby is doing. The baby is a much more active member of the pair
in breast-feeding. This is illustrated in table 1 which shows that talking
to the baby, and touching are importantly influenced by the baby's
sucking: talking being more likely to take place during gaps between
sucking bouts, touching during sucking. In the bottle-feeding situation
mothers' touching and talking, occurred more randomly through the
observation. A particularly interesting point was the difference in re-
sponsibility for ending sucking bouts: in the bottle-feeding situation it
was overwhelmingly the mother who ended the bout, and with breast-
feeders it was equally likely to be the mother or baby. These differences
are still significant where class differences between the 2 groups were
controlled. They were more marked on the days 8 to 10 than earlier in
the first week so are unlikely to be explained by the delay in the coming-
in of the milk with breast-feeding.

All these observations suggest that not only does feeding play a rather
different part in all social interactions for breast and bottle-feeding pairs
but that the feeding interactions themselves are somewhat distinct. To
confirm this we need observations or early non-feeding social situations
for both groups but unfortunately these are not available.

The important question then is, do these early interactive differences
between the two groups have long-term developmental consequences for
the children? There is little hint of this in the data from the Cambridge
Longitudinal Study. However, analysis of the follow-up data (to school
age) is not complete and the measures of intellectual performance used
are relatively crude so may miss more subtle effects. In addition, the
sample size is small for control of all the relevant variables.

Table 1. *Breast-fed/bottle-fed differences (2nd babies).*

| | Days 2 and 3 (N = 35) | | Days 8–10 (N = 49) | |
	Bottle-fed	Breast-fed	Bottle-fed	Breast-fed
Probability mother touch if baby sucking	0.02	0.09 $p<0.01$	0.02	0.12 $p<0.01$
Probability mother talk in gaps between sucking bouts	0.30	0.47 $p<0.05$	0.36	0.49 $p<0.05$

There are, however, reasons for thinking there could be connections between the early interactive differences and later performance. In recent years much stress has been laid on the importance of the development of reciprocal interchange in the first year of life for later cognitive development and language acquisition (12, 13). It has been suggested that give and take that is seen between parents and children towards the end of the first year is a direct precursor of aspects of symbolic functioning as well as being a forum in which rules of social relations are developed and learnt. If one accepts this point of view, the more equal distribution of power and initiation in the breast-feeding situation could have an important bearing on the development of later dialogue (turn-taking) and reciprocal interchange. However, it could also be that the feeding differences are more apparent than real and what the bottle-fed babies appear to miss in the feeding situation is simply transposed to other social situations. As is so often the case in developmental work, at present we can merely speculate and await the result of detailed longitudinal investigation.

There is another line of work which is at least compatible with these speculations. This is research on the later consequences of the early (neonatal) separation of parents and newborns. Following the pioneer studies of KLAUS and KENNELL (14), there is now considerable evidence that neonatal separation has influences on social and cognitive development that persist for several months if not a great deal longer (15). A major process involved in these separation effects is the influence on the parents of the early separation which then has persisting effects on the relationship with the baby and the baby's development (16). WINNICOTT (17) drew attention to the rather special features of the first stage of parental relationships, the phase he called primary maternal preoccupation. Early separation inhibits or prevents the development of this phase which in turn disturbs the succeeding phases of the relationship. It is plausible to argue that the ideal conditions for the initiation and resolution of the primary maternal preoccupation are provided by breast-feeding and the kind of social situation it involves. But once again, we lack any direct evidence on this point. However, it does seem fruitful to explore the consequences of the choice of feeding method in terms of parental feelings and their influence on the social, cognitive and emotional development of the child.

The beginnings of parenthood are a time of considerable emotional upheaval and change (18). Feelings dormant since childhood are re-evoked. Unresolved conflicts often come to the surface. The ways in which this emotional change-point is negotiated might not only influence the choice of feeding method but, in turn, be influenced by it. Breast-feeding creates strong feelings in most women and contains complex elements of sexuality. It is also the one aspect of child-care which cannot be undertaken by men. For all these reasons it is likely to have an effect on parental feelings in general and in particular on feelings towards the baby. And as we are beginning to discover, initial feelings and attitudes towards a child seem to correlate closely with many aspects of development.

CONCLUSIONS

The one safe generalisation one can make about developmental psychology is that the close examination of any question changes what we thought to be relatively simple into something much more complex. So it is with the effects of breast- and bottle-feeding. We certainly cannot say that one is better than the other nor at this point do more than speculate about the general effects. However, even if we had much more data available we would only be able to discuss the problem in very general terms. Because of the complexities of developmental processes and because of their dependence on social and cultural as well as individual factors, the effects of breast-feeding may well vary widely for different individuals. In Europe and America samples of breast-fed and bottle-fed children do show some differences. As I have tried to indicate in this paper, some of these differences could be a consequence of the differences in social interaction that may arise with the choice of each feeding method. However, it must also be said that in these countries, the development of the two groups of children is very similar. There are many reasons for encouraging breast-feeding in all countries (2) but this aim would not be served by stressing the possibility of negative developmental consequences of bottle-feeding.

ACKNOWLEDGEMENTS

The Cambridge Longitudinal Study is supported by a grant from the Social Science Research Council.

REFERENCES

1. CALDWELL, B.M. (1964) In: Review of Child Development Research, vol. 1, Russell
   Sage Foundation, New York.
2. RICHARDS, M.P.M. (1974) Unpublished paper presented at a joint meeting of the
   British Paediatric Association Council and the Medical Education and Information
   Unit of the Spastics Society, Farnham, England.
3. QUINBY, G.E., J.F. ARMSTRONG and W.F. DURHAM. Nature 207:726.
4. DOHERTY, R.A., A.H. GATES and G.E. SEWELL. (1975) In: Milk and Lactation,
   Kretchmen, N. and E. Rossi eds.. Karger. Basel.
5. TAITZ, L.S. (1971) Brit. Med. J. 1:315.
6. RODGERS, B. (1978) Develop. Med. Child Neurol. 20:421.
7. MENKES, J.H. (1977) Develop. Med. Child Neurol. 19:169.
8. RICHARDS, M.P.M. and J.F. BERNAL, (1972) In: Ethological Studies of Child
   Behaviour, Blurton Jones, N. ed., Cambridge University Press, London.
9. RICHARDS, M.P.M. (1975) In: Milk and Lactation, Kretchmen, N. and E. Rossi
   eds., Karger, Basel.
10. DUNN, J.F. (1975) In: Parent-Infant Interaction. Ciba Foundation Symposium No.
    33, Elsevier, Amsterdam.
11. DUNN, J.F. and M.P.M. RICHARDS, (1978) In: Studies of Mother-Infant Interaction,
    Schaffer, H.R. ed., Academic Press, London.
12. RICHARDS, M.P.M. (1974) In: The Integration of a Child into a Social World,
    Richards, M.P.M. ed., Cambridge University Press, London.
13. SCHAFFER, H.R. (ed.) (1977) Studies of Mother-Infant Interaction, Academic Press,
    London.
14. KLAUS, M.H. and J.M. KENNELL. (1976) Maternal-Infant Bonding, Mosby, St.
    Louis.
15. RICHARDS, M.P.M. (1978) In: Early Separation and Special Care Nurseries. Clinics
    in Develop. Med. Spastics Publications/Heinemann Medical Books, London. In
    press.
16. RICHARDS, M.P.M. (1978) In: The First Year of Life. Schaffer, D. and J.F. Dunn
    eds., Wiley, London.
17. WINNICOTT, D.W. (1958) Collected Papers, Tavistock, London.
18. DEUTCH, H. (1947) The Psychology of Women, vol. 2, Research Books, London.

DISCUSSION

PAPER BY L. HAMBRAEUS

M. Gabr: I am particularly interested in your studies on the effects of maternal malnutrition on the protein concentration of milk. I have two short questions. It is not quite clear to me that in your low social class Ethiopians the protein concentration was not markedly affected, while your experimental data, based on Swedish mothers on a low protein diet for 4 days, showed a significant drop in the protein concentration of milk. How do you explain this?

The second question: In your study on Ethiopian mothers you found no decrease in the lactoferrin concentration. You postulated that this was a reflection of the high iron content present in the diet of those low social class mothers in Ethiopia. Do you have similar data on IgA, lysozyme or other proteins involved in immunological properties of breast milk?

L. Hambraeus: As to your question: I think this very odd finding must be an indication that in a short study   these Swedish mothers had been put on a diet for just 4 days before we made our analyses – well-nourished mothers used to a high protein intake will react. They haven't been able to adapt to the situation. On the other hand, those Ethiopian mothers have adapted. This is in accordance with the fact that people who have had a low protein intake utilize the protein more efficiently than those on a high protein diet. This was, of course, a pilot study. You will understand the problems involved in conducting such a study, but I think it's worth continuing.

With respect to your other question, we could say that we are almost certain, that why the lactoferrin is not behaving like the other factors is due to the fact that these mothers have experienced a diet with an extremely high iron content. We have also studied the IgA and some of the immunoglobins, but I cannot give the data.

M.P.M. Richards: I would just like to make a comment about the species differences in the composition of the milk and the relationship with growth rates in young. A very important thing one has to take into account is the pattern of feeding within different species. Very roughly, you can divide mammals into those that carry their young with them and feed frequently, like rats or some of the ruminants; and the other extreme, species that hide their young or leave them in a nest and feed them maybe only once a day, like the rabbit. In those species, you get very highly concentrated milks, as compared with the others. What is quite interesting is then to look at it the other way around, looking at human milk compostion and asking what sort of pattern of interaction would you infer from the milk. And if you do that, you get a picture of virtually continuous feeding – at least something very different from what we would see in hospitals in Europe. And indeed, there is some direct observational data from the bush people in the Kalahari desert which suggests that, where a baby is being carried around by the mother and sleeps with her at night, the interval between feeds is something in the order of 20 minutes.

R. Eeckels: You could say the same thing of every African village, Dr. Richards. I don't think you have to go to the Kalahari.

L. Hambraeus: I think that is a very relevant observation but it seems to me to be more a question for a pediatrician in a university hospital than for me.

N.P. Fernando: You lightly dismiss lactose as a non-essential nutrient and yet looking at the composition of sugars in the milk, we find that human milk has the highest lactose content. I wonder if one is in a position to dismiss it so easily. I am particularly interested because, in recent times, there are many babies who are being fed lactose-free formula for gastroenteritis and following gastroenteritis and sometimes they have to be on this formula for a long time. I wondered whether being on a lactose-free diet would not in any way interfere with cerebral maturation?

L. Hambraeus: One of the reasons why I had to omit it was the time factor. But I think we have to accept that lactose is not an essential component, in that respect that we can synthesize it in the body and grow up normally on a lactose-free diet. We know this also from such in vivo experiments by nature as galactosemia, when we have to start a complete lactose-free diet almost from birth.

So, from that aspect, it is a non-essential nutrient, but that does not imply that it is not an optimum nutrient for the human being. That is what I wanted to stress: we know that it influences the mineral absorption although we don't exactly know how. We know that it has an influence on the most optimal protein utilization. We can't explain that either, but in animal experiments we have certain evidence for that. I think it's a question of definition, but if it means that you cannot synthesize an essential nutrient by yourself, then lactose is not an essential nutrient.

PAPER BY B. CARLSSON

G.B.A. Stoelinga: You said it was presumed that intact T-cells can be absorbed by the neonatal gut. I wonder if these cells are active in the neonate, for they are as antigens different for the child and will be destroyed. And if not, these immuno-competent cells can have harmful effects on the child, for instance graft versus host reaction.

B. Carlsson: I did not say that they were absorbed but that some activity was transferred to the child. I don't think there is much information on this – at least to my knowledge.

G.B.A. Stoelinga: Could it be an effect of the transfer factor? Is the transfer factor present in human milk?

B. Carlsson: It might be, but is not shown.

J. Bande-Knops: You told us that tuberculin positive mothers who breast feed their children could transfer a tuberculin-positive reaction to the newborn. Do you have any percentages on this? Does it mean that every positive mother who is breast feeding will have a baby who will show a positive tuberculin test?

B. Carlsson: I don't know the percentage, this is not our own study. But it has been shown in a couple of studies that there is a transfer.

M. Gabr: The problem of breast feeding is a crucial problem in developing countries. I know it is becoming a problem in your country.

What I am afraid of is that our young doctors who go to Western countries to learn medicine think that the safety of breast milk in our developing countries is related to these various immunological factors you referred to. The main factor of safety with breast milk in developing countries is the fact that it's much less exposed to contamination. This should be very clearly pointed out whenever students from developing countries should be present in your classrooms.

PAPER BY J.D. BAUM

J.G. Koppe: When are you doing a bacterial control? When the milk comes in, before you deep-freeze it in your own freezer? When do you reject it? When does the milk have too many E-coli bacteria?

J.D. Baum: We have found no guideline on which to judge how many of which bacteria we should give babies.

Our own rules are that we look for known pathogens – which we have defined – and, provided there are none of these present, then we allow the babies to have the milk. So we ask our bacteriologists to look at the batch of milk after pasteurization for E-coli, staphoids and streptococcus.

R.D.G. Milner: Can you go on from there and tell us how many batches you've analyzed and how many batches you've rejected, please.

J.D. Baum: I can't give you exact figures, but I can give you approximate figures, because it is greatly influenced by such variables as climatic conditions. During the first 3 months of this year, taking milk which had been in the mothers' home refrigerator – not deep freezers – about 1 in 4 of those batches had to be discarded post-pasteurization. In the May-June-July part of this year, we found that this went up to something like 50%, 2 in 4, and it was at that stage that we started to pressure the mothers into using a freezer or a next-door neighbour's freezer. Since doing that, it's been more like 1 in 10 batches that had to be discarded.

D. Nicolopoulos: I have a practical question. How did you manage, with mothers of prematures, to get their milk for 1 or 2 months without suckling the baby? This seems very difficult to me.

J.D. Baum: I think it is difficult. It requires the devotion of the nursing staff. It requires human-milk pumps and I think these are essential. We have 5 in our unit. They require the same kind of priority as incubators and other pieces of intensive-care equipment. They're expensive. It is only through that kind of support that we find the mothers can maintain their lactation.

B.S. Lindblad: You said that it was impractical to give the milk from the mother to her own child. This is what some people have been doing without treating the milk.

J.D. Baum: May I defend that, because I think that is a most important question. I think that in the United Kingdom the social class distribution of the mothers whose babies come into special-care baby units is skewed to the left. There are more disadvantaged mothers, unmarried mothers, mothers who don't have their own means of transportation, etc. These mothers have in common, at the present time, less motivation to continue lactation and more difficulties in coming backwards and forwards to the nursery for 10 weeks while the baby goes through intensive care. It is for this reason that I think that it is very difficult to produce enough fresh milk from each baby's own mother for each day. I certainly would go along with this as an ideal, which we do achieve in some mothers. But my premise was that if we want to give human milk to the whole nursery, we are therefore committed, for unfortunately a majority, to have some milk-banking system.

A. Pardou: Do you pasteurize the mother's own milk when you give it to the premature baby?

J.D. Baum: If it is expressed or pumped on the ward, then we give it raw to the baby. If the mothers brings it in within – we say 24 hours, but it depends on how we're feeling and how the mother's feeling – approximately 24 hours, we give it untreated to the baby. If it's the mother's own milk but it's a week old and it's the middle of the summer and it's been under non-frozen conditions, we would pasteurize it.

G.E. Gaull: Pigs can receive sow colostrum for about 3 days and then be put on a milk substitute. What is the evidence that we need anything more than the colostrum, which you could give from each mother to each infant, and then forget about what you referred to as the "goodies."

J.D. Baum: Well, I don't know. The whole thing is bristling with questions. We have yet to test whether these immune proteins are biologically active -- all of them, in vivo or in milk in vitro. One has yet to test what they actually do to the immune function of the baby's gut. And one has yet to test whether it is essential to give the immune-rich milk for three days, for 3 weeks or throughout the period of intensive care. I think these are just open questions. I have no information.

R.A. McCance: I will just add one point. You selected pigs, but the amount of time required to get the colostral and other antibodies into animals varies enormously. In some, the process begins before birth and continuous after birth for 3 weeks or so. In pigs and in cows, it takes place in a very short time.

A.G.L. Whitelaw: Could I ask you if your pasteurization will kill viruses. Because there are two worries: firstly because of the rota virus in infantile gastroenteritis and secondly because of the very theoretical risk that things like leukemia and other malignancies might be transmitted with raw breast milk, as they are for example in some animal species.

J.D. Baum: We haven't any data of our own on this. One knows that cytomegaly virus is very heat-labile and Australia antigen is very heat stable, so I guess if Australia antigen is in the milk, it is there in the pool. We take some comfort in our pooling system that we are pooling out the dose of any viral contaminants and I wonder if I could ask Dr. Carlsson to help me on this. If a mother is excreting a virus, whether she is also excreting IgA with that virus and so is protecting the pool with an equivalent dose of IgA?

B. Carlsson: I know there are antibodies to virus, also in milk, especially rota virus. But I don't know if the virus itself is excreted.

PAPER BY P.A. DAVIES

J.D. Baum: Were you not surprised not to find a predominance of lactobacilli in the fresh human milk fed group? Do you think that the antibiotic courses were responsible for the changing flora?

P.A. Davies: Yes, I suppose we were surprised. But not all of the infants had antibiotics. There were 27 babies studied and I have to admit that 14 of them had the drugs. But the findings where lactobacilli and bifidus bacteria were concerned were really irrespective of whether antibiotic treatment had been given or not.

M. Orzalesi: Looking into your data, did you have the impression that those infants that were colonized with lactobacillus were also those who were less colonized with enterobacteria? The reason I'm asking this is that we, in Italy and also in the unit where I used to work, very often used Parmesan cheese for these very small babies when they had diarrhea or when there was babies' diarrhea around. The overall clinical impression – I don't have control trials myself, although there are trials that show this – is that it has preventive value and it shortens the course of the diarrhea episode and it anticipates the time when you can feed them by mouth. But, as I say, mine is only a clinical impression, there are other studies which show the same thing and I would be curious to know if, within your group, those which are colonized with lactobacillus are also the babies that are less or least colonized with enterobacteria.

P.A. Davies: Again, I'd like to be able to say that. But I don't think it was the case. Again, Dr. Gothefors really should be here to answer that question, because he has absolutely all these details in his head. I think I'm right in saying that, no, this advantage really was not there. As for Parmesan cheese, we shall have to start importing this a little bit more into England!

M. Gabr: Dr. Davies, did you measure pH in the stools of these infants and did you find any relation between the acidity and the presence of lactobacillus or E-coli. The reason I am asking is that maybe an explanation for your low incidence of lactobacillus in premature infants is the lactase deficiency with less acid stools as compared with full-terms.

P.A. Davies: Yes, I can see that. The pH of the stools was measured, but I don't have the information you want yet.

A.G.L. Whitelaw: Could I ask you if there was usually a short delay between the admission of the baby and the starting of feeding orally?
In many units, babies get dextrose for a variable period of time, until

the condition of the baby stabilizes. It just occurred to me that if the baby, say, had 36–48 hours nothing by mouth, then there might be an opportunity for the organisms in the intensive care unit to gain access to the gut, without there being any milk of any kind to alter the flora. I would also like to know if any of the babies got necrotizing enterocolitis.

P.A. Davies: Yes, certainly some of the infants did have a short period of dextrose or dextrose-electrolytes before being given human milk. But this really didn't make any very great difference. I'm sure that environmental contamination is one of the reasons – it surely must be in a unit like this – why this disappointing result has come forth. This is our practical problem, is it not?

About necrotizing enterocolitis: one infant developed it. He was in the group fed heat-sterilized human milk, and he developed it 5 days after going back from our hospital to his hospital of origin, where the heat-sterilized milk was continued. Blood cultures were always drawn before starting antimicrobial therapy, and although 14 of the 27 infants had such therapy, proven bacterial infection was only confirmed in three. These were in the human-milk fed groups. One of the smallest infants – 700 g at birth – had two episodes of septicaemia. He was in the group fed raw-milk.

PAPER BY M.P.M. RICHARDS

J.C. Sinclair: Dr. Richards, are you arguing that there is something inherent in the feeding episode itself, whether it be breast or bottle, that determines synchronous or asynchronous behaviour between mother and infant and lays the potential for long-term effects on development? Or are you arguing that it is the original maternal characteristics or attitudes that lead to the choice of feeding, and that determine also the mother's behaviour interaction with her infant and long-term development?

M.P.M. Richards: We don't know because at the present time you can't distinguish those two. I find it very hard to think of experimental situations one could use to pull those two things apart. What we can say is: they are different interactional situations and if in our own work we, for example, reorganize the comparisons so we keep social class constant and various other social factors constant, the differences persist. And they still persist. In fact, we look at various measures we took during pregnancy, of the women's attitudes towards the coming baby, having a baby and what they felt about feeding it and so on. So, I think we are talking about things that probably – at least in part – are products of that choice of feeding and that choice of feeding alone. We do indeed have anecdotal data, but I won't go into that. I would argue though that a major thing is the feeding method itself and it isn't simply a product of choice.

J.C. Sinclair: I recognize that it's impossible to randomly allocate the method of feeding, but, if in the course of breast feeding, breast feeding has to be interrupted for some reason, then you have the opportunity to observe bottle feeding episodes in a baby whose mother has chosen to breast feed. I'd be interested to know about maternal behaviour in that situation.

M.P.M. Richards: That's really what I was aluding to when I said "anecdotal evidence." By and large, in those situations, you can find differences as it were that a breast-feeding mother who bottle feeds will do it somewhat differently than a mother who has never breast-fed. But the overwhelming thing seems to be the technique, at least on the basis of the kind of observational data we have. We are talking about something that shows very great individual differences and that's why I mentioned the particular breast-feeding mother who said she didn't do it for emotional reasons. It is possible to be very mechanical about breast feeding. It is also possible to bottle feed in a way that is very similar to that I have described for breast feeding. But that is not what people do in general. It may be if we launched a great educational programme and tell mothers that it was important to talk to their babies when they weren't sucking, that you could convert one pattern to the other. We are talking about patterns that the people, involved in creating them, are usually not aware of. So, what would happen if we tried to educate people, I don't know.

R. Eeckels: If you ever have tried to let nurses talk to children they are bottle feeding then you'll know that it is very difficult to obtain that. There is a beautiful study by Peter De Chateau. He studied two groups of 20 mothers, all of them breast feeding, from the same socio-economic group. One group of 20 mothers received their children immediately after birth, before the expulsion of the placenta. At that moment the child was given to the mother during 15 minutes – 10 minutes on the belly, 5 minutes at the breast. That changed their behaviour in a significant way and their contact with the child too. That would mean that indeed the way of doing it might already change the whole of your behaviour, without there being any prior difference. Am I right in putting it that way?

M.P.M. Richards: Yes. What I would emphasize about our studies is that it was carried out at home, with a sample of mothers who had delivered at home and indeed all had their babies immediately. I have done a few observations of breast feeding in hospitals in Britain and the United States. That suggests that breast feeding in hospital, whether or not you've had early contact, is a very different kind of experience. For example, most hospitals in Britain still make it very hard for mothers to feed more often than every 4 hours. Mothers are often forced to breast feed not only in public but with a nurse who may not be very skilled, who is there ostensibly to help them. I would, for example, mention another study by Peter De Chateau where he shows that one of the best ways of increasing the rate of lactation in a hospital was to stop test-weighing babies. That produced an immediate increase. What I'm trying to say is that breast feeding is often very difficult in a hospital. The kind of patterns I'm talking about may be partially destroyed by the social environment of the hospital. I feel we are in a rather dangerous situation at the moment where pediatricians quite likely are encouraging breast feeding, but not noticing often the extreme difficulty the mothers have in the usual sort of social situation that exists in hospitals, at least in Britain and I would suspect in many other parts of the world.

R.D.G. Milner: May I just ask you to carry on with what I thought was an implicit comment. Do you think that current pediatric practise in the United Kingdom may be engendering disatisfaction, neurosis and unhappiness in mothers?

M.P.M. Richards: No.

R.D.G. Milner: I'm not posing this question provocatively, I'm posing it sincerely, because as a practitioner in a hospital of the type you described, I am not active. I kowtow to the principle of supporting breast feeding, but I am very sensitive that I may be creating more problems on a day-to-day basis in the wards if I'm going around saying, "now look, my dear, you should be breast feeding", than I may be solving. I would like you to expand a little on that if you would.

M.P.M. Richards: Let me take the issue of frequency of feeding. Our data shows very clearly that it's very hard, if not impossible, to establish lactation if you don't feed a baby much more often than every 4 hours for the first few days. Now, I know many hospitals in Britain still only allow contact between parents and children every 4 hours. So, in that situation, if you tell everyone they ought to be breast feeding but you don't let them have their babies often enough to establish lactation, you are going to have many women who are going to feel like failures at the first signifi-cant thing they would like to do for their own child. I think there are much more subtle effects than that. But the first thing, it seems to me, that is required in a hospital if we're dealing with normal full-term babies is that you do not limit contact between them and their mothers and indeed their fathers. That is a pre-condition for successful lactation. I might just add to that that there are people who believe that nipples become sore and all sorts of other things. There is a very nice study by Illingworth in the 1950's that showed that nipples become sore when you restrict the amount of sucking in the first few days of life – not, as is often believed, when you allow free contact.

J.D. Baum: I have observed a mother with twins of different size, and breast feeding both twins. Her attitude was apparently, to a non-scien-tific observer, different towards the two babies.

I wonder if you had any more carefully designed observations on twins and perhaps there might even be a chance of a mother with twins, one breast-fed, one bottle-fed.

M.P.M. Richards: We haven't directly worked on twins, but you prob-ably know the study by Ann Stewart at University College Hospital (UCH) in London. That is a follow-up study of a group of very small babies all around 1000 g. What she shows essentially is that most of the behavioural problems are confined to the groups of multiple birth children. The evidence, when put together, suggests very strongly that if you do treat twins differently at the beginning – for example, you discharge one that is healthier than another earlier – parents very often begin to treat them differently and that almost invariably seems to lead to behavioural problems later. I think that, ethically, one should be rather careful. It might be rather important to make sure that parents, early on, are not given the opportunity to treat their twins too differently, or you may be bringing on quite serious problems later. It doesn't entirely answer your question, but it is something people haven't thought about a great deal. Very often, the attitude is: if one twin is healthy, at least the parents can have that twin at home and that's so much better. You may then find you set up a situation where the parents aren't fully going to accept the other twin ever.

GENERAL DISCUSSION

J. Senterre: Dr. Hambraeus, in your written summary, you advised to supplement human milk with Vitamin D. More recently, it has been demonstrated that there is quite a lot of hydroxyl derivative of Vitamin D in human milk. Do you think this is not enough? Calcium balances with human milk, not supplemented with Vitamin D, demonstrate a very good calcium absorption. I wonder if it is necessary to supplement human milk with Vitamin D – for full-term infants, of course.

L. Hambraeus: I am not quite sure that there is a need for supplementation. We are also looking at this problem of different kinds of Vitamin D. There are lots of methodological problems involved, so I can't give you the answer. My feeling is that it might not be necessary.

M. Young: Is the development of the enzymes for gluconeogenesis in the newborn related to the concentration of protein in the milk?

L. Hambraeus: That is a difficult question. I'm afraid I can't answer that. This is one of the many factors that should be studied further.

H.M. Berger: The concentration of non-protein nitrogen in human milk is not less than 25%. Now, if we allow that an important part of it would be the free amino acids, there still seems to be a great deal of other nitrogens present. Could you comment on their role? They seem to be a neglected factor.

L. Hambraeus: Free amino acids are not the major part of this non-protein nitrogen. So I don't think they are the major problem. I would stress that we should not talk about protein requirement all the time; we should rather talk about nitrogen requirement. I still feel that if we have 20 to 25% non-protein nitrogen, this is not necessarily unused. On the contrary it might be usable.

Furthermore, I think there are components in the non-protein nitrogen which may occur in very small amounts, but can still have a significant physiological goal. So my answer to you would be, that there is a great need for further study of these components to see what their physiological role is. However, we should stress that the protein requirement is one thing and the nitrogen requirement is another.

R. Eeckels: I must confess I have never rightly understood why there is lactose in the milk of almost all mammals. We live on glucose and mothers transform it into lactose, give it to their children and they can have a lot of trouble with it and, again, have to transform it into glucose. This seems to me a very complicated way of handling things.

L. Hambraeus: First, you know there is a great difference in the lactose content of the milk in various mammals, for instance, this odd finding that the sea lion and the seal have no lactose in their milk is very interesting. This has probably to do with the need for a high caloric, low volume milk. Your question is very difficult. One can speculate in all directions. One possibility is that the lactose intolerance which develops when the child gets older, could be one of the ways to get the infant to stop sucking.

B. Friis Hansen: May I return to the last question and ask whether the – so to speak – advantage of lactose is not that it is slowly absorbed. If milk had been rich in glucose, the baby would get severe hyperglycemia when it had a good meal. Lactose is more slowly absorbed and it is also carried further down in the intestines, thereby presumably helping to get a more acid content of the gut and thereby maintaining lactobacillus.

R. Eeckels: I must say I always wondered if the advantage wasn't bacteriological. But the human infant is a constant suckler, so I don't think the slower absorption is very important. Under physiological circumstances the infant is getting his meal during 24 hours a day.

K. van Acker: Dr. Carlsson, you didn't mention the complement system in the defense against infection. What about the complement system in the milk?

B. Carlsson: I didn't mention it in my paper. We haven't been studying it so much. We have been looking mostly into the antibody system. Of course, you have the complement system also.

Antibodies are mainly IgA and they are not supposed to activate complement to such an extent as the other immunoglobins. But there are some instances that it could be activated by the alternative pathway.

R. Eeckels: From work in my laboratory we know that complement is present in human milk and is active and functioning, as in serum.

H.K.A. Visser: Dr. Baum, did you study the effect of your milk-bank system on the children in any way? I am asking this particularly after we heard Dr. Davies paper.

J.D. Baum: No, we did not. I think we are determined to set up such a study, once we can agree on which variables of the human milk-bank composition we will choose to hold stable, so that we can do a substantial study. It won't be learned quickly; we're not going to suddenly wipe out an epidemic of necrotizing enterocolitis. It's a big undertaking.

B.S. Lindblad: It is evident that some of the secretory IgA immuno-globulins in human milk are specific to bacteria from the mother. So, it may be possible to study the ecology, or the frequency in the community of the different antigens, by studying human milk. Perhaps one should also realise that, by putting up a milk bank in England, that milk would not necessarily provide prevention of diarrhea in human infants in, let us say, North Africa. The milk should probably come from the endogenous population. We may eventually also improve human milk by vaccination of the mothers before storing it into a milk bank.

P.J.J. Sauer: Does freezing for a long period of time – you mentioned 3 months – affect your opsonin and complement activity and also the IgA factor? Can you measure the quantity of IgA or the quality, after 3 months' freezing?

J.D. Baum: Among the five studies that I showed on that complicated slide, three of them had looked at IgA and lactoferrin after freezing – in addition to the figures I showed you – and showed no major loss during the period of storage, which varied from a week (the lowest) up to three months. However, in one experiment that we did we were worried to find that the pasteurized frozen stored milk allowed much more growth of E-coli than the pasteurized unfrozen stored milk. So it could be that there are intricate effects which one doesn't see by doing a simple Mancini immune diffusion assay.

R. Eeckels: I wonder, Dr. Davies, if you have a comment on that freezing problem. I thought you said that there was no difference in your study.

P.A. Davies: Our bacteriologist examined specimens that had been deep-frozen but it was for a rather short period of time – less than a week – and he also found that there had been no change in IgA, lactoferrin or lyzozyme.

R. de Meyer: It has been mentioned many times that there are macro-phages and lymphocytes in the milk. Is it possible that these cells are still active when they are going through the stomach where the pH is at about 1? Do they play some role afterwards?

M. Gabr: In breast-fed infants usually the pH in the stomach is much higher than 1 – about 4 or 4½ – but I don't know the answer. I want to come back to Dr. Carlsson because she mentioned that challenging the mother with oral polio vaccine did not result in an increase in the IgA secreted in her milk, if I got it correctly. This would mean that the IgA in the milk is not specifically directed against the polio vaccine, or do you think the polio vaccine did not reach the target organ in the intestine of the mother? Because if the IgA secreted in human milk is not active against polio, then we don't have to worry so much in our country where most of the babies are breast-fed, and where we vaccinate them orally against polio. We are very cautious to do it 2 or 3 hours after the breast feeding.

B. Carlsson: I said that the IgA in the milk decreased after oral vaccination of the mother.

M. Gabr: How they would decrease, you have no idea?

B. Carlsson: Probably by binding to the virus.

M. Gabr: Locally, in the breast.

B. Carlsson: I don't know where.

R.G. Pearse: Is there any good evidence that giving bacteria with the milk to these babies, especially the bacteria that are being collected with the milk in the home, is harmful? We all assume that giving them a culture of E-coli or staphylococcus epidermidis is harmful. But, is there any evidence to show that that's so?

P.A. Davies: I think the situation is possible a little more complicated than that, because although the preterm infant must be colonized with some E-coli from his mother, he must pick up other E-coli from the environment. His mother, as we know, has antibodies to the E-coli that are in her gut, but she may well not have antibodies in her milk to the E-coli which are in the intensive care nursery environment. I think this is really as far as I can go. When in our study raw human milk had E-coli in it, it was discarded if the organisms were greater than 10^3 per liter.

R.G. Pearse: My original question was quite simple: Is there any evidence that giving more than so many organisms per liter is harmful? Especially as it's organisms from the mother who has got antibodies to her own organisms.

P.A. Davies: I don't think I can answer that, I'm sorry.

B. Friis Hansen: Can the human breast produce antibodies to bacteria it is exposed to, so to speak, directly? I know that is the case in animals. Twenty years ago, I was interested in the possibility that the newborn infant could absorb antibodies. In order to get milk with a high content of antibodies, we injected heat-killed bacteria into the mammary gland (the ducts of the mammary gland) of a cow. The cow started to produce milk with a very high titre of antibodies against these bacteria.

If the human breast reacts the same way, when the baby has a certain strain of coli in his mouth, then regardless of whether the mother's blood contains antibodies, the human breast itself could start to produce antibodies and thereby help to protect the baby.

R. Eeckels: Thank you. I'm sure Professor Ballabriga has a comment on that point.

A. Ballabriga: We now have some experience with cow-whey protein antibodies. We have used coli vaccine with many strains of enteropathogenic coli, that has been injected into the cows during pregnancy. After the birth of the calves, we have made an ultrafiltrate of colostrum that we call cow-whey protein, with a very high content of IgG_1. The problem is the difference with mother's milk, as the antibody in human milk is secretory IgA and in cow's milk IgG_1. This cow-whey protein has been fed to newborn infants in artificial formula, and we have studied the passage of these antibodies through the gastrointestinal tract. We have observed some destruction in the stomach as a result of the action of pepsin and trypsin. It is possible to identify part of the antibodies that act locally and may increase the local immunity. They are not absorbed, because we can recover part of these antibodies in the stools of the infants.

When this cow-whey protein was used in a nursery during more than one year, we observed that the number of the positive stool cultures in infants receiving these antibodies was lower than in the control series. Does the IgG_1 act as antibody against enterotoxin or against the pili with the possibility of stopping the adhesion of the pili of the E-coli to the mucosa surface? Of course, the production of this kind of cow-whey protein antibody is terribly expensive. It's more an academic problem than a practical problem.

PARENTERAL NUTRITION OF THE NEWBORN AND INFANT

THE INTRAVENOUS AND PERORAL
REQUIREMENTS OF AMINO ACIDS
DURING EARLY INFANCY

B.S. LINDBLAD, G. ALFVÉN and B.E. GINSBURG*

Optimal intake does not just mean a safe margin, but avoiding undesirably large intakes. An amino acid imbalance may cause a multitude of toxic effects (1) and negative effects on protein synthesis rate (2). High tyrosine levels of plasma have been correlated to specific learning disabilities later in life (3, 4). The fact that up to 14 times normal concentrations of amino acids in brain tissue have been registered during parenteral nutrition of pups, in spite of near-normal plasma levels (5) means that the monitoring of plasma levels does not in itself guarantee against toxic effects. Theoretically, there is a relative intolerance to phenylalanine, tyrosine and methionine in the immature newborn human infant (6). This has been confirmed during parenteral nutrition of newborn infants (7, 8, 9, 10). In particular, the methionine levels increase during parenteral nutrition (7, 8) and during peroral overload (11).

A. THE INTRAVENOUS AMINO ACID REQUIREMENTS

In a recent study of 20 young infants under total parenteral nutrition (7), our conclusion based on the amino acid levels obtained in peripheral blood, was that we were providing minimal rather than optimal amounts of amino acids. This was in spite of our having provided 4 kcal/kg/hr and 2.4 g amino acids/100 kcal. The requirements of infants being less than 1.7 g/100 kcal when fed perorally (12), it seems that the "protein", or amino acid solution we used (Vamin, Vitrum, Sweden) was inadequate, in spite of the fact that the pattern was made according to the composition of whole egg -- an "ideal" protein when fed perorally to adults. The low efficiency of the intravenous amino acid solution has been observed by other authors (5, 8, 13, 14, 15).

* From the Paediatric Clinic of Karolinska Institutet at St. Göran's Children's Hospital, Stockholm, Sweden.

H.K.A. Visser (ed.), Nutrition and Metabolism of the Fetus and Infant, 325-339. All rights reserved.
Copyright © 1979 *Martinus Nijhoff Publishers b.v., The Hague/Boston/London.*

However, it is possible that the intravenous requirements of amino acids are quite different from those of peroral feeding, as parenteral nutrition means infusing nutrients directly into a deep vein, by-passing the regulatory mechanisms of the gut and the liver. The amino acid pattern of plasma obtained from the hepatic vein would represent the result of those intestinal and hepatic regulatory mechanisms. Since the amino acid pattern in peripheral blood plasma seems to mimic the amino acid pattern of the intravenous intake (13) an intake pattern resembling that of the hepatic vein plasma should result in a more normal amino acid pattern in peripheral plasma. We, therefore, decided to investigate the free amino acid levels of hepatic venous plasma during infancy.

Material and methods

Blood was collected into heparinized tubes from the hepatic vein during diagnostic heart catheterization of 5 children, 2 months to 6 years of age. The heart catheterizations were performed after an overnight-fast. The samples were centrifuged immediately and plasma deproteinized with crystalline sulphosalicylic acid, 50 mg/ml, and the supernatant stored in --72 °C until analyzed for the individual amino acid concentrations (16). A lithium buffer system (17) was used, allowing for the separation of serine, glutamine and asparagine. Cysteine was oxidized to cystine by allowing the sample to stand in room temperature at pH 7 for 4 hr (18). The methionine-sulphone and methionine-sulfoxide peaks were added to the one representing methionine during the estimation of the methionine concentration. Reproducibility was mean 4.9 ± 0.5 (SE) % for the 23 parameters determined by ion-exchange chromatography, ranging from 1.2% (glutamine) to 9.4% (cystine).

Results

The results are given in table 1. The Vamin R solution (Vitrum, Sweden), based on the composition of hydrolyzed whole egg protein and representing a balanced protein ideal for the peroral alimentation of adults, showed no correlation with the composition of the hepatic venous plasma (fig. 1). There was a close correlation between the hepatic venous and the peripheral *arterial* (19) amino acid concentrations during infancy.

Table 1. *The amino acid concentrations of deproteinized plasma collected from the hepatic vein of infants.*

	Hepatic vein (n = 5) μmol/l $\pm$ SE
Glutamine	512 ± 54
Alanine	181 ± 49
Lysine	239 ± 43
Glycine	162 ± 20
Threonine	85 ± 12
Valine	219 ± 26
Taurine	51 ± 6
Proline	202 ± 43
Serine	106 ± 17
Leucine	96 ± 12
Histidine	78 ± 17
Ornithine	44 ± 10
Glutamic acid	88 ± 35
Phenylalanine	45 ± 4
Arginine	Tr
Isoleucine	50 ± 8
Tyrosine	42 ± 5
Asparagine	46 ± 6
Tryptophan	Tr
Cystein	82 ± 13
a-NH$_2$-butyric acid	24
Methionine	15 ± 3
Aspartic acid	23 ± 5
Citrulline	Tr

Discussion

There seems to be a general agreement on both sides of the Atlantic as to the rates of total amino acid supply during parenteral nutrition of young infants (20, 21, 22, 23). The suggestions in table 2 are derived from our recent publication (7). 312 mg/kg/day of nitrogen seems to be minimal at this level of calorie intake, which agrees well with the fact that 310–350 mg is being stored per kilogram per day in the human fetus towards the end of pregnancy (21).

The most obvious difference between the pattern of amino acids in a protein hydrolysate of an "ideal" protein versus the hepatic venous plasma (fig. 1) is the predominance of *glutamic acid* in the hydrolysate, while *glutamine* dominates the plasma composition. This is mainly because glutamine is converted to glutamic acid during acid hydrolysis.

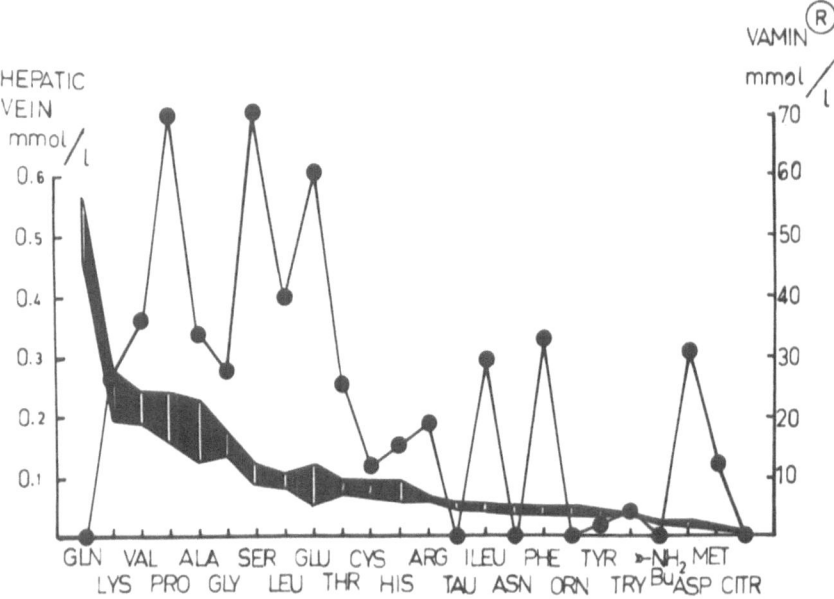

Fig. 1. A comparison between the free amino acid pattern of the hepatic venous plasma of infants and the composition of the Vamin^R (Vitrum, Sweden) amino acid solution for intravenous use. The black area, with the white vertical lines, represent mean ± 2 SE for the free amino acid concentrations of the hepatic venous plasma and the filled circles represent the Vamin^R composition.

In the natural state, milk contains equal amounts of glutamine and glutamic acid (24).

Glutamine participates in a variety of enzymatic transformations; it is required for purine biosynthesis, and is essential to mammalian cells (25). It is normally mainly produced by muscle tissue in the adult, but is, like alanine, most efficiently consumed by tumor and fetal tissues (26, 27, 28). During parenteral nutrition, the plasma levels of glutamine tend to decrease (8). All these facts speak in favor of the hypothesis that glutamine is "essential" to rapidly growing tissues. It is worth noting that the 5 non-essential amino acids found to be "essential" to mammalian cells in tissue culture: arginine, glutamine, tyrosine, cystine and histidine (25), have all been found to be essential to the newborn immature child. Thus, histidine is essential to human infants and growing children (29), tyrosine and cystine are probably essential to the immature human newborn infant due to enzymatic immaturity (6, 30), and parenteral

Table 2. *Suggested rate of nutrient supply during total parenteral nutrition of young infants (7, 62).*

	per kg/hr	
Glucose	0.56 g (57 kJ%)	
Amino acids	0.10 g (8 kJ%)	(2.4 g/kg/day)
Fat	0.15 g (35 kJ%)	
Nitrogen	13 mg	(312 mg/kg/day)
Energy	17 kJ (4 kcal)	

Molar relationship glucose/nitrogen   3.4.

alimentation without arginine causes hyperammoniemia and seizures (31). A low supply of tyrosine, glutamine and taurine during total parenteral alimentation leads to a lowering of the plasma levels of these amino acids (7, 8, 22). The tendency of the amide glutamine to convert to ammonia and pyroglutamate during storage of an amino acid mixture has been an obstacle to its inclusion in amino acid solutions.

It is known that glutamic acid is largely converted to alanine, ammonia, glutamine and glutathione in the small intestinal mucosa (32). It might therefore be highly unphysiological to infuse large amounts of glutamic acid, which actually leads to increased glutamic acid levels (7, 9, 15) of plasma. High intakes of aspartic acid, glutamic acid and cysteine are known to lead to retinal degeneration and hypothalamic damage in rats (33). Furthermore, even if glutamic acid is essential to intracellular processes (26), cells are somewhat impermeable to this particular amino acid. Thus, glutamic acid is not transported across the placenta to any larger extent (34), but seems to be synthesized by the fetus (35). It seems that not only the gut converts a considerable amount of glutamic acid to alanine, but there is a hepatic control as well, as the portal venous plasma of the pig contains 480 μmol/l, as compared to 80 μmol/l of glutamic acid in the peripheral venous plasma (13). There is considerably lower alanine level in arterial (19) than in cubital venous plasma (36) and this confirms the hypothesis of an "alanine-glucose" cycle with peripheral release and a hepatic extraction of, mainly, alanine (37). If alanine is the main non-essential nitrogen carrier in infants, it seems that it should be well represented in an intravenous mixture.

On the basis of the facts mentioned above it is suggested that a major part of the glutamic acid in the infusate is replaced by alanine.

Taurine seems to play a major role in brain development (38) and low activity of cystein-sulphinic acid decarboxylase in fetal and mature liver (39) indicates that this amino acid is essential. There is a fetal accumulation of taurine (40, 41) and taurine is effectively accumulated by ascites carcinoma cells (42), which suggests that taurine is essential during intensive growth. It is, therefore, suggested that taurine should be included in the intravenous solution: in the relative amounts as found in the hepatic vein (table 1).

B. THE PERORAL AMINO ACID REQUIREMENTS

The most logical standard for the peroral optimal requirements of the different amino acids is the composition of hydrolyzed human milk, a food made exclusively for the human infant. There is a lack, in the literature, of reliable normal values obtained from studies of the milk of healthy women where the infant has also been shown to thrive normally at the breast. The amino acid content of hydrolyzed human milk was therefore determined with a thorough clinical correlation.

The optimal peroral protein requirement, or *total* requirement of amino acids, is not well defined during early infancy. It has been proposed, on the basis of experimental growth studies, that it is no more than 1.7 g/100 kcal (12), but the optimal amounts are not known.

The changes in the postabsorptive levels of plasma free amino acids seen in malnutrition are highly consistent and characteristic in all age groups. A survey of the extensive literature with a tentative explanation of the characteristic changes has recently been published (43). Thus, subclinical protein deficiency is characterized by a decrease in the concentrations of the branch-chained amino acids valine, isoleucine and leucine and an increase in the glycine levels. An overload is characterized by the opposite changes and it therefore seems possible to use the fasting plasma levels of free amino acids to evaluate the protein content of different milk formula in relation to protein requirements. A study was therefore made of the free amino acid levels of peripheral venous plasma during ad libitum feeding of human milk to young infants (36), in order to compare the results with that obtained during different levels of cow milk formula feeding (44).

Material and methods

Twenty mothers, of a mean age of 24 years, who were selling their excess breast-milk to the Stockholm milk distribution center were hospitalized with their healthy 1-5 month old (mean 80 day old) infants. The total milk volumes were 1244 ± 381 ml/24 hr, according to test-weighing and mechanical pumping of excess milk at home before admission. Breast-milk was expressed by mechanical pumping 5 times during 24 hr, a sample withdrawn each time for analysis and the rest given to the infant. The 5 samples were pooled before analysis. Diluted milk was hydrolyzed with equal amounts of concentrated HCl under vacuum for 72 hr at 105 °C before analysis for total amino acids on a Bio-Cal 200 (München) automatic amino acid analyzer according to the method of Spackman et al. (16). Cysteine was determined as cysteic acid and methionine as methionine-sulfone and -sulfoxide after oxidation with performic acid (45). Tryptophane was determined, after hydrolysis with BaOH and separation on Sephadex G-25, with ninhydrine according to Slump and Schreuder (46).

Table 3. *The amino acid concentrations of hydrolyzed human milk in g/d. Mean ± SE are given.*

Amino acid	The present investigation n = 20	Saito et al. (47) n = 65	Soupart et al. (48)
Isoleucine	0.53 ± 0.02	0.54 ± 0.01	0.54
Leucine	1.02 ± 0.04	1.01 ± 0.03	1.00
Lysine	1.37 ± 0.08	0.66 ± 0.01	0.64
Methionine	0.11 ± 0.01	0.26 ± 0.01	0.20
Cystine	0.25 ± 0.01	0.14 ± 0.01	0.23
Phenylalanine	0.36 ± 0.02	0.37 ± 0.01	0.41
Tyrosine	0.23 ± 0.02	0.38 ± 0.01	0.46
Threonine	0.49 ± 0.02	0.45 ± 0.01	0.48
Tryptophan	0.18 ± 0.01	0.19 ± 0.01	0.19
Valine	0.53 ± 0.02	0.65 ± 0.01	0.54
Arginine	0.28 ± 0.02	0.32 ± 0.01	0.31
Histidine	0.26 ± 0.02	0.23 ± 0.01	0.21
Alanine	0.34 ± 0.02	0.41 ± 0.01	0.38
Aspartic acid	0.86 ± 0.04	0.89 ± 0.01	0.93
Glutamic acid	1.64 ± 0.05	1.80 ± 0.03	1.98
Glycine	0.23 ± 0.01	0.21 ± 0.01	0.23
Proline	0.95 ± 0.03	0.93 ± 0.01	0.86
Serine	0.45 ± 0.02	0.56 ± 0.01	0.49
Total	10.06	10.00	10.08
Taurine	0.05 ± 0.01		
Ornithine	0.22 ± 0.01		
a-NH$_2$-Bu	0.27 ± 0.03		

Table 4. *The venous plasma free amino acid and urea concentrations of breast-fed infants 1–5 months of age (36).*

Amino acid	μmol/l	S.D.	n
Taurine	90	34	19
Aspartic acid	15	7	19
Threonine	108	50	19
Serine	156	56	19
Glutamine	663	208	19
Asparagine	43	18	18
Glutamic acid	63	27	19
Citrulline	23	13	6
Proline	195	90	19
Glycine	187	66	19
Alanine	269	96	19
½ Cystine	98	39	19
Valine	113	47	18
Methionine	21	8	18
Isoleucine	45	16	19
Leucine	89	23	19
Tyrosine	49	25	19
Phenylalanine	31	15	17
Ornithine	102	38	16
Lysine	119	61	19
Histidine	84	22	19
Arginine	83	29	16
Urea	2984	1613	19

The infants of these women, 10 boys and 10 girls, were all full term and showed a normal growth from normal birth weights and heights and were healthy with a normal development. They had all been fed ad libitum from the breast. Blood was collected from the cubital vein in a heparinized tube before a morning feed. The blood was centrifuged immediately and the plasma deproteinized and analyzed according to the description under Section A above.

Results

The composition of hydrolyzed human milk is given in table 3. The plasma free amino acid concentrations of breast-fed infants, 1–5 months of age, are given in table 4 (see also Ref. 36).

Discussion

There are only two previous investigations of human milk known to the authors where the total amount of amino acids determined adds up to the known protein concent of human milk (49). The results of these investigations are given in table 3 and are remarkably consistent with those of the present investigation. The only difference is that of the lysine concentration. Lysine is very easily lost during the hydrolysis in the presence of sugar. The hydrolysis in the present investigation (49) produced higher lysine levels. However, the actual lysine concentrations should probably be considered as minimal. The taurine levels are consistent with those of two available studies (39, 50).

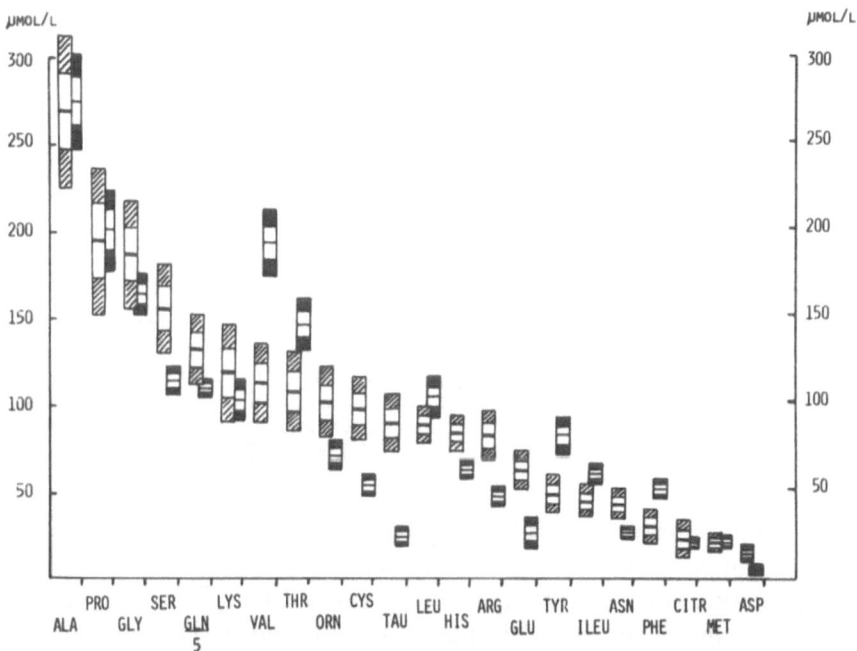

Fig. 2. Peripheral venous plasma free amino acid concentrations of 1–5 months old human infants. Partly striped bars indicate brest-fed infants (mean ± 2 S.E., n = 19) (36), partly filled bars cow-milk-formula fed infants, 3–3.5 g protein/kg (mean ± 2 S.E., n = 29) (44). The glutamine concentrations have been divided by 5 before being included in the diagram. The levels during formula-feeding of glutamine, glutamic acid and aspartic acid are those of infants 1–2 years of age (13).

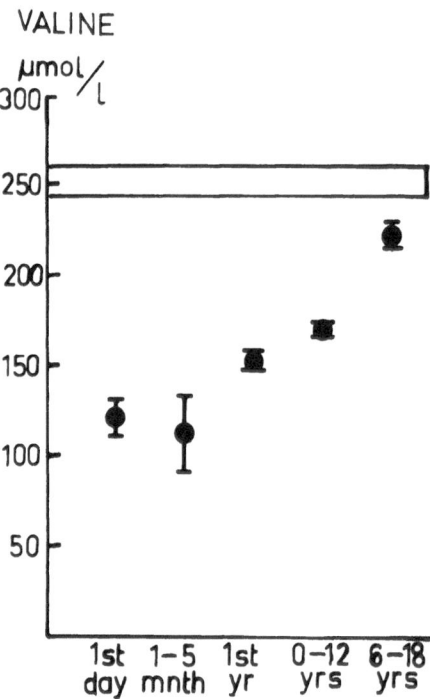

Fig. 3. Fasting peripheral venous plasma free valine concentrations at different ages. The horizontal bar represents mean + 2 SE of the fasting valine levels of normal adults (51). From left to right the filled circles represent the valine levels of newborn infants during the first day of life, before the first feed (52), the valine level of wholly breast fed young infants (36), the fasting valine levels during the first year of life and during the first 12 years of life (53) and the fasting levels of normal children 6–18 years of age (51).

A comparison of the peripheral venous plasma free amino acid levels of 3 g protein/kg cow milk formula fed infants (44) with the results of the investigation of breast-fed infants (36) shows as main differences almost doubled valine levels, a low glycine/valine ratio and low cystine and very low taurine levels of plasma from the cow milk formula fed infants (fig. 2). This indicates a protein overload (43, 44) and a lack of taurine in these formula fed, normal infants.

A survey of the literature as regards the valine level of plasma shows that it is a remarkably constant variable with small inter-individual variation and that it is related to age (fig. 3). In each age group there is also a strong dependence on the protein intake (fig. 4). It is evident from figure 4 that the cow milk protein intake during infancy should be

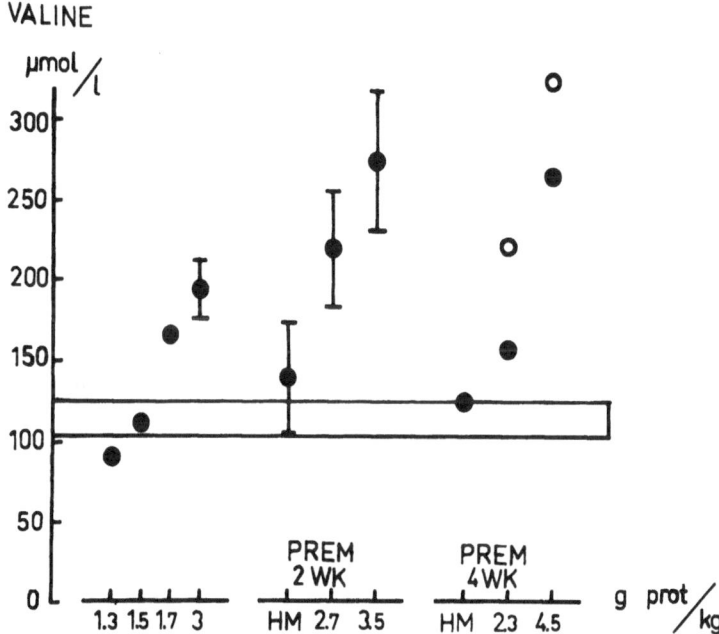

Fig. 4. Fasting peripheral venous plasma valine concentrations during different levels of protein intake. The horizontal bar represents the valine levels of the wholly breast fed young infants (36) (table 4), mean ± 2 SE. From left to right the filled circles represent the different valine levels upon increasing protein intake in normal full term young infants (44), the levels found in 2 week old premature infants fed human milk and a 'humanized' (lactalbumin/casein ratio of 60:40) formula containing 2 different amounts of protein (54) and the valine levels of premature infants at 4 weeks of age given human milk and 2 different levels of protein intake (55). The open circles represent the valine levels during feeding with a 'non-humanized' formula (lactalbumin/casein ratio of 18:82).

between 1.5 and 1.7 g/kg/day when provided in "humanized form" (with the lactalbumin/casein ratio of human milk) in order to give the same valine levels of plasma as that of human milk feeding. This is considerably less than that provided by the cow milk formulas in current use but consistent with the earlier recommendation of maximum 1.7 g/100 kcal (12).

The difference shown between normal breast-fed Swedish young infants consuming 0.82 g protein/100 ml (49) (fig. 2) and normal cow milk formula fed American young infants (44) consuming 2–2.3 g protein/100 ml could be of importance, as there are indications that the branch-chained amino acid (valine, leucine, isoleucine) levels in particular influence insulin metabolism. The branch-chained amino acid levels of plasma seem to be especially sensitive to exogenous and endogenous insulin (56, 57, 58, 59, 60). These amino acids are also significantly elevated in obese subjects (57) and inversely correlated with immunoreactive insulin levels. The branch-chained amino acid levels are also significantly elevated in patients with diabetic keto-acidosis (61).

A low taurine level of plasma from the formula fed infants is consistent with the low amounts of taurine in cow milk as compared to human milk (39, 50). As taurine seems to be essential and to play a major role in brain development (38, 39) it is suggested that taurine is added to cow milk formulas in the relative amounts present in human milk (table 3).

SUMMARY AND CONCLUSIONS

A.   Amino acid solutions for *intravenous* use mostly have an amino acid composition modeled after proteins which are "ideal" when fed per-orally to adults. This is unsatisfactory, as total parenteral nutrition bypasses the regulatory mechanisms of the gut and the liver, and it has led to an inbalance of the amino acid composition of the peripheral blood, with an inefficient utilization and possible toxic effects. In order to define a standard for the intravenous amino acid intake we have analyzed hepatic venous plasma obtained from infants during diagnostic· heart catheterization. The rational for this being that the amino acid pattern of the hepatic venous plasma represents the result of both the intestinal and hepatic regulatory mechanisms. The solution used by us during total parenteral alimentation of infants (Vamin, Vitrum, Sweden, with a composition like that of hydrolyzed whole egg protein) showed a poor correlation with the composition of the hepatic venous plasma. On the basis of this investigation it is our intention to decrease the glutamic acid concentration and to increase the alanine and taurine content of the intravenous solution. The total amounts will be held constant at 0.10 g amino acids/kg/hr during an energy supply of 4 kcal/kg/hr.

B.   The requirements of the individual amino acids during *peroral* feeding of young infants is probably best defined by the amino acid composition of human milk. These concentrations have been investigated, with a thorough clinical correlation, and the results were found to compare well with those of two earlier studies using similar methods.

The fasting peripheral venous plasma free amino acid levels of wholly breast-fed infants were determined in order to define the optimal protein intake during early infancy. This "normal" plasma aminogram shows considerably lower valine levels and higher cystine and very much higher taurine levels than those of formula-fed infants of the same age. A reveiw of the literature shows that the fasting valine levels of peripheral venous plasma are related both to age and to protein intake. It is demonstrated how the protein intake with a "humanized" formula should be between 1.5–1.7 g protein/kg in order to give the same fasting blood plasma valine concentrations as those of infants fed human milk ad libitum. This is considerably less than what is usually given during cow milk formula feeding. A possible consequence of this protein overload (and the high plasma valine levels) during early infancy could be a higher level of insulin release with an increased risk of lasting obesity. It is suggested that a formula, when used during early infancy, should be "humanized" not only with regard to the lactalbumin/casein ratio, but also to the cystine and taurine content and that the protein content should be no higher than 1.0–1.2 g/100 ml.

ACKNOWLEDGEMENT

This investigation was supported by Grant No. 2583 from the Swedish Medical Research Council.

REFERENCES

1. HARPER, A.E. (1964) In: Mammalian Protein Metabolism, Munro H.N. and J.B. Allison eds. Academic Press Inc., New York, vol. 2, p. 87.
2. WONG, P.W.K. and P. JUSTICE. (1972) In Advances in Experimental Medicine and Biology. Volk, B.W. and S.M. Aronson eds. Plenum Press, New York, p. 163.
3. MENKES, J.H., D.W. WELCHER, H.S. LEVI, J. DALLAS and N.E. GRETSKY. (1972) Pediatrics 49:218.
4. MAMUNES, P., P.E. PRINCE, N.H. THORNTON, P.A. HUNT and E.S. HITCHKOCK. (1976) Pediatrics 57:675.
5. HEIRD, W.C., D. RASSIN and G.E. GAULL. (1977) Pediatr. Res. 11: 1028.
6. LINDBLAD, B.S. (1976) In The Fetus: Physiology and Medicine, Beard R.W. and P.W. Nathanielsz eds. W.B. Saunders Co.. Ltd, Londen, 80.
7. LINDBLAD, B.S., G. SETTERGREN, H. FEYCHTING and B. PERSSON. (1977) Acta Paediatr. Scand. 66:409.
8. ABITBOL, C.L., D.B. FELDMAN, P. AHMANN and D. RUDMAN. (1975) J. Pediatr. 86:766.
9. DALE, G., M. PANTER-BRICK, J. WAGGET a/ G. YOUNG. (1976) J. Pediatr. Surg. 11:17.

10. Wong, P.W.K. and R.S. Pildes. (1974) Biol. Neonate 25:300.
11. Levy, H.L., V.E. Shih, P.M. Madigan, V. Karolkewicz, J.R. Carr, A. Lum, A.A. Richards, J.D. Crford and R.A. MacCready. (1969) Am. J. Dis. Child. 117:96.
12. Fomon, S.J., E.E. Ziegler, L.N. Thomas and L.J. Filer, Jr. (1971) In: Metabolic Processes in the Foetus and Newborn Infant, 3rd Nutricia Symposium. Jonxis J.H.P., H.,A. Visser and J.A. Troelstra eds, H.E. Stenfert Kroese, Leiden, Holland p. 144.
13. Stegink, L.D. and G.L. Baker. (1971) J. Pediatr. 78:595.
14. Pohlandt, F. (1975) Monatsschr. Kinderh. 123:448.
15. Higgs, S.C., A.F. Malan and H. De V Hesse. (1977) South Afr. Med. J. 51:5.
16. Spackman, D.H., W.H. Stein and S. Moore. (1958) Anal. Chem. 30:1190.
17. Benson, J.V., Jr., M.J. Gordon and J.A. Patterson. (1967) Anal. Biochem. 18:228.
18. Stein, W.H. and S. Moore. (1954) J. Biol. Chem. 211:915.
19. Settergren, G., B.S. Lindblad and B. Persson. (1976) Acta Paediatr. Scand. 65:343.
20. Børresen, H.C. (1974) In: Parenteral Nutrition in Acute Metabolic Illness, Lee, H.A. ed., Acadmic Press, London and New York, p. 221.
21. Shaw, J.L.C. (1974) Proc. Nutr. Soc. 33:103.
22. Winters, R.W. (1975) Pediatrics 56:17.
23. Ghadimi, H. (ed.) (1975) Total Parenteral Nutrition, John Wiley & Sons, New York.
24. Mercien, J.C., F. Grosslande, and B.R. Dumas. (1972) Milchwissenschaft 27:402.
25. Eagle H. (1955) Science 122:501.
26. Roberts, E. and T. Tanaka. (1956) Cancer Res. 16:204.
27. Levintow, L. (1954) J. Nat. Cancer Inst. 15:347.
28. Yamamoto, H., T. Aikawa, H. Matsutaka and E. Ishikawa. (1974) Metabolism 23:1017.
29. Holt, L.E., Jr and S.E. Snyderman. (1961) J.A.M.A. 175:100.
30. Gaull, G., J.A. Sturman and N.C.R. Räihä (1972) Pediatr. Res. 6:538.
31. Heird, W.C., J.F. Nicholson, J.M. Driscoll, J.N. Schullinger and R.W. Winters (1972) J. Pediatr. 81:162.
32. Elwyn, D.H., H.C. Parikh and W.C. Shoemaker. (1968) Am. J. Physiol. 215:1260.
33. Olney, J.W. and O.L. Ho. (1970) Nature 227:609.
34. Lemons, J.A., E.W. Adcock II, M. Douglas Jones, Jr., M.A. Naughton, G. Meschia and F.C. Battaglia. (1976) J. Clin. Invest. 58:1428.
35. Smith, R.M., I.G. Jarrett, R.A. King and G.R. Russell. (1977) Biol Neonate 31:305.
36. Lindblad, B.S., G. Alfvén and R. Zetterström, (1978) Acta Paediatr. Scand. 67:659.
37. Felig, P. (1973) Metabolism 22:179.
38. Sturman, J.A., D.K. Rassin and G.E. Gaull. (1977) Pediatr. Res. 11:28.
39. Gaull, G.E., D.K. Rassin, N.C.R. Räihä and K. Heinonen. (1977) J. Pediatr. 90:348.
40. Lindblad, B.S. and A. Baldensten. (1967) Acta Paediatr. Scand. 56:37.
41. Lindblad, B.S. and A. Baldensten. (1969) Acta Paediatr. Scand. 58:252.
42. Christensen, H.N., B. Hess and T.R. Riggs. (1954) Cancer Res. 14:12.
43. Lindblad, B.S., R.J. Rahimtoola, H. Ur-Rehman, R. Shamim Ahmad, K. Fancy, L. Singha and S. Sajjad Mussian. (1978) Acta Paediatr. Scand. 67:335.

44. SNYDERMAN, S.E., L.E. HOLT, Jr., P.M. NORTON, E. ROITMAN and S.V. PHANSALKAR. (1968) Pediatr. Res. 2:131.
45. SOUPART, P., S. MOORE and E.J. BIGWOOD. (1954) J. Biol. Chem. 206:699.
46. SLUMP, P. and H.A.W. SCHREDER. (1969) Anal. Biochem. 27:182.
47. SAITO, K., E. FURUICHI, W. KONDO, Q. KAWANISHI, I. NISHIKAWA, H. NAKAZATO, Y. NOGUCHI, T. DOI, A. NOGUCHI and S. SHINGO. (1965) Studies on Human Milk, Snow Brand Milk Products Co., Ltd., Tokyo.
48. SOUPART, P., S. MOORE and E.J. BIGWOOD. (1954) J. Biol. Chem. 206:699.
49. LINDBLAD, B.S. and R.J. RAHIMTOOLA. (1974) Acta Paediatr. Scand. 63:125.
50. GHANDIMI, H. and P. PECORA. (1963) Am. J. Clin. Nutr. 13:75.
51. ARMSTRONG, M.D. and U. STAVE. (1973) Metabolism 22:549 and 571.
52. MESTYÁN, J., GY. SOLTÉSZ, K. SCHULTZ and M. HORVATH. (1975) J. Pediatr. 87:409.
53. NICOLAIDOU, M., C.C. LUND and R.H. McMENAMY. (1962) Arch. Biochem. Biophys. 96:613.
54. RIGO, H. and J. SENTERRE. (1977) Biol. Neonate 32:73.
55. RASSIN, D.K., G.E. GAULL, K. HEINONEN and N.R.C. RÄIHÄ. (1977) Pediatrics 59:407.
56. CROFFORD, O.B., P.W. FELTS and W.W. LACY. (1964) Proc. Soc. Exp. Biol. Med. 117:11.
57. FELIG, P., E. MARLISS and G.F. CAHILL, Jr. (1969) N. Engl. J. Med. 281:811.
58. FELIG, P., O.E. OWEN, J. WAHREN and G.F. CAHILL, Jr. (1969) J. Clin. Invest. 48:584.
59. POSEFSKY, J., P. FELIG, J.D. TOBIN, J.S. SOELDNER and G.F. CAHILL, Jr. (1969) J. Clin. Invest. 48:2273.
60. ZINNEMAN, H.H., F.Q. NUTTALL and F.C. GOETZ. (1966) Diabetes 15:5.
61. FELIG, P., E. MARLISS, J.L. OHMAN and G.F. CAHILL, Jr. (1970) Diabetes 19:727.
62. OLEGÅRD, R. (1974) Metabolism of Blood Lipids in Newborn Infants. Academic Thesis, Dept. of Pediatrics I, University of Gothenburg, Sweden.

STUDIES ON THE REQUIREMENT OF AMINO ACIDS IN NEWBORN INFANTS RECEIVING PARENTERAL NUTRITION

FRANK POHLANDT*

The quality of nutrition influences the development of the fetus and the infant. Disturbances in the morphologic development of the brain and some impaired mental abilities should be emphasized as consequences of deficient nutrition. These disturbances arise predominantly during the spurt in cerebral growth (1). This vulnerable phase of cerebral development covers the period from the middle of pregnancy until after the end of the second year of life. This means 80% of growth spurt occurs after birth.

Isolated hyperaminoacidemias, as well as deficient nutrition, effect irreversible disturbances of physical growth and central nervous functions during the growth spurt. For example, newborn infants of mothers who were not treated for phenylketonuria are small for their gestational age and show microcephaly (2, 3). Hyperphenylalaninemia, induced into the fetus by the mother, is considered a cause of this. That this damage is irreversible is illustrated by the fact that the physical and intellectual development of these infants is impaired also after birth. The studies made by MENKES et al. (4) on premature infants and by MAMUNES et al. (5) on term newborn infants demonstrate the probability, that even transitory hypertyrosinemia of more than 14 mg% can cause permanent limitations of some mental abilities. The incidence of transitory hypertyrosinemia is increased in newborn infants fed protein rich milk (6). Goldman et al. undertook follow-up studies on 204 premature infants weighing less than 2000 g at birth (7). Those children who were fed protein rich milk (6.0 – 7.2 g/kg/day) during the neonatal period yielded remarkably often low intelligence quotients.

In cases of oral nourishment the liver absorbes the greater part of the amino acids out of the portal vein blood and this prevents strong variations in the amino acid concentration in the blood after a meal (8). But in

* Zentrum für Kinderheilkunde, University of Ulm, Fed. Rep. Germany.

H.K.A. Visser (ed.), Nutrition and Metabolism of the Fetus and Infant, 341-364. All rights reserved.
Copyright © 1979 Martinus Nijhoff Publishers b.v., The Hague/Boston/London.

the case of parenteral nutrition the nutrients are infused directly into the general circulation and the homeostatic function of the liver is almost completely switched off.

During parenteral nutrition it is especially important for newborn babies and infants who are in the vulnerable phase of cerebral development to have an amino acid solution which on the one hand meets the requirement for growth and on the other hand, does not cause any imbalances in the plasma amino acid concentrations. This paper reports on studies aimed at developing the correct composition of an amino acid solution which meets the both above-mentioned requirements.

Our studies were based on the assumption that the intrauterine supply of nutrients to the fetus represents an ideal model of parenteral nutrition. This model is characterized by a steady state of nutrients in the blood of the fetus. The level of steady state is determined by that concentration provided by the umbilical cord vein blood and the amount of nutrients consumed by the fetus. The model gives the opportunity to determine in two different ways the amino acid consumption by the fetus and newborn infant:

1. The amount of amino acids which is extracted from the blood in the umbilical cord vein and which is presumably consumed by the fetus, can be calculated from the differences between the amino acid concentrations in the umbilical cord vein and artery if the rate of blood flow in the umbilical cord vessels is known.

2. If the amino acid concentrations of newborn infants can be kept at the intrauterine steady state level by constant infusion of amino acids, the consumption of amino acids by the infant can be established from the amounts of amino acids which were infused.

Theoretically it is possible, that the level of steady state changes after birth. Breast-fed newborn infants seem to be the most appropriate model for the study of amino acids in steady state after birth. By our studies we tried in both ways to answer the question about the amino acid requirement of newborn infants receiving parenteral nutrition.

MATERIAL AND METHODS

To solve the problem by the first method we measured the amino acid concentrations in the plasma of the umbilical cord vein and artery of 23 infants born spontaneously (table 1). To study the possible influence of labour on the amino acid concentrations in the plasma of the umbilical

Table 1. *Data of 24 newborn infants delivered spontaneously.*

	Minimum	10th percentile	Median	90th percentile	Maximum
Birthweight (g)	2550	2720	3200	4100	4550
Gestational age (weeks)	35	36.7	40.0	41.3	42
APGAR Score 1 min (n = 7)	7	7	8	9	9

Table 2. *Data of 23 newborn infants delivered by elective caesarean section.*

	Minimum	10th percentile	Median	90th percentile	Maximum
Birthweight (g)	2730	2820	3450	3900	4580
Gestational age (weeks)	38	38.0	40.0	42.0	42
APGAR Score 1 min	8	8	9	9	10
Umbilical cord artery pH	7.20	7.24	7.30	7.35	7.37

Table 3. *Data of 40 newborn infants breastfed ad libitum.*

	Minimum	10th percentile	Median	90th percentile	Maximum
Birthweight (g)	2430	3100	3595	3940	4110
Gestational age (weeks)	38	38.8	40	42	43
Age (days)	0.7	3.4	4.4	7.5	20.9
Milk volumen (g/kg/day)	25	72	103	137	168

cord vessels, we measured additionally the amino acid concentrations in
the umbilical cord vessels of infants who were born by elective cesarean
section i.e. without preceding labour (table 2). The differences between
the concentrations of each amino acid in the umbilical cord vein and
artery were established for each patient. The median differences between the concentration were multiplied by the rate of blood flow in the
umbilical cord vessels in order to calculate the fetal retention of amino
acids. A haematocrit of 49% was taken into account in the calculation.

Fetal retention (mmol/kg body weight/day) =

$$\Delta_{V-A} \text{ (mmol/l)} \times \text{blood flow (108 l)} \times 0.51.$$

The steady state level of amino acids after birth was determined in the
venous plasma of 40 newborn infants who were breast-fed ad libitum
(table 3) (9). All infants were healthy and born at term in the University
Hospital.

The amino acid concentrations at steady state were determined,
during the years 1972 to 1977, in 264 plasma samples of 118 mostly
premature infants receiving parenteral nutrition (table 4). During this
period 2 commercial solutions of crystalline l-amino acids and 5 of our
own (ASP1-ASP5) were used in intravenous nutrition (tables 5 and 6)
(9). The median concentration of each amino acid was calculated and
related to the median infused dose.

The plasma amino acid concentration were measured from an 0.1 ml
aliquot by ion exchange column chromatography (9).

Table 4. *Parenteral nutrition in newborn infants during the years 1972–1977: birth weight and gestational age of the studied infants, dosage of amino acids and energy.*

	Aminofusin^R L-forte	AS-KH-E for pediatrics	ASP1	ASP2	ASP3	ASP4	ASP5
Birthweight (g)							
Minimum	1030	1000	1640	1490	840	1100	605
10th percentile	1070	1024	1670	1490	876	1100	750
Median	1525	1940	2400	1710	1590	1650	1880
90th percentile	2890	2600	3060	2093	2757	3050	3030
Maximum	3510	3350	3060	2450	3000	3900	3710
Gestational age (weeks)							
Minimum	24	28	32	31	27	28	25
10th percentile	27	28	32	32	28	28	28
Median	30	33	33	32	32	32	33
90th percentile	36	36	37	33	37	40	41
Maximum	39	38	43	34	38	40	41
kJ/kg/day							
Minimum	100	213	113	205	151	109	241
10th percentile	222	339	176	239	234	218	269
Median	276	360	213	289	260	330	381
90th percentile	347	398	255	402	410	414	442
Maximum	373	523	352	448	481	594	465
Amino Acids (g/kg/day)							
Minimum	1.5	2.4	1.2	2.3	1.5	1.6	1.6
10th percentile	2.9	2.4	1.2	2.3	1.5	1.6	2.1
Median	3.0	2.5	2.5	2.5	1.6	1.8	2.3
90th percentile	3.8	2.6	2.7	2.8	1.7	2.0	2.5
Maximum	4.0	2.7	2.8	2.8	2.2	2.4	2.6
Number of patients	26	12	17	6	21	17	19
Number of plasma samples	59	23	33	22	53	37	38

Table 5. *Standardized parenteral nutrition in newborn infants during the years 1972 – 1977.   Doses per kg bodyweight per day.*

Type of amino acid solution	AMINOFUSIN L-forte	AS-KH-E-F·P	ASP1	ASP2	ASP3	ASP4	ASP5
Amino acids (g)	3– 4	2.6	2.5	2.5	1.63	1.87	2.33
Glucose (g)	6–12	8–14	8–14	8–14	8–17	8–17	8–17
Fructose (g)	6– 8	–	–	–	–	–	–
Sorbitol (g)	1.5– 2	5	1.7	1.7	–	–	–
Xylitol (g)	1.5– 2	5	–	–	0 or 5	0 or 5	0 or 5
Lipid (g) (INTRALIPID)	–	–	–	–	–	0–2	0–4
Na (mmol)	2	4	2	2	3.3	3.3	4.0
K (mmol)	1.5	3	1.5	1.5	2.5	2.5	2.5
Ca (mmol)	1	1	1	1	1.25	1.25	0.35
Mg (mmol)	0.2	0.125	0.2	0.2	0.75	0.75	0.75
Zn (mmol)	–	–	–	–	–	–	0.09
Cl (mmol)	1.7	4	1.7	1.7	3.9	3	3
P (mmol)	0.2	–	0.2	0.2	–	2	2
Heparin (I.E.)	100	100	100	100	100	100	100
Retinol (I.E.)	–	500	–	–	500	500	500
Thiaminechloride·Hydrochloride (mg)	–	2.5	–	–	2.5	2.5	2.5
Riboflavin-5'-phosphoric acid ester Sodium salt (mg)	–	0.5	–	–	0.5	0.5	0.5
Nicotinamide (mg)	–	5	–	–	5	5	5
Pyridoxin Hydrochloride (mg)	–	0.75	–	–	0.75	0.75	0.75
Ascorbic acid (mg)	–	25	–	–	25	25	25
α-Tocopherolacetate (mg)	–	0.25	–	–	0.25	0.25	0.25
Panthenol (mg)	–	1.25	–	–	1.25	1.25	1.25
Volumen (ml)	130–160	134–154	130–160	130–160	167–335	124–154	136–156
kJ/kg/day	221–347	351–456	209–310	209–310	167–335	167–481	280–511

Table 6. Composition and dosage of different amino acid solutions which were used in newborn infants during parenteral nutrition.

Amino acid	AMINOFUSIN L forte		"AS-KH-E"		ASP1		ASP2		ASP3		ASP4		ASP5	
Median dosage of amino acid mixture (g/kg/day)	3.0		2.5		2.5		2.5		1.61		1.87		2.33	
	1*	2*	1*	2*	1*	2*	1*	2*	1*	2*	1*	2*	1*	2*
L-Threonine	20	504	32	664	51	1070	51	1075	126	1700	108	1700	61	1202
L-Serine	—	—	—	—	41	980	—	—	—	—	—	—	—	—
L-Aspartic acid	—	—	79	1489	—	—	—	—	—	—	—	—	—	—
L-Glutamic acid	—	—	257	4381	—	—	—	—	—	—	—	—	—	—
L-Proline	60	1565	79	1643	24	530	24	530	21	300	18	300	18	374
Glycine	260	10400	79	2520	122	4060	122	4080	93	2000	80	2000	32	1000
L-Alanine	260	8767	135	3787	285	8000	286	8022	276	5000	238	5000	305	8000
L-Valine	32	821	40	846	63	1340	63	1350	51	700	44	700	50	1000
L-Cystine	—	—	4	42	—	—	35	733	24	158	20	158	15	150
L-Methionine	48	966	18	302	22	380	22	376	18	200	16	200	19	302
L-Isoleucine	28	641	47	908	32	620	33	622	33	400	80	1143	64	1145
L-Leucine	48	1099	55	1061	41	770	41	779	49	600	96	1372	90	1603
L-Tyrosine	—	—	7.9	110	12	170	12	166	9	80	11	110	9	110
L-Phenylalanine	44	800	36	539	45	680	45	685	41	400	35	400	33	460
L-Tryptophan	10	147	18	221	20	250	20	250	25	196	21	196	35	410
L-Ornithine	—	—	—	—	—	—	—	—	—	—	—	—	—	—
L-Lysine	40	822	44	760	81	1390	82	1397	101	980	96	1228	125	2000
L-Histidine	30	580	14	226	61	980	61	987	58	600	50	600	53	800
L-Arginine	130	2241	72	1034	102	1460	102	1471	76	700	86	918	90	1201

1* : Composition of the amino acid mixture (mg amino acid/g mixture)
2* : Dosage (µmol/kg bodyweight/day) with regards to the median infused dose

RESULTS AND DISCUSSION

No differences were found between the amino acid concentrations of spontaneously and operatively born infants (9). Both samples, therefore, could be combined. More precise values of the 10th, 50th and 90th percentile would thereby be achieved (fig 1). This kind of statistical description was chosen because the distribution of the data was mostly skewed. With the exception of taurine, glutamic and aspartic acid all amino acids showed lower concentrations in the umbilical cord artery than in the vein. This means that all but these 3 amino acids are extracted from the blood of the umbilical cord vein and are presumably consumed by the fetus. The amounts of the amino acids extracted are recorded in table 7.

Newborn infants breast fed ad lib show very similar amino acid concentrations in venous plasma to those observed in the plasma of the umbilical cord artery (fig. 1). Only taurine, lysine (-93 μmol/l, 37%) and threonine (-89 μmol/l, 46^0_0) show a marked decrease of concentration compared with the umbilical cord vessel level. The decrease of histidine and phenylalanine is also significant but rather small. The concentrations of the rest of the amino acids do not decrease after birth in

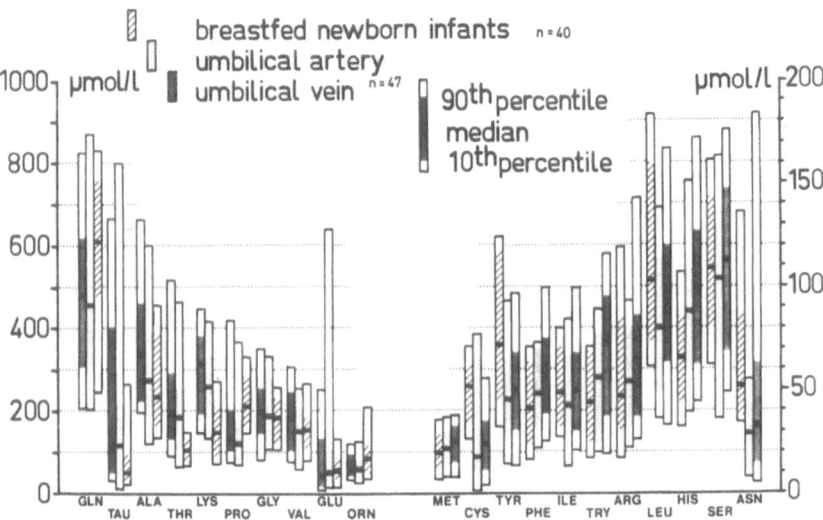

Fig. 1. Amino acid concentrations in the plasma of the umbilical cord vein and artery and of newborn infants breast-fed ad libitum.

Table 7. *Retention of amino acids by the fetus and dosage recommendations of amino acids in newborn infants receiving parenteral nutrition.*

| | Intrauterine retention of amino acids by the fetus (mmol/kg/day) | Dosage of amino acids in newborn infants during p.n. | |
		mg /kg/day	mmol
LYS	2.30	175–(330)	1.2 –(2.3)
THR	1.11	60–130	0.5 –1.1
VAL	1.60	180	1.6
LEU	0.93	130–210	1.0 –1.6
ILE	0.45	60–100	0.5 –0.75
TRY	0.61	80–120	0.4 –0.6
PHE	0.36	59– 76	0.36–0.46
TYR	0.30	20	0.1
MET	0.15	22– 45	0.15–0.3
CYS	0.16	40	0.16
HIS	0.77	50–120	0.32–0.7
ARG	0.46	210	1.2
ALA	3.58	320–700	3.6 –8.0
GLY	0.06		
SER	0.43	50	0.5
ORN	0.32	0	0
PRO	1.05	120	1.05
ASP	–0.88	0	0
ASN	0.14	0	0
GLU	–0.09	0	0
GLN	0.5	0	0

newborn infants who are breast-fed ad libitum. Because of this parity in amino acid concentrations in the plasma of the umbilical cord artery and in venous plasma or breast-fed infants, we were prompted to use this data as reference values which should be kept during parenteral nutrition in premature babies as well as in infants.

The median plasma amino acid concentrations of newborn infants receiving parenteral nutrition made up, at any one time, of one of 7 different solutions of crytalline l-amino acids, are illustrated in figures 2–7. Based on these data and the retention of amino acids from the umbilical cord vein blood the following recommendations for amino acid dosage are given in cases of parenteral nutrition of newborn infants.

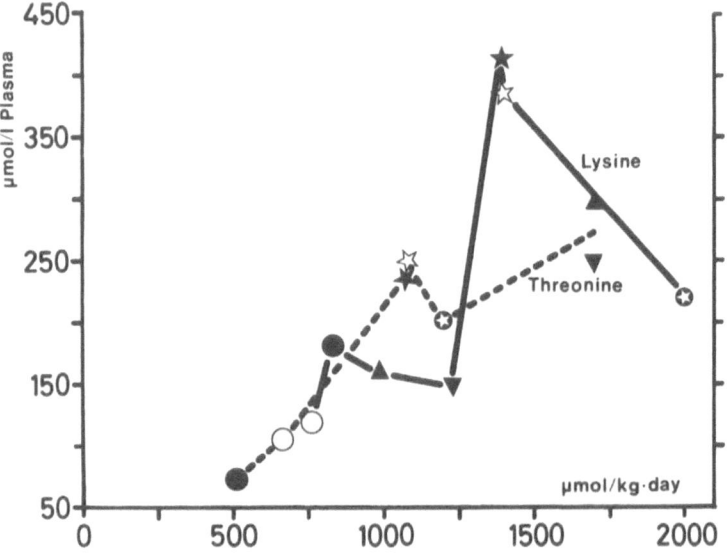

Fig. 2. Plasma concentrations (median) of threonine and lysine in newborn infants receiving parenteral nutrition with different amino acid solutions ● AMINOFUSIN[R]-L-forte, ○ Aminosäuren-Kohlenhydrate-Elektrolyte für die Pädiatrie, ★ ASP1, ☆ ASP2, ▲ ASP3, ▼ ASP4. ◐ ASP5, ✳ ASP5 proline-free.

Aspartic acid, asparagine, glutamic acid, glutamine

Aspartic acid, glutamic acid and their respective amides, asparagine and glutamine, are dispensable (non-essential) amino acids and therefore do not need to be included in solutions of amino acids for parenteral nutrition. The main argument, however, against the usage of the amides in parenteral nutrition is that they decompose in aqueous solution and release ammonia. The fetus at term certainly extracts glutamine and asparagine from the umbilical cord vein blood but it could be shown that also in cases of parenteral nutrition without glutamine and asparagine these amino acids show plasma concentrations at the level of those in the umbilical cord artery (9).

Apartic and glutamic acid are released by the fetus into the placenta (table 7). The administration, therefore of these amino acids during parenteral nutrition is not necessary. In cases of parenteral nutrition without aspartic and glutamic acid, the plasma concentrations of these amino acids remain at the level of the reference value.

Table 8. Dosages of amino acids which are recommended for the parenteral nutrition of newborn infants (per kg bodyweight per day). Review of the literature.

	Fetal		ASP5		GHADIMI (ref. 20)		STEGINK (ref.32)		BÜRGER (ref.21)		POHLANDT	
	mg	retention mmol	mg	mmol	mg	mmol	mg	mmol	mg	mmol	mg	mmol
Taurine	0	0	–	–							0	0
Hydroxyproline	0	0	–	–							0	0
Aspartic acid	-12	-0.88	–	–	12.5	0.09	71	0.540	135	1.01	0	0
Asparagine	8.5	0.06	–	–			71	0.540	–		0	0
Glutamic acid	-14	-0.09	–	–	12.5	0.09	72	0.480	490	3.33	0	0
Glutamine	81	0.5	–	–			578	3.960			0	0
Threonine	132	1.11	143	1.20	60	0.50	143	1.200	150	1.26	60-130	0.5-1.1
Serine	45	0.43	–	–	100	0.95	98	0.936	80	0.76	50*	0.5*
Proline	121	1.05	43	0.37	50	0.43	132	1.152	135	1.17	120	1.05
Glycine	4.5	0.06	75	1.0	100	1.33	203	2.700	255	3.40	50*	0.5*
Alanine	319	3.58	712	8.0	100	1.12	282	3.168	290	3.26	320-700	3.6-8.0
Citrulline	12	0.07	–	–			–	–			0	0
α-aminobutyric acid	5.0	0.05	–	–			–	–			0	0
Valine	187	1.6	117	1.0	200	1.71	188	1.612	80	0.68	180	1.6
Cystine	40	0.16	36	0.15	85	0.35	84	0.336	50	0.21	40	0.16
Methionine	22	0.15	45	0.3	15	0.1	54	0.360	40	0.27	22-45	0.15-0.3
Isoleucine	59	0.45	149	1.14	200	1.53	127	0.972	70	0.53	60-100	0.5-0.75
Leucine	122	0.93	238	1.6	400	3.05	216	1.644	125	0.95	130-210	1.0-1.6
Tyrosine	55	0.30	20	0.11	12.5	0.07	79	0.432	50	0.28	20	0.1
Phenylalanine	59	0.36	76	0.46	100	0.61	104	0.638	95	0.58	59-76	0.36-0.46
Tryptophan	124	0.61	84	0.41	30	0.15	43	0.216	30	0.15	80-120	0.4-0.6
Ornithine	42	0.32	–	–			–	–	45	0.34	0	0
Lysine	336	2.30	292	2.0	120	0.82	334	2.280	160	1.10	175-(330)	1.2-(2.3)
Histidine	119	0.77	124	0.8	50	0.32	74	0.480	110	0.71	50-120	0.32-0.77
Arginine	80	0.46	209	1.20	250	1.44	187	1.080	110	0.63	210	1.2
Sum	1971	16.11	2363	19.74	1897.5	14.66	3069	27.19	2500	20.62	1576-2451	12.64-20.49

* Combined doses of glycine and serine

Moreover, the value of glutamic acid for the purpose of intravenous nutrition is controversial. Firstly, a favourable effect of glutamic acid on the mental function was described (10, 11). Later, a destruction of certain brain areas was found in monkeys and mice (12–14). These observations, however, were not been confirmed by others (15) and they seem to occur only in certain species (16) and after high doses (17). On the other hand glutamate was recognized as the cause of the "chinese restaurant syndrome" which occurs after eating glutamate rich meals (18). These different observations argue against the use of glutamic acid in parenteral nutrition.

Dosage recommendation

Aspartic acid	0
Asparagine	0
Glutamic acid	0
Glutamine	0

Threonine

Threonine is an indispensable (essential) amino acid which acts as a "brick" in protein synthesis. The fetal plasma concentration of threonine is remarkably higher in comparison with those of breast-fed newborn infants. The significance of these high concentrations in utero is unknown. The high fetal retention rate of threonine corresponds to the transfer rate which was measured by BÜRGER et al. (19) in premature infants. Being in agreement with our results, GHADIMI's data (20) indicates, that a daily dose of 1.1 mmol threonine per kg will give a plasma concentration of about 250 μmol/l. Breast-fed newborn infants show threonine concentrations of about about 100 μmol/l, which can be kept during parenteral nutrition by a daily dose of 60 mg (700 μmol) (fig. 3). Accordingly, the turnover of threonine seems to decrease by half after birth.

Dosage recommendation

60–130 mg or 0.5 – 1.1 mmol/kg/day.

Glycine and Serine

Glycine is a non-essential amino acid which is formed from serine by cleaving off formaldehyde. In utero, glycine is hardly extracted from the umbilical cord vein blood (fig. 1, table 7). Figure 3 illustrates that the daily dose must be smaller than 1 mmol to prevent undesirable

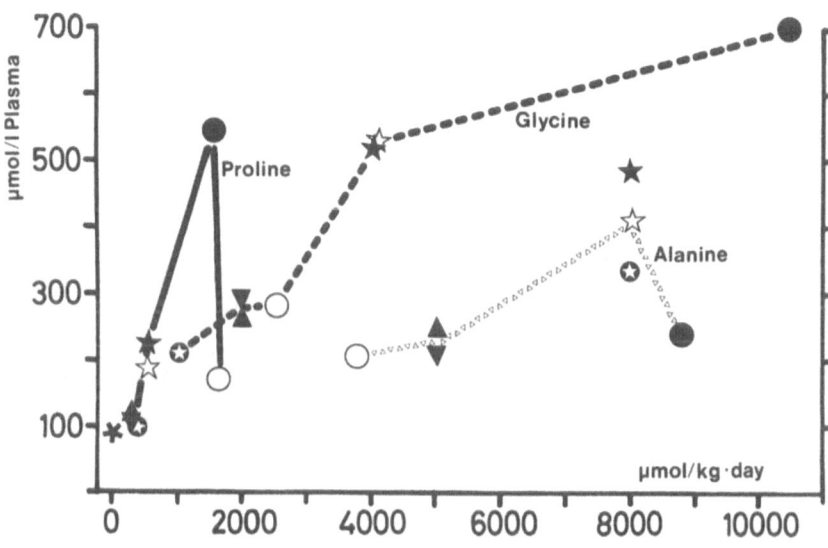

Fig. 3. Plasma concentrations (median) of glycine, alanine, and proline in newborn infants receiving parenteral nutrition with different amino acid solutions. For legend see figure 2.

high plasma concentrations. The dosage of 3.4 mmol recommended by BÜRGER and WOLF (21) would give concentrations 2 or 3 times higher than the reference value.

Serine is also a non-essential amino acid which can be synthesized from glycine and activated formaldehyde. The plasma concentration of serine remains constant despite the infusion of serine-free amino acid solution. Infusions rich in glycine cause not only hyperglycinemia but also increased concentrations of serine (9). Accordingly, the mutual metabolism of serine-glycine seems to happen so quickly that the requirement of serine can be met by synthesis from glycine in cases of serine-free intravenous nutrition.

Dosage recommendation
    Glycine: 0–0.5 mmol
    Serine: 0–0.5 mmol   0.5 mmol or 50 mg/kg/day

Alanine

Alanine is a non-essential amino acid closely associated with carbohydrate metabolism. Activated acetic acid which flows into the pool of metabolism is formed from alanine by transamination and subsequent decarboxylation. The versatility of this amino acid emphazises the fact that the fetal consumption of alanine is the highest one on a molar basis in comparison with all other amino acids (fig. 1, table 7).

The fact that the plasma alanine concentrations only vary slightly despite different dosages, indicates a fast metabolism of this amino acid (fig. 3). In contrast, GHADIMI (20) mentioned a very low tolerance to alanine during intravenous nutrition. This statement, however, was not supported by figures nor details about his studies. On the other hand, our studies demonstrate that alanine does not accumulate in plasma despite a high dosage. Alanine, therefore, seems to be a suitable source of non-specific nitrogen during parenteral nutrition.

Dosage recommendation
320 – 700 mg or 3.6 – 8 mmol/kg/day.

Proline

Proline is a non-essential amino acid which can be synthesized from glutamic acid via glutamic acid semialdehyde and pyrrolincarboxylic acid. Its break down takes the opposite course or hydroxyproline is formed in an irreversible reaction.

The fetus extracts 1.1 mmol/kg/day from the umbilical cord blood. Dosages between 0 and 1.6 mmol/kg/day result in plasma concentrations within the range of the reference values. Only infants who showed a markedly distorted pattern of plasma amino acids during the infusion of Aminofusin[R]-L-forte had greatly increased concentrations although the dose of 1.1 mmol/kg/day is usually appropriate. We consider the marked imbalances of plasma amino acids as a cause of the hyperprolinemia which results from an impaired metabolism of proline.

JÜRGENS et al. (22) believed they had evidence in favour of a limited synthesis of proline and alanine in adults. These authors enriched the amino acid solution with proline to improve the nitrogen balance in their patients. Heine (23), however, could not demonstrate any effect of proline on the nitrogen retention in 6 infants. We ourselves, infused a proline-free variant of the solution ASP5 to 3 newborn infants. The proline concentration in 5 plasma samples of these infants were at the reference value level (figure 3). In addition, this observation does not support the hypothesis that proline synthesis is so limited to become of clinical importance.

Dosage recommendation

120 mg or 1.05 mmol/kg/day.

Valine, leucine and isoleucine

Valine, leucine and isoleucine are essential amino acid due to their branched carbon chain. The break down of valine and partly of isoleucine leads via proprionate to succinate, which can serve for gluconeogenesis. From leucine and partly from isoleucine acetoacetate originates together with activated acetic acid which can be used for different synthetic purposes and the production of energy via the citric acid cycle. The fetus at term extracts 0.45 mmol isoleucine, 0.93 mmol leucine, and 1.6 mmol valine/kg/day from the umbilical cord vein blood in proportion to their concentrations in the umbilical cord vessels. The retention of isoleucine and leucine corresponds quite well to their turnover which was calculated by Bürger et al. (19) from the transfer rate in premature infants. During parenteral nutrition there are only slight variations in the plasma concentrations of isoleucine and leucine, when the dose is increased from 0.4 to 1.15 and from 0.6 to 1.6 mmol (fig. 4). In contrast, the requirement of valine, calculated from pharmacokinetical studies (19), amounts to less than half the fetal retention rate. The mutual influence of leucine on the one hand and isoleucine and valine on the other hand on the plasma concentrations are not known in cases when there is an overdosage or a lack of these amino acids (24, 25). The experimental design of Bürger et al. (19) who used bolus injections in studying the amino acid transfer, probably also alters the transfer rate.

In contrast to the results of GHADIMI (20) our study demonstrates that the plasma concentrations of valine exceed the reference values if an amount corresponding to the fetal retention rate is infused during parenteral nutrition (fig. 4). This could be a consequence of an otherwise inappropriately composed amino acid solution.

L-leucine, l-isoleucine, and l-valine can be recommended as a source of nonspecific nitrogen in addition to alanine, because there is a wide range of possible dosages of these branched chain amino acids without resulting variations in their plasma concentrations. Furthermore, with regards to insulin secretion which is especially stimulated by leucine (26, 27), it seems rational to give a leucine dose which exceeds the requirement for growth. It is unknown, however, whether the secretion of

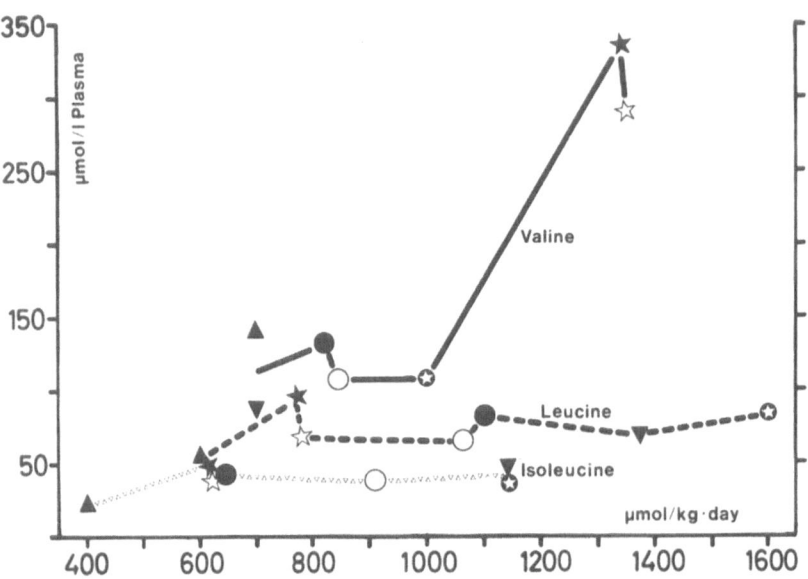

Fig. 4. Plasma concentrations (median) of valine, leucine, and isoleucine in newborn infants receiving parenteral nutrition with different amino acid solutions. For legend see figure 2.

insulin is stimulated by an increased turnover of leucine with normal plasma concentrations.

Dosage recommendation

Valine:	180 mg or 1.6 mmol/kg/day
Isoleucine:	60 – 100 mg or 0.5 – 0.75 mmol/kg/day
Leucine:	130 - 210 mg or 1.0 – 1.6 mmol/kg/day

Methionine and Cystine

Methionine contains sulphur and is an essential amino acid. It is the substrate for the synthesis of the other sulphur containing amino acids. Due to a low activity of the enzyme cystathionase the synthetic capacity of the fetus and the newborn infant for cystine is limited (28). This enzyme cleaves cystathionine which is formed from methionine via homocysteine, forming homoserine and cysteine. Newborn infants receiving parenteral nutrition without cysteine often showed decreased plasma concentrations (29). Based on these observations it was concluded that cysteine or cystine should be supplied to infants receiving

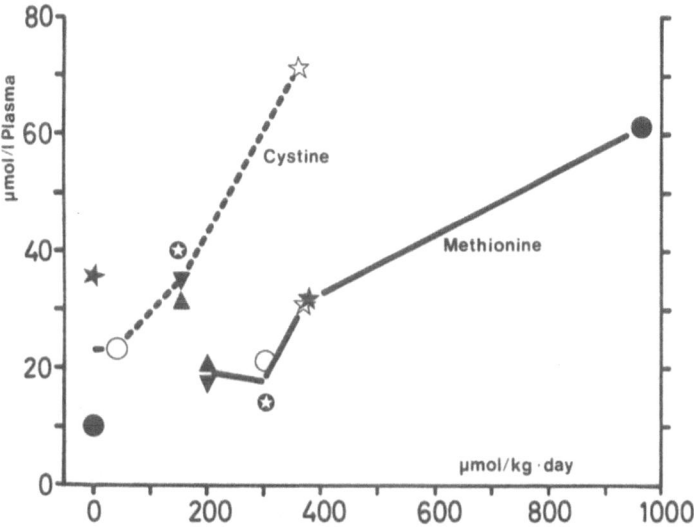

Fig. 5. Plasma concentrations (median) of methionine and cystine in newborn infants receiving parenteral nutrition with different amino acid solutions. For legend see figure 2.

parenteral nutrition (29). There is a lack, however, of clinical studies which demonstrate the favourable effect of a cystine supply on the growth or on the nitrogen balance of parenterally fed infants. SNYDER-MAN (30) who noticed a reduced growth rate in infants being fed a cystine-free diet provided the only clinical evidence that this amino acid is essential in infants.

The low cystine concentrations as reported in our study (29) were observed in small premature infants (median of birth weight 1243 g). In 18 plasma samples of 8, more mature infants (median of birth weight 1640, of gestational age 32.5 weeks) belonging to the same study group, the median of cystine concentrations was 21 μmol/l. Six premature infants (median of birth weight 2030 g, of gestational age 33 weeks), receiving a cystine-free ASPl-infusion showed in 19 plasma samples a median concentration of 28 μmol/l. These concentrations are in the upper range of the reference value. A limited biosynthesis of cysteine is not supported by these data.

The fetus at term extracts 0.16 mmol cystine and 0.1 mmol methionine/kg/day from the umbilical cord vein blood. The infusion of 0.16 mmol l-cystine results in plasma concentrations at the reference value level (fig. 5). Cystine has a low solubility, but the amount to meet its requirement can be dissolved in 100 ml of aqueous amino acid solution. Physiologic concentrations of methionine can be achieved with a dose of 0.2 – 0.3 mmol/kg/day (fig. 5). Bürger et al. (19, 21) and GHADIMI (20) gave similar dosage recommendations.

Dosage recommendation
    Methionine: 22–45 mg or 0.15 – 0.3 mmol/kg/day
    Cystine: 40 mg or 0.16 mmol/kg/day

Phenylalanine and Tyrosine

Both amino acids contain a benzene ring as a part of their carbon frame work, but only phenylalanine is essential. Tyrosine can be formed in man from phenylalanine by a hydroxilase. Both amino acids are protein elements. Tyrosine, in addition, is important as a substrate of the synthesis of different hormones (adrenalin, noradrenalin and thyroid hormones) and of melanin. The break down of phenylalanine and tyrosine is via homogentesic acid and ends in fumaric and acetoacetic acid. The enzymes involved in the metabolism of phenylalanine have a low activity rate in the liver of the fetus (31). On the one hand this can mean, that newborn infants can not synthesize tyrosine in sufficient amounts, but on the other hand, can mean that tyrosine supplied in excess of its requirement accumulates due to a limited rate of metabolism.

The fetus at term extracts 0.3 mmol tyrosine/kg/day. Tyrosine, however, is accumulated in premature infants receiving an infusion of 0.17 mmol/kg/day (fig. 6). This seemingly conflicting fact can be understood when different enzymatic activities due to different gestational ages are taken into account. Figure 6 illustrates different plasma tyrosine concentrations despite equal tyrosine dosages. This may be related to different gestational ages as well as different phenylalanine dosages.

The fetus at term extracts 0.36 mmol phenylalanine/kg/day. Dosages of 0.4 to 0.46 mmol/kg/day provide plasma concentrations at the reference value level (fig. 6). The administration of tyrosine decreases the requirement of phenylalanine. These amino acids should be considered together when working out the dosage. We recommend a total dose of 0.56 mmol/kg/day. GHADIMI's dosage (20) is similar and amounts to 0.68 mmol. The recommendations of BÜRGER and WOLF (0.86 mmol) (21) and of STEGINK (1.07 mmol) (32) seem to be too high.

Dosage recommendation
    Phenylalanine: 59–76 mg or 0.36 – 0.46 mmol/kg/day
    Tyrosine: 20 mg or 0.1 mmol/kg/day

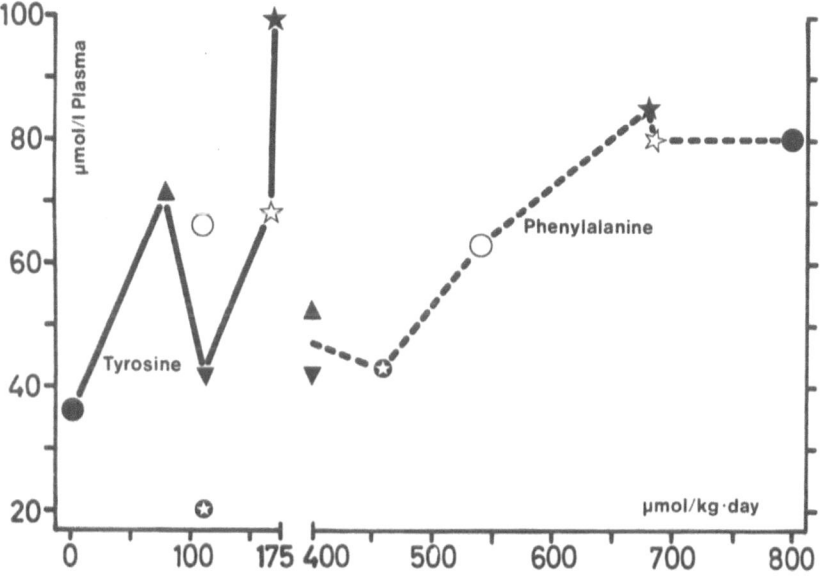

Fig. 6. Plasma concentrations (median) of tyrosine and phenylalanine in newborn infants receiving parenteral nutrition with different amino acid solutions. For legend see figure 2.

Tryptophan

Tryptophan is an essential amino acid due to its heterocyclic indolring. Tryptophan is important as a protein element and substrate for the synthesis of serotonin and the vitamin nicotinic acid. At term, the fetus extracts 0.61 mmol/kg/day from the umbilical cord vein blood. Based on our studies the dosage recommendations of GHADIMI (0.15 mmol), STEGINK (0.22 mmol), and BÜRGER et al. (0.15 mmol) can not provide plasma tryptophan, concentrations at the reference value level (fig. 7).
   Dosage recommendation
      80 – 120 mg or 0.4 – 0.6 mmol/kg/day

Lysine

Lysine is an essential amino acid of great importance in protein synthesis. The high lysine concentrations of the fetus markedly decrease after birth. This occurs to a similar degree only in the case of threonine. The metabolic importance of this characteristic is unknown. The high

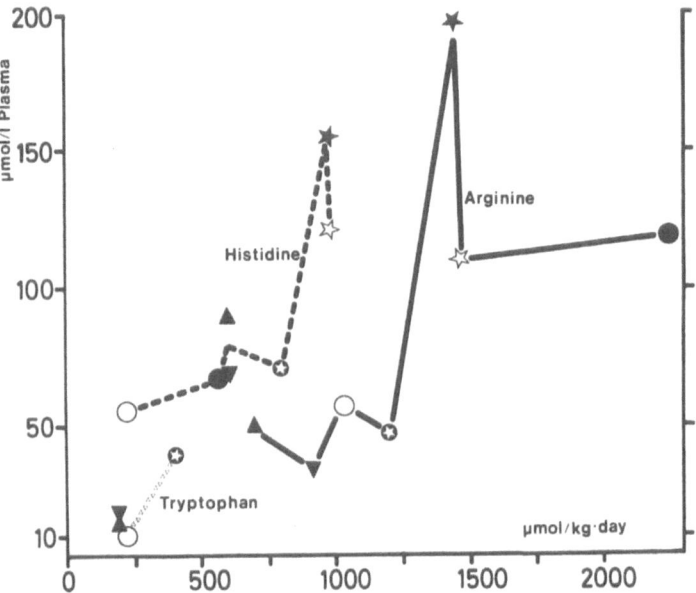

Fig. 7. Plasma concentrations (median) of tryptophan, histidine, and arginine in new-born infants receiving parenteral nutrition with different amino acid solutions. For legend see figure 2.

intrauterine lysine concentrations correspond to the high rate of fetal retention of 2.3 mmol/kg/day. A lysine requirement of 1.2 mmol/kg/day was extrapolated from the relation between plasma concentrations and lysine infusion rate (fig. 2) in order to maintain lysine concentrations of breast-fed infants during parenteral nutrition. GHADIMI recommended a daily dose of 0.84 mmol/kg/day but aimed at lower plasma concentrations than we do in regard of the mental damage in patients with hyperlysinemia, which may develop even when the concentrations are only moderately increased. The factor of high intrauterine lysine concentration was not considered an argument against this.

Dosage recommendation

175 (330) mg or 1.2 - (2.3) mmol/kg/day

Histidine

Histidine is not considered essential in adults. But following a short congress abstract made by SNYDERMAN et al. (33) histidine is regarded to be essential at least in infancy. Histidine acts as protein element and substrate for histamine.

The fetus at term extracts 0.77 mmol/kg/day. If the relation between plasma concentrations and infused dose is taken into account, its requirement during parenteral nutrition amounts to 0.8 mmol/kg daily. GHADIMI achieved physiologic concentrations in newborn infants receiving parenteral nutrition when he used only 0.32 mmol.

Dosage recommendation

50 – 120 mg or 0.32 – 0.77 mmol/kg/day

Arginine and Ornithine

Alongside the function as protein and peptide elements arginine and ornithine are particularly important as intermediates in the urea cycle. In this cycle, arginine is cleaved into urea and ornithine from which citrulline is formed by binding carbondioxide and ammonia. A further binding of citrulline with ammonia forms arginine again. According to BRAUNSTEIN (cited after 14) the formation of at least half the urea nitrogen takes a course via free ammonia. The infusion of great quantities of amino acids has probably also a toxic effect due to hyperammonia which arises as a result of the desamination of part of the amino acids. The simultaneous infusion of arginine, as shown in experiments in animals and human beings, protects against this toxity (35–44). The infusion of arginine probably increases the turnover of the urea cycle and thereby the elimination of ammonia.

At term, the fetus extracts 0.46 mmol argininc/kg/day. During parenteral nutrition this dose can be increased threefold without increasing plasma concentrations (fig. 7). GHADIMI (20) found no rise in plasma concentrations up to a daily dosage of 0.86 mmol. He recommended, however, 1.4 mmol because of the good tolerance to arginine in intravenous stimulation tests and because of the basic pH of this amino acid which increases the otherwise acid pH of the amino acid mixtures. Furthermore, the stimulating effect of arginine on the secretion of insulin is welcomed in order to raise the postnatally low assimilation rate of glucose (45–47). Administration of ornithine is not necessary where there is a sufficient arginine dosage.

Dosage recommendation

210 mg or 1.2 mmol/kg/day

There is much agreement between our and GHADIMI's dosage recommendations. At a level of 1.9 g amino acids/kg body weight/day they are considerably lower than other recommendations and approach the protein supply of breast-fed newborn infants (1.6 g/kg/day) (48). Our total dose exceeds that of GHADIMI by 460 mg, because of the high alanine dosage which was choosen greatly above the growth requirement in order to serve as a source of non-specific nitrogen. As a result of our studies a dosage recommendation could be given for each individual amino acid which is administered to newborn infants during parenteral nutrition. Continuous infusions on the basis of this recommendation probably meet the requirements and certainly prevent imbalances between plasma amino acids.

SUMMARY

The nutrition of the fetus via the umbilical vein is considered as a natural model of parenteral feeding. Corresponding to this model the amino acid concentrations in the plasma of newborn infants, who are nourished parenterally, should be maintained by continuous infusion at the level found either in the umbilical cord vessels or in newborn infants who are breast-fed ad libitum.

To illustrate the natural model quantitatively, the amino acid concentrations were studied in the plasma of the umbilical cord vein and artery of infants born either spontaneously or by elective cesarean section, and in the venous plasma of newborn infants breast-fed ad libitum. Based on these data labour does not significantly influence the amino acid concentrations of the plasma in the umbilical cord vessels and except for lysine and threonine, in breast-fed infants there is no decrease in plasma amino acid concentrations. The amount of amino acids, which is extracted by the fetus, was calculated from the differences between the plasma amino acid concentrations in the umbilical cord vein and the artery, and the bloodflow in the umbilical cord vein.

Plasma amino acid concentrations were studied in newborn infants receiving a continuous infusion of synthetic crystalline amino acids during parenteral nutrition. On the basis of the data obtained from the natural model and the studies on parenterally fed infants, the dosage of amino acids for parenteral nutrition is recommended. The total dose amounts to 1.9 g/kg body weight/day, which is significantly less than the current recommendations. This dose approaches the protein ingestion of breast-fed infants (1.6 g/kg body weight/day).

REFERENCES

1. DOBBING, J. (1974) In: Scientific Foundations of Paediatrics, Davis, J. and J. Dobbing eds., W. Heinemann Medical Books Ltd., London, p. 565.
2. FRANKENBURG, W.K., B.R. DUNCAN, R.W. COFFELT, R. KOCH, J.G. COLDWELL and C.D. SON. (1968) J. Pediatr. 73:560.
3. GAUDIER, B., C. PONTÉ, C. DUQUENNOY, G. CALLENS, M. CALLENS, and L. BALLESTER. (1972) Ann. Pédiat. 19:269.
4. MENKES, J.H., D.W. WELCHER, H.S. LEVI, J. DALLAS and N.E. GRETSKY, (1972) Pediatrics 49:218.
5. MAMUNES, P., P.E. PRINCE, N.H. THORNTON, P.A. HUNT and E.S. HITCHCOCK (1976) Pediatrics 57:675.
6. AVERY, M.E., C.L. CLOW, J.H. MENKES, A. RAMON, C.R. SCRIVER, L. STERN and B.P. WASSERMAN (1967) Pediatrics 39:378.
7. GOLDMAN, H.I., J.S. GOLDMAN, I. KAUFMAN and O.B. LIEBMAN (1974) J. Pediatr. 85:764.
8. ELWYN, D.H. (1968) In: Protein Nutrition and Free Amino Acid Patterns, Leathem. J.H. ed., Rutgers University Press, New Brunswick, N.J., p. 88.
9. POHLANDT, F. (1978) Habilitationsschrift, Medizinisch-klinische Fakultät, Universität Ulm.
10. ALBERT, K., P. HOCH and H. WAELSCH. (1946) J. Nerv. Ment. Dis. 104:263.
11. ZAMENHOF, S., E. VAN MARTHENS and F.L. MARGOLIS (1968) Science 160:322.
12. OLNEY, J.W. (1969) Science 164:719.
13. OLNEY, J.W. and L.G. SHARPE (1969) Science 166:386.
14. OLNEY, J.W. and O.L. Ho (1970) Nature 227:609.
15. OSER, B.L., S. CARSON, E.E. VOGIN and G.E. Cox (1971) Nature 229:411.
16. REYNOLDS, W.A., V. BUTLER, and N. LEMKEY-JOHNSTON (1976) J. Toxicol Environ. Health 2:471.
17. STEGINK, L.D., J.A. SHEPHERD, M.C. BRUMMEL and L.M. MURRAY (1974) Toxicology 2:285.
18. KWOK, R.H.M. (1968) N. Engl. J. Med. 278:796.
19. BÜRGER, U., H. WOLF and S. MEISZNER (1975) Z. Kinderheilk. 120:87.
20. GHADIMI, H. (1975) In: Total Parenteral Nutrition, H. Ghadimi ed., Wiley & Sons, New York, p. 393.
21. BÜRGER, U. and H. WOLF. (1976) Europ. J. Pediat 122:169.
22. JÜRGENS, P., D. DOLIF, C. PANTELIADIS and C. HOFERT. (1973) Z. Ernährungswiss., Suppl. 15:69.
23. HEINE, W. (1972) In: Parenteral Nutrition, Wilkinson, A.W. ed., Edinburgh-London, Churchill Livingston, p. 299.
24. CLARK, A.J., Y. PENG and M.E. SWENSEID. (1966) J. Nutr. 90:228.
25. CLARK, A.J., C. YAMADA, M.E. SWENSEID. (1968) Am. J. Physiol. 215:1324.
26. FLOYD, J.C., Jr., S.S. FAJANS, R.F. KNOPF and J.W. CONN. (1963) J. Clin. Invest. 42:1714.
27. GRASSO, S., G. PALUMBO, A. MESSINA, C. MAZZARINO and G. REITANO. (1976) Diabetes 25:545.
28. GAULL, G., J.A. STURMAN and C.R. RÄIHÄ. (1972) Pediatr. Res. 6:538.
29. POHLANDT, F. (1974) Acta Paediatr. Scand. 63:801.
30. SNYDERMAN, S.E. (1974) In: Nutricia Symposium Metabolic Processes in the Foetus and Newborn Infant, Stenfert Kroese, Leiden, Holland, p. 128.
31. KRETCHMER, N. (1959) Pediatrics 23:606.

32. STEGINK, L.D. (1975) In: Intravenous Nutrition in the High Risk Infant, Winters, R.W. and E.G. Hasselmeyer, John Wiley & Sons, New York, 1975, p. 411.

33. SNYDERMAN, S.E., P.H. PROSE, L.E. HOLT, Jr., E. ROITMAN and A. BOYER. (1959) Am. J. Dis. Child 98:459.

34. FURUYA, H. and D. MAEHARA. (1969) J. Jap. Obstet. Gynaecol. Soc. 11:167.

35. FAHEY, J.L. (1957) J. Clin. Invest. 36:1647.

36. GREENSTEIN, J.P., J.P. DU RUISSEAU, M. WINITZ and S.M. BIRNBAUM. (1957) Arch. Biochem, Biophys. 71:458.

37. GREENSTEIN, J.P., M. WINITZ, P. GULLINO, S.M. BIRNBAUM and M.C. OTEY. (1956) Arch. Biochem. Biophys. 64:342.

38. GREENSTEIN, J.P., M. WINITZ, P. GULLINO and S.M. BIRNBAUM. (1955) Arch. Biochem. Biophys. 59:302.

39. GULLINO, P., M. WINITZ, S.M. BIRNBAUM, J. CORNFIELD, M.C. OTEY, J.P. GREEN-STEIN. (1956) Arch. Biochem. Biophys. 64:319.

40. GULLINO, P., M. WINITZ, S.M. BIRNBAUM, M.C. OTEY, J. CORNFIELD and J.P. GREENSTEIN. (1975) Arch. Biochem. Biophys. 58:255.

41. KAMIN, H. and P. HANDLER. (1951) J. Biol. Chem. 193:873.

42. NAJARIAN, J.S. and H.A. HARPER. (1957) Surg. Forum 7:438.

43. SETNIKAR, I. (1957) Boll. Soc. Ital. Biol. Sper. 33:1636.

44. WINITZ, M., J.P. DU RUISSEAU, M.C. OTEY, S.M. BIRNBAUM and J.P. GREENSTEIN. (1956) Arch. Biochem. Biophys. 64:368.

45. FALORNI, A., F. MASSI-BENEDETTI, S. GALLO and S. ROMIZI. (1975) Pediatr. Res. 9:55.

46. KING, K.C., P.A.J. ADAM, K. YAMAGUCHI and R. SCHWARTZ. (1974) Diabetes 23:816.

47. PONTÉ, C., B. GAUDIER, B. DECONINCK and J.C. FOURLINNIE. (1972) Ann. Endocrinol. 34:66.

48. WIDDOWSON, E.M. (1974) In: Scientific Foundations of Paediatrics, Davis, J.A. and J. Dobbing eds., Medical Books, Ltd., London 1974, p. 44.

BRAIN COMPOSITION OF BEAGLE PUPPIES
RECEIVING TOTAL PARENTERAL NUTRITION*

WILLIAM C. HEIRD* MD and MICHAEL H. MALLOY*, MD

The concept that inadequate nutrition during the period of rapid central nervous system growth may exert an adverse effect on subsequent central nervous system development (1, 2) coupled with the fact that intact neurological survival of low birth weight infants does not seem to be improving as fast as overall survival (3) has focused attention upon the nutritional management of low birth weight infants during the neonatal period. The implication is that better nutritional management might further improve the quality of survival.

Considering the usual difficulties of feeding these infants enterally, the possibility of providing all nutrient requirements by the parenteral route (4) was received with much enthusiasm. Thus, this practice with various modifications over that initially described by WILMORE and DUDRICK (5) has found its way into most special care nurseries throughout the world. After approximately 10 years, it is obvious that the technique of total parenteral nutrition, although fraught with problems, permits delivery of more nutrients than would be possible by more conventional feeding methods (6). In even the sickest infants, in fact, it is usually possible to produce at least some growth, albeit at times subnormal. Certainly, the technique has permitted survival of many infants who otherwise would have succumbed to simple starvation.

Whether parenterally delivered nutrients adequately support growth of the developing central nervous system, however, has not been established. The one study in which children who received only parenteral nutrients during a part of the neonatal period were evaluated at 5 years of age suggests that parenteral nutrition does not affect subsequent intellectual capacity adversely (7). On the other hand, an advantage in terms of improved intellectual capacity was not demonstrated.

Over the past several years, we have been involved in studies of brain

*Department of Pediatrics, Columbia University College of Physicians and Surgeons, New York, N.Y.

H.K.A. Visser (ed.), Nutrition and Metabolism of the Fetus and Infant, 365-375. All rights reserved.
Copyright © 1979 Martinus Nijhoff Publishers b.v., The Hague/Boston/London.

growth and development of animals nourished only by the parenteral route during the neonatal period. While these studies are not likely to provide the total answer with respect to the role of parenteral nutrients in supporting growth and development of the human brain, they should be useful in establishing principles of brain growth and development during parenteral nutrition thereby permitting factors which might allow further improvements of such regimens for the human infant to be identified.

As with all animal studies, our initial problem concerned the choice of a relevant model. Obviously, the biochemical brain growth and development of the model chosen should resemble that of the human infant. Further, it was necessary that the animal chosen be large enough at birth to permit catheter insertion and subsequent delivery of parenteral nutrients. The puppy was an ideal choice with respect to size; however, little was known concerning the biochemical growth and development of the puppy brain. On the other hand, animals for which this information was available (e.g., the rat (8), guinea pig (9), monkey (10)) were either too small or otherwise unsuitable. Our initial studies, therefore, were directed toward defining the biochemical growth and development of the puppy brain.

GROWTH AND DEVELOPMENT OF THE BEAGLE BRAIN

Brain growth and development is characterized by a period of cellular proliferation followed by a period of cellular enlargement and outgrowth of axons and dendrites and, finally, myelination (11). Biochemically, the phase of cellular proliferation can be monitored by increases in DNA content (12). Calculation of the protein to DNA or various lipid to DNA ratios allows biochemical monitoring of cellular hypertrophy. Since the outgrowth of axons and dendrites is associated with establishment of synapses, the determination of gangliosides, a class of lipid concentrated in synaptic membranes (13), allows this phase to be monitored. Myelination has been monitored by the concentration of glycolipid or cholesterol (9).

Summarizing a considerable amount of data obtained in our laboratory over the past several years, the development of the beagle brain is characterized as follows:

a. the phase of cellular proliferation begins prenatally and continues for the first several weeks to months of life.

b. Cellular hypertrophy (increasing protein: DNA ratio) begins at approximately 7 days of age.
c. Ganglioside concentration begins to increase at approximately 14 days of age, signalling the outgrowth of axons and dendrites and establishment of synapses.
d. Myelination as detected by an increasing concentration of glycolipid, begins at approximately 21 days of age.

Given the problems with all animal models, it would appear that development of the beagle brain over the first 2 weeks of life is similar to that of the human brain during the last trimester of pregnancy (14). Thus, the beagle model of brain growth and development is a reasonable model for the growth and development of the brain of prematurely born human infant.

BRAIN COMPOSITION OF BEAGLE PUPPIES RECEIVING ONLY PARENTERAL NUTRIENTS

Having validated the model chosen, studies of the effect of total parenteral nutrition on brain growth and development of the beagle puppy were begun. After various periods of parenteral nutrition the brain was removed, separated into its component parts, weighed and immediately frozen for subsequent analysis of DNA and protein content as well as the content of the lipid fractions chosen as markers for the various phases of development. These data from parenterally nourished puppies were compared to those from normally suckled animals. In all groups, parenteral intake consisted of 6 gm/kg/day of amino acids and approximately 180 cal/kg/day plus electrolytes, vitamins and minerals. Some animals received only glucose as the caloric source while others received a combination of glucose and fat. The quality of caloric intake made no difference with respect to brain composition; thus, the data from groups receiving only glucose and those receiving glucose and fat have been combined. With this regimen, the gain in body weight of animals that received only parenteral nutrients was equal to or greater than that of control animals.

Figure 1 shows the cerebral weight of control animals at birth and at 10, 21, and 28 days of age as well as the weight of the cerebrum of animals studied after receiving only parenteral nutrition over the first 10 days of life, between 10 and 21 days of age and between 21 and 28 days of age. Total parenteral nutrition during the first 10 days of life did not affect

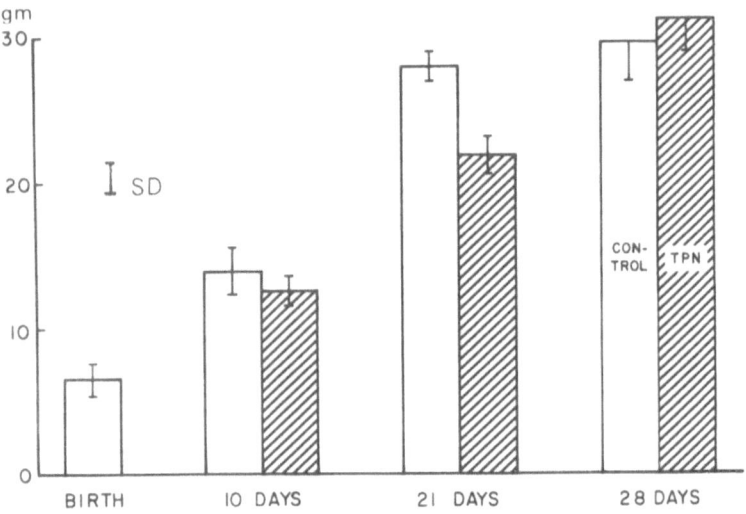

Fig. 1. Cerebral weight (Gm) of control animals (clear bars) and animals receiving only parenteral nutrients (hatched bars) for the first 10 days of life, between 10 and 21 days of age and between 21 and 28 days of age.

cerebrum weight nor did total parenteral nutrition between 21 and 28 days of age. However, the cerebrum of animals that received only parenteral nutrients between 10 and 21 days of age weighed significantly less than that of control animals.

The DNA content of the cerebrum of both control animals and animals that received TPN over the various periods is shown in figure 2. Total parenteral nutrition during any period over the first 28 days of life did not affect cerebral DNA content.

In contrast (fig. 3), parenteral nutrition from either 10 to 21 or 21 to 28 days of age, but not during the first 10 days of life, resulted in a decreased protein content. The differential effects of parenteral nutrition on DNA content and protein content resulted in marked differences in the protein to DNA ratio, or the size of individual cells. While this ratio was not affected by parenteral nutrition over the first 10 days of life, parenteral nutrition during either of the other two periods resulted in a decreased cell size.

These data indicate that parenteral nutrition does not support normal cellular hypertrophy of the cerebrum of beagle puppies during the period from 10 to 28 days of age which is the period in normally-fed animals of

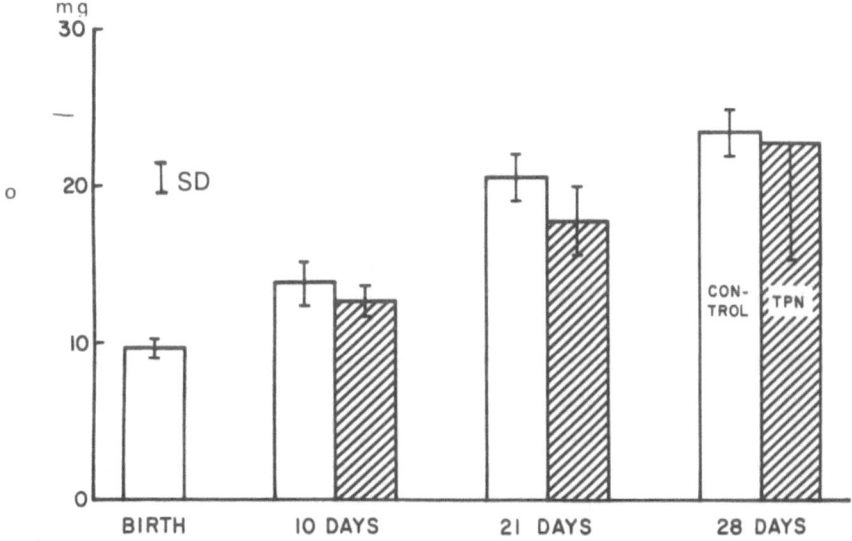

Fig. 2. Cerebral DNA content (Mg) of control animals (clear bars) and animals receiving only parenteral nutrients (hatched bars) for the first 10 days of life, between 10 and 21 days of age and between 21 and 28 days of age.

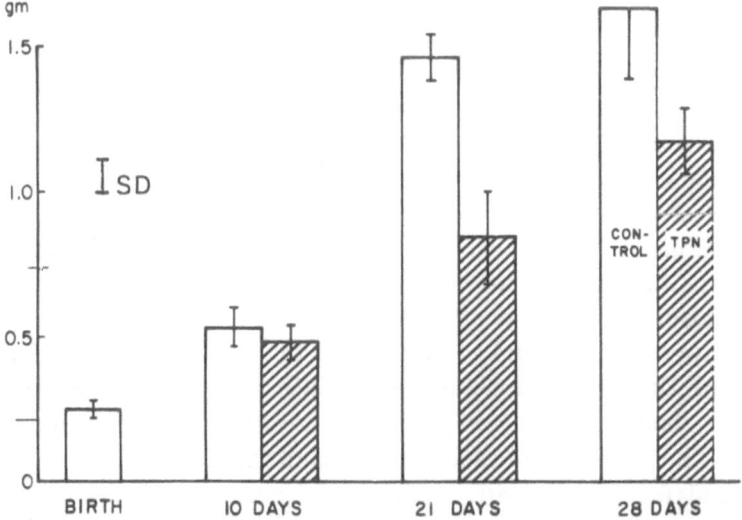

Fig. 3. Cerebral protein content (Gm) of control animals (clear bars) and animals receiving only parenteral nutrients (hatched bars) for the first 10 days of life, between 10 and 21 days of age and between 21 and 28 days of age.

the most rapid increase in both DNA and protein content. During the first 10 days of life, when neither DNA nor protein are increasing at very rapid rates, parenteral nutrition does not appear to exert a profound effect on brain growth. Thus, the concept emerges that parenteral nutrition may not fully support normal growth, particularly when this growth is rapid.

The low protein content of the cerebrum of animals that received parenteral nutrition during periods of rapid protein deposition is likely to be due to one of two general possibilities. The first such possibility is that nitrogen intake was inadequate. The second possibility is that the nitrogen delivered was not utilized efficiently. Nitrogen intake was on the low side of recommended allowances (15). However, amino acids accounted for approximately 15% of the total caloric intake; in general, a diet in which metabolizable nitrogen provides 10–12% of metabolizable energy is considered adequate for the growing puppy. Therefore, rather than an inadequate total nitrogen intake, per se, the more likely explanation is an inadequate intake of metabolizable, or utilizable, nitrogen.

PLASMA AND CEREBRAL AMINO ACID PATTERNS

One possible explanation for the apparent decreased utilization of the administered nitrogen concerns the mixture of amino acids provided. Decreased utilization of a less than optimal mixture (e.g., an 'unbalanced' mixture or a mixture deficient in one or more essential amino acids) would be expected. Further, the overall quality of the amino acid mixture should be reflected by the plasma and tissue amino acid patterns. Both plasma and cerebral amino acid concentrations of 21 day old control animals and animals that received only parenteral nutrients between days 10 and 21 of age have been determined in collaboration with Drs. Gerald E. Gaull and David K. Rassin. Both patterns, in fact, are abnormal when compared to control animals (figs. 4 and 5).

The plasma amino acid pattern of all parenterally nourished animals tends to reflect the pattern of the amino acid intake. The plasma concentration of some amino acids are elevated compared to control while the concentrations of others are decreased.

Two different patterns of cerebral free amino acids are observed. In some animals (fig. 4), the usual similarity between the amino acid pattern of the plasma and the free amino acid pattern of the cerebrum is

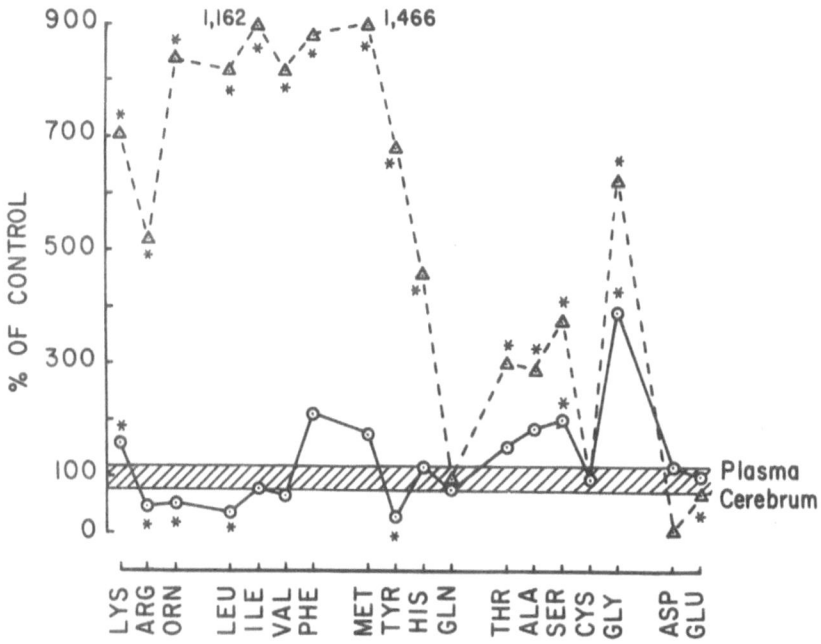

Fig. 4. Relative plasma and cerebral free amino acid concentrations of animals receiving only parenteral nutrients between 10 and 21 days of age. Both plasma and cerebral amino acid concentrations of control animals (21 days of age) are expressed as 100% (hatched horizontal bar) while those of animals receiving only parenteral nutrients are expressed as a percentage of either the plasma concentration (⊙) or cerebral concentrations (▲) of control animals.

not apparent (16). The cerebral concentrations of the basic amino acids as well as the large neutral amino acids are some 8–14 times the concentrations observed in control animals whereas the cerebral concentrations of the smaller neutral amino acids as well as the acidic amino acids tend to mimic the plasma amino acid pattern. In other animals, the cerebral pattern of free amino acids tends to mimic the amino acid pattern of the plasma (fig. 5).

This apparent discrepancy between the two sets of results in identical animals has been extremely confusing. However, comparison of the DNA and protein contents of the cerebrum of the two sets of animals provides a possible explanation. As shown in figure 6, the cerebral DNA content of animals with the cerebral free amino acid pattern that can not be predicted from the plasma pattern is significantly less than that of

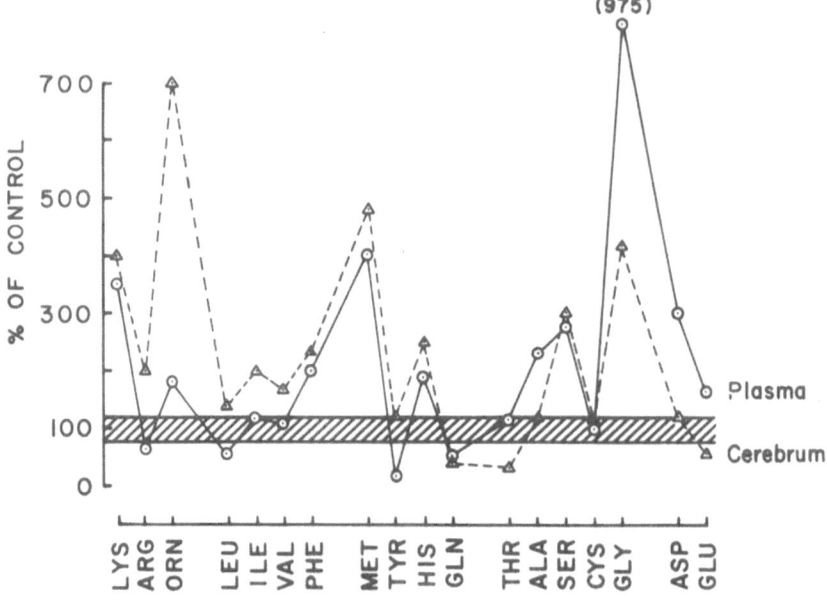

Fig. 5. Relative plasma and cerebral free amino acid concentrations of animals receiving only parenteral nutrients between 10 and 21 days of age. Both plasma and cerebral amino acid concentrations of control animals (21 days of age) are expressed as 100% (hatched horizontal bar) while those of animals receiving only parenteral nutrients are expressed as a percentage of either the plasma concentrations (⊙) or cerebral concentrations (▲) of control animals.

control animals although not less than that of animals with the predictable cerebral amino acid pattern. While the protein content of the cerebrum of either group of animals is significantly different from that of controls, the protein content of the animals with the unpredictable cerebral amino acid pattern is significantly less than that of animals with the predictable pattern. These data suggest that protein accretion, while, reduced in both groups of animals compared to control animals, is reduced to a greater extent in the animals with the more abnormal cerebral free amino acid pattern.

Based on these observations, it seems reasonable to conclude that net synthesis of protein is reduced in the cerebrum of animals receiving only parenteral nutrients, possibly as a result of the quality of the amino acid mixture provided. Further, it appears that some animals are more susceptible to this deficient intake than others; in these, protein accretion is

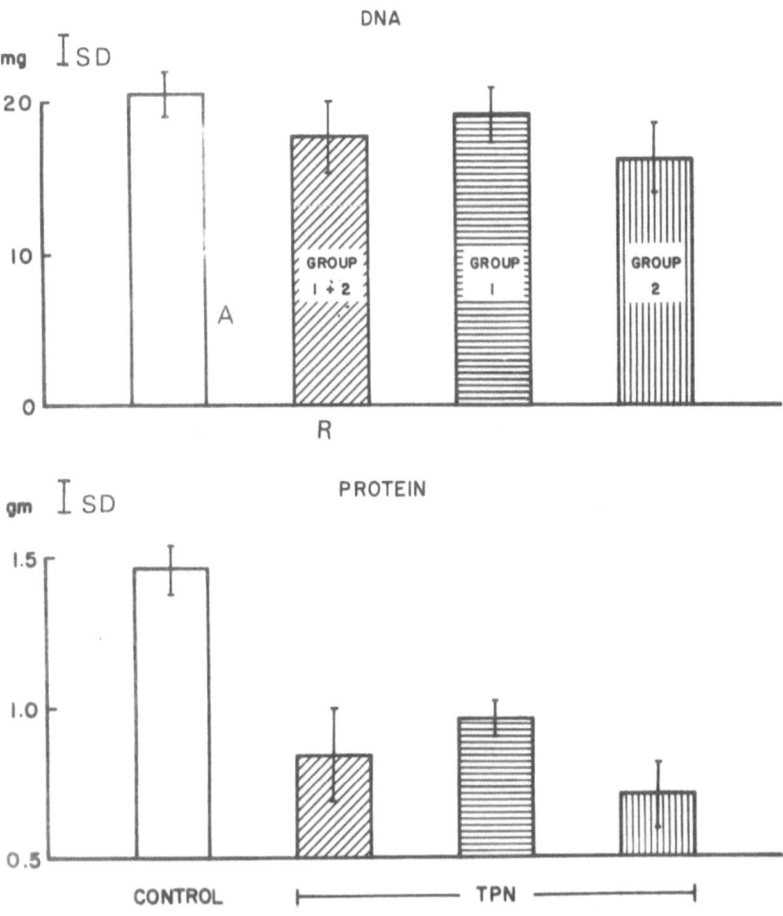

Fig. 6. Cerebral DNA and protein content of groups of animals receiving only parenteral nutrients from 10–21 days of age. Group 1 is composed of animals with the predictable cerebral pattern of free amino acids (fig. 5); Group 2 is composed of animals with the unpredictable cerebral pattern of free amino acids (fig. 4).

slowed to an even greater extent. With the more marked inhibition of net protein synthesis in the face of continued amino acid infusion, free amino acids seem to accumulate within the intra and extracellular fluid of the cerebrum. Obviously, this is an hypothesis and much further work will be required to establish its validity.

CONCLUSION

Regardless of the explanation of the different patterns of cerebral free amino acids in animals receiving identical nutrient regimens, several facts are obvious. First, under the conditions of parenteral nutrition in the puppies for which data were presented, cerebral protein content is decreased. Further, both the plasma and cerebral patterns of amino acids of all parenterally nourished animals are deranged compared to control animals. What remains to be established is the relationship between the decreased protein on the one hand and the abnormal amino acid patterns on the other.

If the two observations are related, as seems likely, these animal studies may be particularly relevant to the situation of total parenteral nutrition in the human infant. For example, the plasma amino acid pattern of infants receiving the mixture of amino acids used in these animal studies is very similar to the pattern observed in the puppies (17). Thus, to the extent that abnormal plasma and presumably also tissue amino acid patterns are related to a decrease in net protein synthesis, there is reason to expect that amino acid utilization by the human infant who receives only parenteral nutrients may also be less than optimal. Perhaps it is for this reason that improvement in subsequent intellectual capacity has not accompanied what has been assumed to be improved nutritional management during the neonatal period.

ACKNOWLEDGEMENT

The original research of the authors is supported by a grant from the National Institutes of Health (HD-08432).

REFERENCES

1. WINICK, M and P. ROSSO. (1969) Pediatr. Res. 3:181.
2. DOBBING, J., J.W. HOPEWELL and A. LYNCH. (1971) Exp. Neurol. 32:439.
3. PATE K.E., R.J. BUNCIC, S. ASHLY and P.M. FITZHARDINGE. (1978) J. Pediatr. 92:253.
4. DRISCOLL, J.M., Jr., W.C. HEIRD, J.N. SCHULLINGER, R.D. GONGAWARE and R.W. WINTERS. (1972) J. Pediatr. 81:145.
5. WILMORE, D.W. and S.J. DUDRICK (1968) J.A.M.A. 203:860.
6. HEIRD, W.C. and R.W. WINTERS (1975) J. Pediatr. 86:2.
7. TEJAMI, A., R. MADADEVAN, B.C. NANGIA, B. DOBIAS and P.M. VARMA. (1978) Pediatr. Res. 12:376.
8. WINICK, M. and A. NOBLE. (1965) Dev. Biol. 12:451.

9. DAVISON, A.N. and J. DOBBING. (1968) Applied Neurochemistry, Blackwell Scientific Publications, Oxford, p. 253.
10. CHEEK, D.B., D.E. MELLITUS, D.E. HILL and A.B. HOLT. (1975) In: Fetal and Post-Natal Cellular Growth, Cheek, D.B. ed., John Wiley & Sons, New York, p. 75.
11. WINCICK M. (1976) Malnutrition and Brain Development, Oxford University Press. New York, p. 35.
12. ENESCO, M. and L.P. LEBLOND. (1962) J. Embryol. Exp. Morph. 10:530.
13. WIEGARDT, H. (1967) Neurochem. 14:671.
14. BIEBER, M.A., J.A. BASSI, J.A. BRASEL and W.C. HEIRD. (1977) Fed. Proc. 36:1108.
15. Nutrient Requirements of Dogs. (1977) National Academy of Sciences, Washington.
16. HEIRD, W.C., D.K. RASSIN and G.E. GAULL. (1977) Pediatr. Res. 11:1028.
17. WINTERS, R.W., W.C. HEIRD, R.B. DELL and J.F. NICHOLSON. (1977) In: Clinical Nutrition Update: Amino Acids, Greene, H.L., M.A. Holliday and H.N. Munro eds., American Medical Association, Chicago, Ill., p. 147.

TRACE ELEMENTS IN PARENTERAL FEEDING
OF INFANTS

HARRY L. GREENE, DOENA VAN DER VORM, GERARD L. HELINEK
and GEORGE NICHOALDS*

Infants delivered prematurely may be at high risk to develop zinc and/or copper dificiency in the absence of dietary or intravenous supplementation. WIDDOWSON et al. (1) have shown that copper and zinc stores accumulate during the last trimester; DAUNCEY et al. (2) have noted that most low birth weight infants are in negative zinc and copper balance during the first days to weeks of life.

Although there are 14 trace metals known to be of nutritional importance in animals, only five have been clearly identified as being required for normal human nutrition (table 1). Two of these, iron and iodine, have been studied extensively and will not be discussed. Until this decade, zinc and copper deficiencies were only seen in association with malnutrition. However with the development of ultra-pure dietary constituents for total parenteral nutrition (TPN), zinc deficiency has become relatively common in patients receiving non-zinc supplemented

Table 1. *Trace elements (each < 0.01% of T.B.W.).*

Iron	Cobalt
Iodine	Molybdenum
Copper	Silicon
Zinc	Vanadium
Chromium	Tin
Manganese	Fluorine
Selenium	Nickel

Elements found in concentrations of less than 0.01% of total body weight (T.B.W.) which have been identified as necessary nutrients in animals. Elements underlined have been identified as required in man.

*Dept. of Pediatric, Vanderbilt Medical Center, Nashville, Tn. 37203, U.S.A.

H.K.A. Visser (ed.), Nutrition and Metabolism of the Fetus and Infant, 377-389. All rights reserved.
Copyright © 1979 Martinus Nijhoff Publishers b.v., The Hague/Boston/London.

TPN for more than 2 months. Copper deficiency is seen less commonly but may also develop within 4–6 months of non-copper supplemented TPN.

The purpose of this paper is to review briefly the important functions, deficiency disorders and results of studies which led to dosage recommendations for these two elements in parenteral feedings. Emphasis will be placed on studies relevant to the infants with birth weights less than 1250 g. In addition, 4 other elements, chromium, manganese, selenium and molybdenum have been implicated as essential in human nutrition. These elements will be discussed briefly.

ZINC

Function

The biologic importance of zinc appears to be related primarily to its role in many enzyme systems. Over 40 zinc-containing enzymes have been identified and an additional number are activated by the metal. The identification of key enzymes in nucleic acid metabolism such as thymidine kinase, DNA polymerase and RNA polymerase, which are zinc dependent, may explain the vital importance of zinc for normal growth and development (3, 4).

Approximately 20–30% of dietary zinc is usually absorbed, although this percentage can be influenced by the amount of zinc ingested and dietary source of zinc. For example, zinc is adsorbed better from meat than vegetables.

The distribution of zinc indicates that it is very high in concentration in tissues such as hair, nails, bone and semen (approaching 100 μg/g tissue), whereas it is somewhat lower in liver, kidneys and muscle (about 50 μg/g tissue) and lower in blood. In the blood about 80% is carried on the erythrocyte (about 12 to 14 μg/g) and only 20% is present in the plasma (about 80 μg/100 ml).

Zinc circulates primarily bound to albumin and alpha$_2$ macroglobulin with less amounts on amino acids and transferrin. The mechanism of absorption of zinc has not been clearly defined although there appears to be a zinc binding factor (zinc binding ligand) which is present in the bowel lumen, and secreted from the pancreas. The zinc binding ligand combines with intralumenal zinc which transports it into the epithelial cell. There it is released to a membrane-bound zinc binding protein.

This second stage of zinc transport then releases the zinc into the circulation to be transported primarily by albumin to the liver (5). The major excretory route of zinc is the intestine by way of sloughed mucosal cells, bile, and pancreatic secretions. Approximately $1-1\frac{1}{2}$ mg are lost daily by this route. Two other routes of excretion are the kidneys and sweat glands, each of which secrete approximately 0.5 mg/day.

Deficiency

The major clinical features of zinc deficiency are listed in table 2. As plasma zinc levels decrease, diarrhea may be the only sign of deficiency. Dermatitis usually develops as the deficiency worsens and alopecia and changes in finger nails develop as the deficiency becomes severe. With chronic zinc depletion, growth retardation, delayed wound healing and mental lethargy develop. Other symptoms which may be present are delayed sexual maturation, hypoguesia, and increased susceptibility to infection.

Table 2. *Zinc. Common clinical features of depletion.*

Acute	Chronic
Diarrhea	Growth retardation
Dermatitis	Delayed sexual maturation
Alopecia	

Although other features have been noted in zinc deficiency the above manifestations are the more common and more easily recognized.

Recommended intake

Term infants: In 1973 HENKIN et al. (6) noted that the plasma zinc levels fell within the normal adult range during the first 24–48 hr of age. However, zinc levels declined to reach a mean low of about 40 μg/100 ml by 3–5 months of age. By the 6 month of life, plasma levels returned to normal adult levels. A second depression occurred at about 1 year of age to 50 μg/100 ml. Finally, by 15 months of age zinc increased to adult levels of between 75 and 110 mg/100 ml. Thus, during the first 5 months of life there appears to be a physiologic depression of plasma zinc levels. The physiologic significance of this transient depression has not been defined but may represent an actual depletion of total body zinc. This is suggested from balance studies undertaken during the first few weeks of postnatal life and the recent finding by WALRAVENS and HAMBIDGE who found improved growth in males supplemented with dietary zinc (7). While these observations must be confirmed in a larger group of infants they do suggest that zinc nutrition might be improved in a substantial group of infants living in the United States. On the basis of the above observations the Food and Nutrition Board of the National Academy of Sciences recommends 3 mg of zinc per day for the first 6 months of live and 5 mg daily for the remainder of the first year (table 3).

Premature infants, oral recommendations: Since most zinc accumulates in the fetus during the last trimester of intrauterine growth, it is reasonable to expect that infants born prematurely are at a higher risk to develop zinc depletion and clinical signs of zinc deficiency than infants delivered at term. Furthermore, balance studies in very low birth weight infants indicate that a sizeable number of infants may continue to have negative zinc balance during the first few weeks of feeding (2). On the other hand, these same investigators noted that in spite of the negative zinc balance, infants grew at their expected rate.

We have had the opportunity to study 42 infants with birth weights less than 1250 g who were maintained on a formula which supplied between 2.5 and 3.3 g of zinc daily (Similac-Ross). Figure 1 illustrates the initial serum zinc levels which were within normal range for older children in all instances. However, during subsequent weeks, the serum zinc levels declined to reach 'deficient' levels, between 53 and 66 μg/100 ml. In spite of this finding, the infants continued to grow and during the course of the next several months, zinc levels returned to

Table 3. Zinc. (*Recommended intakes.*)

Pregnancy* (mg/d)	Infant[+]		Premature	
	Oral (mg/d)*	Intravenous[++] (μg/kg/d)	Oral	Intravenous
	0 6 mo 7 12 mo			
20	3 5	100–300	1 mg/kg/d	300 μg/kg/d**

* Food and Nutrition Board, NAS.
[+] Human colostrum contains up to 20 mg/l and declines to 2–3 mg/l, and cow's milk 3–4 mg/l. Proprietary formulas usually <2 mg/l unless supplemented.
[++] AMA Advisory Group for Trace Metals in Parenteral Nutrition.
** Based on predicted fetal accretion rate, urinary and fecal losses plus the use of this dose level in all infants for 8 years.

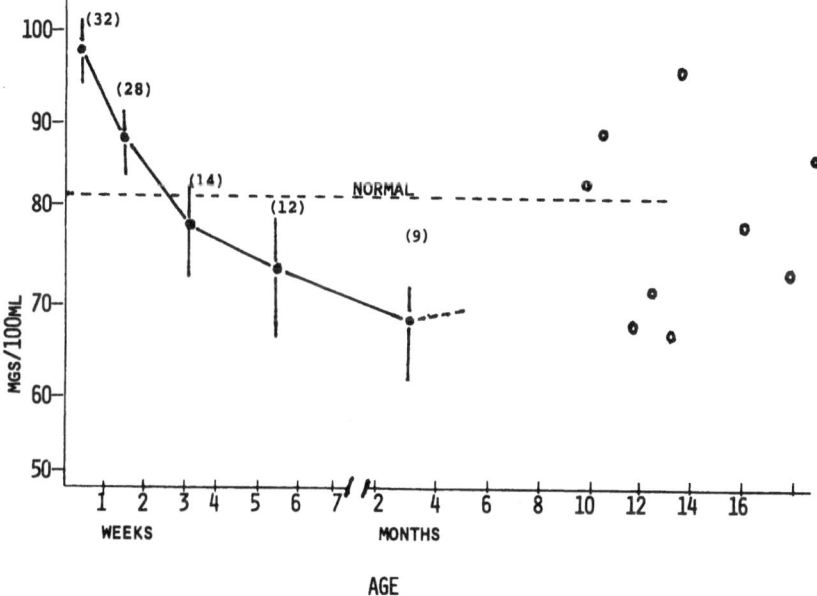

Fig. 1: Serial changes in serum zinc in premature infants (birth weight < 1250 g). Closed circles indicate mean of the number of patients indicated in parenthesis. Open circles indicate individual measurement in nine patients between 9 and 18 months of age.

normal in all but two infants. By 1 year of age, all infants were within the 25th and 60th percentiles for both height and weight. These observations suggest that further trials are necessary to determine the therapeutic efficacy of dietary zinc intakes which exceed that recommended for normal term infants (e.g. 3 mg/d).

Premature infants, intravenous recommendations: Very low birth weight infants (< 1250 g) frequently require TPN for the first weeks of life. Thus, it is extremely important to determine needs of intravenously administered zinc for this very special group of infants. Methods for determining marginal zinc deficiency are not yet defined; but clearly, simple measurement of serum zinc levels do not reflect body content or level of exogenous needs. Balance studies do not necessarily reflect needs but are more likely to provide a better indication than simple serum levels. A series of balance studies for 24–48 hr periods, performed twice on the same infant was recently completed (8). Zero balance was achieved at approximately 100μg/kg/d. Accretion rates for infants in utero who were growing at a similar rate would have accumulated about

200 μg/d. Thus, these investigators felt that between 250–300 μg/kg/d would be necessary to meet the needs of low birth weight infants who received total intravenous feedings.

Infants at our neonatal unit have been receiving 300–400 μg/kg/d during routine intravenous feedings for the past 8 years. The majority receiving this dose have not had serum zinc measurements made. However, 4 premature infants (birth weight 1300–1900 g) who received this dose for between 4 and 6 months showed serum levels between 112 and 131 mg/100 ml. Thus, this dose does not appear excessive. Further studies are in progress to determine the efficacy of supplying zinc at this level versus that of a somewhat lower lever of 150 μg/kg/day.

In summary the recommended intakes of zinc are listed in table 3. While the data upon which these suggested intakes involve a relatively small group of infants, it does suggest that these dosages should meet the needs of most infants. It is also evident that of all the trace minerals, zinc is by far the most important to supply since deficiency symptoms may develop in infants as early as two months without TPN supplementation. In addition to basal needs, data further indicates that under conditions of excessive fecal or enteric fluid losses additional zinc should be given. Measurement of zinc content of enteric losses in adults and older children indicate that between 8 and 12 μg of zinc per gram of enteric fluid lost should be added to the TPN solution in order to achieve positive zinc balance.

COPPER

Function

Copper is an essential part of 3 important enzymes: 1) cytochrome oxidase which is necessary for normal electron transport and therefore synthesis of ATP, 2) tyrosinase which is involved in synthesis of dopa and melanin, and 3) amine oxidase which forms the cross links with elastin. In addition, it is an integral part of ceruloplasmin which is present in plasma. This glycoprotein has 4 important roles (9, 10). 1) As a ferroxidase it facilitates iron absorption and release from body stores, 2) It is apparently the major transport protein for copper, 3) It appears to have some role in regulation of biogenic amines, and 4) With excess copper intake, it may aid in protection of the liver from excessive hepatic accumulation.

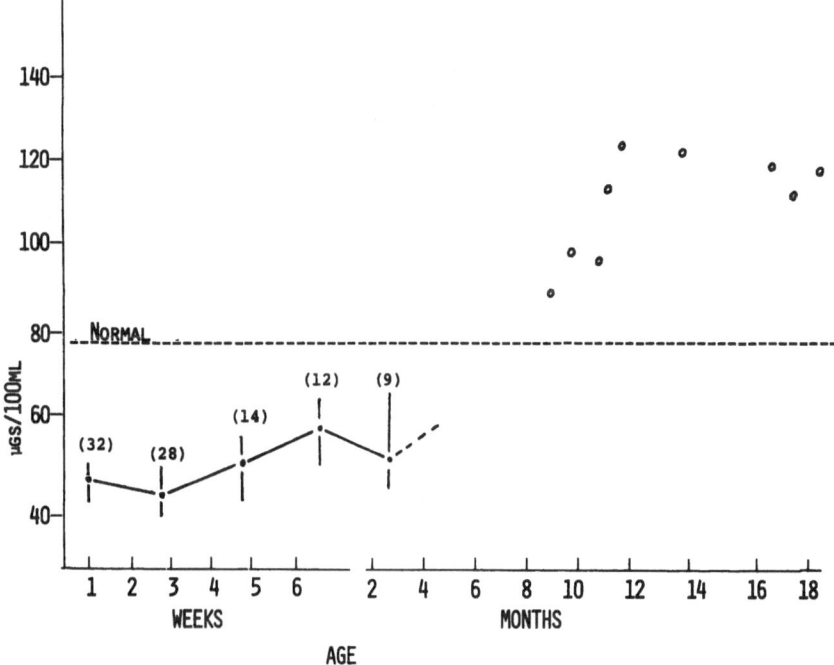

Fig. 2. Serial changes in copper in premature infants (birth weight < 1250 g). Closed circles indicate mean of the number of patients indicated in parentheses. Open circles indicate individual measurements in nine patients between 9 and 18 months of age.

About 30–40% of dietary copper is absorbed in the upper gastro-intestinal tract. The mechnism of absorption is not entirely clear, but at least two separate proteins appear to be necessary; one which binds intraluminal copper for transport into the cell and a second which transports intracellular copper into the portal circulation (11–13).

The primary site of copper excretion is via active secretion in the biliary tract (about 80%), whereas the remainder is excreted via the intestine and about 1% in urine (15).

Deficiency

Clinical manifestations of copper deficiency such as anemia, leukopenia and abnormalities in collagen and elastin (table 4) (15–17) can be appropriately linked to several of its functions. The latter may be manifest radiographically after several weeks of copper depletion and is virtually indistinguishable from the bone lesions produced by vitamin C deficiency (18).

In the developed countries, the most common cause of copper deficiency is from prolonged total parenteral feedings without added copper. Laboratory and clinical evidence of copper deficiency develope somewhat later than zinc deficiency. During a three year period, two infants at Vanderbilt developed clinical signs of deficiency as a result of TPN therapy (18). One, a term infant did so by 6 months of age; the second, a premature of 32 weeks gestation, by 4 months of age.

Table 4. *Major clinical manifestations of copper deficiency.*

Anemia: - unresponsive to iron therapy.
Leukopenia: - absolute neutropenia.
Radiographic bone changes: - similar to scurvy.
   Periosteal elevation
   Osteoporosis - 'ground glass' appearance
   Metaphyseal flaring and spur formation
   Soft tissue calcification

Although other features have been noted, the above manifestations are most commonly noted and easily recognized.

Recommended Intake

Term Infant: The Food and Nutrition Board of the National Academy of Sciences recommends a daily intake of 80 μg/kg for infants and young children. Based on copper content of milk (20–25 μg/100 kcal), it is doubtful that most infants receive this level of intake until mixed feedings are begun. Apparently, the high hepatic stores of copper are able to compensate for this transient period of low copper intake during the first few months of life, and therefore make most standard techniques for determining requirements very unsatisfactory. Nevertheless, experience in infants fed intravenously has led to a recommendation that 20 μg/kg/d be supplied during TPN (22).

Premature infants, intravenous recommendations: Fluids commonly used for total parenteral nutrition have very small to almost undetectable amounts of copper present. As with zinc, if copper needs are to be met during parenteral feedings, additional copper should be supplied. Insufficient copper is present in transfused blood or plasma to meet infant needs also.

Balance studies indicate that virtually all intravenous administered copper is retained (8). Exceptions to this are infants with chronic diarrhea or other causes of excessive losses of enteric fluid or bile. However, most infants receiving total parenteral nutrition have little fecal losses and very littly copper lost via the urine or sweat.

JAMES et al. have performed balance studies in 15 infants less than 1250 g. Their findings indicate that positive balance was achieved with an input of about 8 μg/kg/day (8). The normal accretion rate, had the infants remained in utero, was calculated to be about 60–70 μg/kg/day (1). On the basis of these findings, they have recommended an input of 90–100 μg/kg/day. However we have been more conservative in our recommendation of copper for the premature for 4 reasons: 1) very high hepatic copper levels (59–107 μg/g) have been found in four infants (< 1250 g) on post mortem examination, 2) low ceruloplasmin levels (a suggested 'protector of hepatic copper toxicity') of 6–12 mg/100 ml, 3) the lack of signs of copper deficiency for up to three months of age, and 4) the known hepatotoxicity of excess copper intake. For these reasons the present recommended dose of copper for prematures is the same as for term infants.

Table 5 lists the suggested copper intake during TPN and until more definitive studies are completed to indicate that a higher dose is more efficacious, 20 μg/kg/d for both prematures and newborn infants is recommended for routine TPN solutions. However if excessive amounts of enteric fluid are lost, the dose should be increased to provide an additional 0.07–0.1 μg/ml of intestinal fluid loss, or as much as 1–2 μg/ml of bile loss. In addition, with obstructive biliary disease the dose should be halved.

Table 5. *Copper (recommended intake (μg/kg/d))*

Infants and young children		Premature (?)	
Oral[*]	Intravenous[+]	Oral	Intravenous
80	20	90	20–30 (?)[++]

[*] Food and Nutrition board, NAS.
[+] AMA, Advisory Group for Trace Metals in Parenteral nutrition.
[++] Conservative estimate is based on low serum and extremely high hepatic copper levels in five autopsied infants < 1200 g who survived 7–31 days.

CHROMIUM

Chromium deficiency has been documented in 3 adult patients receiving TPN for extended periods of time. The first patient took about $3\frac{1}{2}$ years to develop symptoms of glucose intolerance (19), but the other 2 patients developed symptoms within the first year of treatment (20). Although no pediatric patients has been documented with symptoms of chromium deficiency, it would seem that if chromium continues to be omitted from the feeding regimen, it will only be a matter of time before it is documented in infants receiving prolonged TPN.

The major recognized role of chromium is as a cofactor for insulin. It appears to initiate formation of disulfide linkages between the intrachain disulfide of insulin and sulfhydryl groups of the cell membrane by precipitating a ternary complex (21).

Deficiency symptoms in man are: 1) insulin-resistent carbohydrate intolerance, 2) hyperglycemia and glucosuria, 3) perpiheral neuropathy, 4) poor growth, and 5) weight loss. Treatment with trivalent chromium causes complete resolution of the abnormalities.

Virtually all intravenously infused chromium is retained. Based on the data in adults and very sparse data in infants coupled with its low level of toxicity, it seems prudent to recommend the addition of chromium to TPN fluids at a dose of 0.14–0.2 $\mu g/kg/day$ (22).

MANGANESE

Pyruvate carboxylase is a manganese metalloenzyme and manganese plays a coenzyme role in several other enzyme systems (23). However, it has been recognized as producing deficiency symptoms in only one individual (24) and in no patients during TPN. Thus, the extent of human risk from manganese deficiency remains uncertain. However, its apparent importance in animal nutrition and the identification of deficiency symptoms in man, led to the recommendation that manganese be included in TPN solutions.

Evidence for a proper dosage is based emperically on normal accretion rates, balance data in eight infants (8), normal dietary intakes, and extrapolation of data from adults on TPN. Since manganese, like copper is excreted almost exclusively in bile, and because of the common association between TPN and cholestasis in premature infants treated with TPN, current recommendations of 2–10 $\mu g/kg/d$ are the same for premature as for term infants (22).

MOLYBDENUM

Molybdenum deficiency has apparently been documented in one adult patient requiring prolonged treatment with TPN. This patient has been studied by Dr. Abdou-Mourad and associates (25). Signs and symptoms were repeatedly induced by amino acid infusion and consisted of tachycardia, tachypnea, headaches, central scotomas, night blindness, and alkalosis. Outstanding laboratory findings included a marked increase in serum and urinary methionine, sulfathionine, xanthurinic acid and low levels of uric acid. Two molybdenum-containing metalloenzymes, xanthine oxidase and sulfite oxidase (23), are important in the metabolism of the two substrates which were elevated in the patient's blood and urine. Treatment with 300–600 μg/day of molybdenum caused reversal of the clinical as well as the biochemical aberrations in the patient.

This finding suggests the importance of molybdenum in human nutrition, but as yet, no recommendations have been made concerning the inclusion of molybdenum in TPN solutions.

SELENIUM

Glutathione peroxidase in human erythrocyres in a selenium-containing enzyme and many of the known actions of selenium in animals are closely linked to those of vitamin E. Although clinical symptoms from selenium deficiency have not been clearly identified in man, improvements in weight gain and anemia have been observed in some malnourished infants treated with selenium (26). Most infants treated with TPN in the U.S. receive low intakes of vitamin E as well as selenium. Although inclusion of selenium in TPN solutions may very well be necessary, the absence of data on therapeutic efficacy has excluded it as routine additive for TPN solutions.

SUMMARY

The content of zinc, copper, and chromium in total parenteral (TPN) solutions are substantially less than the recommended intravenous intake, and a number of patients have developed clinical signs of deficiency during TPN treatment. Therefore, at least these 3 metals should be added to TPN solutions. Of the 3 elements, zinc appears to be the most important. Since the needs for zinc are quantitatively greater than for the other metals and in infants, deficiency symptoms may develop as early as 4 weeks without zinc-supplemented TPN. Copper is second in importance since infants may develop signs of copper by 4–6 months without copper–supplemented TPN. Chromium deficiency appears less critical as an additive than either zinc or copper. The needs are quantitatively less and deficiency has been seen in only three adult patients on parenteral feedings for 1 to $3\frac{1}{2}$ years and chromium deficiency is not recognized in infants. Manganese deficiency has not been recognized in any patients requiring TPN, but suggestive evidence of symptoms from manganese deficiency exists in one adult, and therefore it is probably important to include manganese as an additive. It is recommended that 100–300 $\mu g/kg/d$ of zinc and 20 μg of copper be provided intravenously at the outset of TPN in all infants. Chromium is recommended at 0.14–0.2 $\mu g/kg/d$ and manganese 2–10 $\mu g/kg/d$.

Although selenium and molybdenum are found in several metalloenzymes in man and are probably required nutrients they are less well documented as essential nutrients and until further studies have been completed, no recommendations are made to include them as TPN additives. However one as yet unreported patient who received TPN for several years developed several clinical and chemical abnormalities suggestive of molybdenum defienciency which improved with molybdenum treatment.

ACKNOWLEDGEMENTS

The authors wish to express appreciation to Sandra Bennett and Bella Stringer for laboratory assistance and Martha Hoyle for secretarial assistance.

REFERENCES

1. WIDDOWSON, E.M., M.J. DAUNCEY and J.C.L. SHAW. (1974) Proc. Nutr. Soc. 33:275.
2. DAUNCEY, M.J., J.C.L. SHAW and J. URMAN. (1977) Pediatr. Res. 11:1033.
3. RIORDAN, J.F. and B.L. VALLEE. (1976) In: Trace Elements in Human Health and Disease, vol. I, Prasad, A.S. ed., Academic Press, New York, p. 227.
4. PRASAD, A.S. and D. OBERLEAS. (1974) J. Lab. Clin. Med. 83:634.
5. EVANS, G.W. (1974) In: Trace Elements in Human Health and Disease, vol. I, Prasad, A.S. e., Academic Press, New York, p. 181.
6. HENKIN, R.I., J.D. SHULMAN and C.B. SCHULMAN. (1973) J. Pediatr. 82:831.
7. WALRAVENS, P.A. and K.M. HAMBIDGE. (1976) Am. J. Clin. Nutr. 29:1114.

8. JAMES, B.E., P. HENDRY and R.A. MACMAHON. (1979) Aus. Pediatr. J. (in press).
9. EVANS, G.W. (1973) Physiol. Rev. 53:535.
10. HSIEH, H.S. and E. FRIEDEN. (1975) Biochem. Biophys. Res. Commun. 67:1326.
11. DANKS, D.M., E. CARTWRIGHT, E., B.J. STEVENS and R.R.W. TOWNLEY. (1973) Science 179:1140.
12. HUNT, D.M. (1974) Nature (London) 249:852.
13. BUCHNALL, W.E., H.A. HASLAMM and N.A. HOLTZMAN. (1973) Pediatrics 52:633.
14. CARTWRIGHT, G.E. and M.M. WINTROBE. (1964) Am. J. Clin. Nutr. 14:224.
15. CORDANO, A. and G.G. GRAHAM (1966) Pediatrics 38:596.
16. ASHKENAZI, A., S. LEVIN and M. DJALDETTI. (1973) Pediatrics 52:525.
17. KARPEL, J.T. and V.H. PEDEN. (1972) J. Pediatr. 80:32.
18. HELLER, R.M., S.G. KIRCHNER, J.A. O'NEILL, M.B. HOWARD and H.L. GREENE. (1978) J. Pediatr. 92:947.
19. JEEJEEBHOY, K.N., R.C. CHU, E.B. MARLISS, G.R. GREENBERG and A. BRUCE-ROBERTSON. (1977) Am. J. Clin. Nutr. 30:531.
20. FISHER, F. (personal communication).
21. MERTZ, W., E.W. TOEPFER, E.E. ROGINSKI and M.M. POLANSKY (1974) Fed. Proc. 33:2275.
22. A.M.A. Committee on Trace Elements in Parenteral Nutrition, To be published in Federal Register 1979.
23. UNDERWOOD, E.J. (1977) In: Trace Elements in Human and Animal Nutrition, ed. 4, E.J. Underwood, ed., Academic Press, New York, p. 170.
24. DOISY, E.A. (1974) In: Trace Element Metabolism in Animals, ed. 2, W. Hoekstra, ed., University Park Press, Baltimore, p. 668.
25. ABDOU-MOURAD, N.N., J.A. SCHNEIDER, D.R.N. STEEL and L.S. ROGER. (manuscript in preparation).
26. MAJAJ, A.S. and L.L. HOPKINS, Jr. (1966) Lancet 2:592.

DISCUSSION

PAPER BY B.S. LINDBLAD

F.C. Battaglia: If I understood your talk, I have trouble seeing why you choose as a reference hepatic venous concentrations as a reflection of substrate flow for each amino acid. On what basis are you equating an aminogram on plasma concentrations with the quantities entering the circulation from an organ? It certainly wouldn't apply across the umbilical circulation where we measured substrate flow. The order of amino acids entering in quantities would bear little relationship to the concentration in the blood. Why is that your reference point?

B.S. Lindblad: I am not speaking about the quantities entering the circulation from the liver or a substrate flow; I'm speaking about the amino acid balance, or the pattern of the relative concentrations of the different amino acids as they enter a deep vein, the V. cava, from the enterohepatic circulation. We know quite a lot about how much nitrogen we should give intravenously per unit time, but what I'm looking for is the optimal relative molar concentration of one amino acid as compared to the other.

F.C. Battaglia: But I'm asking why you're interested in that. If I look at drugs, I'm interested in talking about dosage, I'm interested in quantities. Why not be interested in the quantity of each amino acid, rather than its concentration in the plasma.

B.S. Lindblad: I'm interested in the amino acid balance of the solution to be infused into a deep vein during parenteral alimentation, in the same way as the nutritionist is interested in the pattern when he looks at the amino acid composition of proteins for peroral use. An 'ideal' protein, or amino acid solution, has the optimal balance between the different amino acids. From this study I cannot say anything about the total quantity of flow of amino acids.

F.C. Battaglia: Then I'll just make a comment. I think the nutritionists who do that are incorrect. I think the pattern is important, but it is the pattern of uptake of each amino acid that's important, if you wish to compare intake with the needs for growth, that is accretion of each amino acid. I don't think it's their concentration in plasma.

C.T. Jones: To follow on that argument, most people I've heard present amino acid data today have talked about plasma concentrations and effectively ignored the red cell, which is capable of storing a large amount of amino acids in the circulation. It has been demonstrated that the pool of red cell amino acids changes substantially with both nutrition and endocrine status. The question that I would like to ask is: Are the amino acid compositions in plasma, that you have been showing today, indicative of blood as a whole, or are you ignoring a very important factor in blood composition?

B.S. Lindblad: We have dealt with this problem in a study of amino acid and peptide transfer across the small intestine. (LINDBLAD, B.S., A. BAUM, D. BURSTON, L. CHAO, P. FÜRST, B. LINDQVIST, D.M. MATTHEWS, R. TARCHINI and E. TAYLOR. (1979) In: Development of mammalian absorptive processes, O'Connor, M. and J. Whelan eds., Ciba Foundation Symposium No. 70, London.) We examined both portal whole blood and plasma. The patterns of the amino acids in whole blood and plasma were not significantly different. On the other hand, if one wants, like Dr. Battaglia, to have the flow of each amino acid quantitatively across an organ, then you should study whole blood. However, when we studied the cerebral amino acid uptake during infancy and childhood (SETTERGREN, S., B.S. LINDBLAD and B. PERSSON. (1976). Acta Paediatr. Scand. 65:343), the analysis of arterial and venous whole blood did not significantly change the A-V differences as compared to plasma analysis of the same samples.

G.E. Gaull: It seems to me that the question is even more complicated than that. What is the evidence that red cell mass, that pool, is exchanging with the tissue? Is it not itself a kind of tissue? The plasma, in a sense, is the result of a whole host of influxes, effluxes, the kidney, the liver. We are making a static determination at that one time and we are drawing all sorts of conclusions. What we really want to know is something more about the flux through the pools and definition of the pools, if we're really going to understand what we're doing.

B.S. Lindblad: Let me make a general comment applicable to all these remarks. We do not think that we are providing more than one piece of information which could lead us a bit further towards the optimal composition of the intravenous fluid solution. It might tell you something about the pattern or balance of the solution, but I think the quantitative aspects are dealt with in studies like those of Dr. Widdowson. Could you think of any method in which we could actually measure the flux across the enterohepatic unit of healthy human infants?

G.E. Gaull: I want to make very clear that nothing I said was in any way denigrating of the work that you have done, but I think that before we can arrive at a solution of a problem we really have to understand the complexity of the problem. In the field of amino acids in nutrition, we're only just beginning to get a taste of how complicated the problem really is and how really inadequate our present methods are. Perhaps the era of stable isotopes and mass spectrometry will give us some aid over the next generation.

B.S. Lindblad: May I ask how that relates to the present-day widespread use of total parenteral alimentation of very small newborn infants?

M. Young: You were able to measure the plasma amino acids in the hepatic vein blood in these children, were you also able to make a hepatic vein flow measurement?

B.S. Lindblad: No, not at all.

M. Young: That would have helped.

B.S. Lindblad: Yes.

F.C. Battaglia: I guess it's the questions what's complex and what's simple that are bothering me. It's quite simple what you need to measure, to obtain the quantity of amino acids entering an organ; it's not at all complicated. You need whole blood measurements. The difficulties are manifold in measuring flow, especially in men, across any organ. What you need is very simple, and you're not into an elaborate discussion of how red cells exchange.

You're saying blood perfuses organs, the Fick principle applies today as it did many years ago and there's absolutely no ambiguity about the measurements. It's also quite clear in physiology when you need plasma concentrations: whole blood measurements will not tell you concentration gradients across vessels or cells. And so those measurements are equally important to discuss the concentration differences that are driving forces across membranes.

There are many difficulties, as Dr. Lindblad has said, in collecting all the relevant data in man. I admire tremendously these attempts, but we can get ourselves to the point of thinking there is a huge dust storm of complexity about what is needed. And I don't believe there is.

G.E. Gaull: How does that help you with re-utilization of particular amino acids. We don't even know, in some instances, what the precursor pool of the amino acid for the protein is.

F.C. Battaglia: That's a different question.

G.E. Gaull: But it's a relevant question.

F.C. Battaglia: If I tell you that I'm measuring the height of an elephant and you ask me what is his vision, I'll tell you I can't use a ruler to tell you how well he sees. It's a different question. The question we were discussing was; when do you want plasma concentrations, when do you want whole blood concentrations? That to me is not at all ambiguous.

PAPER BY F. POHLANDT

R.M. Pitkin: If I understood you correctly you measured A-V differences in the umbilical cord in normal infants and then these data are utilized in small premature infants. Is there any evidence one way or another relating amino acid requirements at these two gestational ages, to say nothing of the in utero versus ex utero conditions?

F. Pohlandt: You are right, we measured the A-V differences in the umbilical cord vessels in newborn infants at term and then used these data in premature infants. We did so, because there were no data which are more appropriate. In fact, the amino acid dosages derived from term infants generally meet the requirement of premature infants, if you accept the plasma concentrations during continuous infusion as a criterium.

In premature infants, there are only few data on A-V differences, which are hampered by a small number of samples and therefore do not allow to calculate mean differences. (GHADIMI, H. and P. PECORA. (1964) Pediatrics 35:100; YOUNG, M. and M.A. PRENTON. (1969) J. Obstet. Gynaec. Brit. Cwlth. 76:333.)

M. Young: Have you been able to compare your amino acid utilization values with the composition of the human infant's protein made by Dr. Widdowson?

F. Pohlandt: No, I haven't.

E.M. Widdowson: I was very interested in your figures, but I haven't been quick enough to compare them with mine. However, you do show the dangers of taking the figures I presented yesterday and making those relative amounts up into a solution for parenteral administration. I think we are on safer grounds with the essential amino acids, but when it comes to the non-essential ones, and particularly glycine, then I think we have to think very carefully about it and you've shown this very clearly.

F. Pohlandt: I think that in regard to glycine, there is a good agreement between your and our data: glycine is consumed by the fetus and needed during parenteral nutrition only in very low amounts.

J.C. Sinclair: Could Dr. Battaglia tell us from his fetal lamb experiments what the ratio between the fetal uptake and excretion of nitrogen is?

F.C. Battaglia: Of the 1.5 g N/kg/day entering the umbilical circulation as amino acids, 0.36 g N/kg/day are excreted as urea (about 25%). There may be other excretory forms of nitrogen. I think that's implied by the fact that nitrogen uptake as amino acids alone exceeds the urea production rate plus accretion. That's what led us to look at ammonia as a possible

excretory form and we were embarrassed to find in fact that it's transferred to the fetus because of placental synthesis. But I think it's still an
interesting line to pursue: What are other excretory forms of nitrogen? I
don't think we know right now what quantities of each amino acid the
human fetus receives.

That's what we'd all like to know for infants born between 27 weeks
and term, when we deal with viable infants.

B.S. Lindblad: Dr. Wretlind (WRETLIND, A. (1972) Nutr. Metab. 14
(Suppl.): 7.) has shown that you will get the best results, as measured by
nitrogen retention, when including into intravenous alimentation all the
18 amino acids that occur in proteins. May I ask you, is there any reason
to believe that any of the amino acids present in proteins should not be
included in the solution? I am a bit unsure as to what 'essentiality' and
'non-essentiality' mean here. It's interesting to make the comparison
with what is needed in tissue culture. We know that in addition to the 8
essential amino acids, one needs histidine, cystine, arginine, tyrosine
and glutamine. We know that histidine is essential to infants, cystine has
been shown by Dr. Gaull et al. (GAULL, G.E., J.A. STURMAN and N.C.R.
RÄIHÄ (1972) Pediatr. Res. 6:538.) to be essential to the prematurely
born, tyrosine is essential to the newborn due to low oxydation of phenylalanine, and lack of arginine will lead to hyperammoniemia, as shown by
Fahey et al. (FAHEY, J.L., R.S. PERRY and P.F. McCOY. (1958) Am. J.
Physiol 192:311.) The only one remaining, I would say, that we don't
know anything definite about as yet is glutamine. We know about the
essentiality in tissue culture of glutamine. Perhaps someone has an idea
about the essentiality of glutamine in the newborn?

F. Pohlandt: It has been shown in animal experiments, that you can
demonstrate the limited supply of one amino acid by measurement of the
amino acid concentrations. (LONGENECKER, J.B. and N.L. HAUSE (1959)
Arch. Biochem. Biophys. 84:46; McLAUGHLAN, J.M. (1964) Can. J.
Biochem. 42:1353; DEAN, W.F. and H.M. SCOTT. (1966) J. Nutr. 88:75;
McLAUGHLAN, J.M., S.V. RAO, F.J. NOEL and A.B. MORRISON. (1967)
Can. J. Biochem. 45:31; POTTER, E.L., D.B. PURSER and W.G. BERGER.
(1972) J. Anim. Sci. 34:660.) In this way you can determine which
amino acid in a growing animal is the one that is delivered in the smallest
and limited amount. If we apply this system to the human being, we can
see that the glutamine concentration is not decreasing despite glutamine-

free infusions. From that, we would conclude that the body is able to synthesize sufficient amounts of glutamine.

J. Senterre: I am very surprised that you found no differences in the amino acid concentrations of plasma after birth as compared to the amino acid concentrations in cord blood. We have observed a decrease in concentration in term infants on breast milk. Do you think it is a question of methodology? Is it decreasing or not decreasing? Generally, for all amino acids, we observed a decrease after birth.

F. Pohlandt: That has also been reported in the literature, but I think it depends on how these infants have been fed. Are they fed by their own mothers or are they fed by pooled breast milk? This would make a difference, due to the high protein content of the milk in the first days of lactation. I don't know how your infants have been fed.

J. Senterre: When one measures after one week of life, one observes an important decrease in amino acid concentrations. At what time did you measure the amino acid concentrations after birth?

F. Pohlandt: We studied infants between the first and twentieth day of life and the median age of our infants was 6.6 days.

J. Senterre: At that time you are not dealing with colostrum-fed infants.

G.E. Gaull: With regard to the question that Dr. Senterre just raised: Is it possible – if I understood your paper correctly – that you did not follow individual infants sequentially.

F. Pohlandt: That's correct.

G.E. Gaull: Is it possible that this obscured the individual differences between infants because you handled this as a group, this may also have obscured the differences that other people have found.

F. Pohlandt: It is theoretically possible. It seems to me unlikely.

PAPER BY W.C. HEIRD

R.A. McCance: I was very interersted in this paper and I think you've done a good job. How did you nurse these puppies? Were their bladders always distended? At what temperature did you keep them? Because if they weren't in their thermo-neutral environment or very near it and had access to warmth, they were using these amino acids, I'm perfectly certain, to provide themselves with energy.

W.C. Heird: That's a very important consideration. Control animals were left with their mothers in litters limited to five puppies. The animals that received parenteral nutrients were kept at a temperature of approximately 90–92 °F. They were kept in separate cages because of the metabolic studies, but in the cage was a hot-water bottle. It is true that puppies cannot urinate spontaneously until approximately 2 to 3 weeks of age. These studies actually require an around-the-clock puppy intensive-care unit for which we used students who stimulated the puppies to urinate every 2 hours.

R.A. McCance: Who was managing the feces, the mother looks after those too, you know.

W.C. Heird: This was also done by our students. In the animals on parenteral nutrition, however, the stool output was really very small.

A. Ballabriga: What was the kind of parenteral nutrition that you used? Did you use fat and, if so, what kind of fat and in what quantity? When you studied the cerebrum, was it purely the cerebrum or cerebrum plus cerebellum?

W.C. Heird: Let me answer the last question first. All of the DNA and protein analyses were done on the right cerebrum and corrected for the total weight of both cerebral hemishperes. Lipid studies were done on the other half of the cerebrum. Some of the animals received only glucose as the calorie source; other received 3 g/kg of intralipid. With respect to the data that I have presented (protein, DNA and weight) there was no difference between the two groups of animals and they have been grouped together.

M.P.M. Richards: Following on from the point made by Professor McCance, it seems to me that it should be necessary, in studies of this kind, to use a control group which are fed presumably bitches milk, but kept under the conditions that you reared your experimental group. There is a large literature that shows that very small manipulations of weaning animals produce big changes in rates of maturation, growth, brain growth and size, in virtually every other primate that's been looked at.

W.C. Heird: That, of course, is correct. The studies that were presented were difficult enough. To add another group fed artificially with artificially expressed bitch milk—which it would have to be, I think, to be the proper control—would have been very difficult. It is possible to feed the puppies artificially; in other studies we've done that, but not in this study.

R. Eeckels: I would like to remind Dr. Richards of studies by the late Professor Birch of New York on the infants of a certain tribe of Indians in Central America. That particular tribe has the small infants closely bound during the entire day and night, and they even put a black cloth on their faces. They are free in fact only to suckle. After one year, the difference in their psychomotor development as compared with other children is really very small; they are more passive and this is the only difference.

W.C. Heird: The other comment which I suppose is pertinent is that the suckled animal in the animal quarters of any university facility is not in a normal environment.

E.M. Widdowson: Did you rear any of these puppies after you finished your experiments and look at their brains later on or look at any aspect of their development?

W.C. Heird: That comes next summer, Dr. Widdowson.

B.S. Lindblad: You said that not any one of the commercially available mixtures could provide a normal homeostasis in the peripheral blood. Was there a correlation between the composition of these solutions and the derangement of the peripheral blood?

W.C. Heird: In these puppies, we only used one solution and the derangements that you saw were the results of that one solution. I'm not familiar with all of the mixtures that are available in Europe and perhaps that comment was a bit hasty. In our clinical work, however, we can to a great extent relate the plasma pattern of amino acids to the pattern of the infusate. This has been true for the approximately seven such mixtures available in the United States–some investigational, some on the market.

R.D.G. Milner: Excluding your initial pilot experiments, how many infusion experiments have you performed? And of those, how many have you had to discard for technical problems?

W.C. Heird: Somewhat over 50% of the total infusion studies that are started are successful in that the animal survives the entire ten days without mechanical problems related to the catheter or other difficulties.

J.D. Baum: Have you any information on cerebro-spinal fluid amino acid levels? And does this offer a probe to cerebral free amino acid levels?

W.C. Heird: We do have some information but I don't have it at my fingertips now. Unfortunately, we do not have cerebro-spinal fluid data from the group of puppies with marked amino acid derangements. We really have not analyzed the cerebro-spinal fluid data to any great extent. But the data are available and will be forthcoming.

B. Friis Hansen: I wonder if you have analyzed Group I and II as to whether they received any lipids or not. Had the degree of derangement something to do with lipids? How can the brain grow without lipids?

W.C. Heird: We have done that, as a matter of fact. In one group, two animals received lipids; in the other group, three of the five received lipids. The lipid intake did not seem to make any difference at all.

PAPER BY H.L. GREENE

J.G. Koppe: Can small infants be born with a deficiency of trace elements?

H.L. Greene: To my knowledge, clinical signs of zinc depletion have not been noted in any infant at the time of birth. It is possible that a mother with low zinc stores might not provide the usual complement of zinc during the latter stages of pregnancy, and such infants would be more prone to develop zinc deficiency symptoms with subsequent low zinc intake. Such a condition would be further aggrevated if energy–protein intake is sufficient for growth. As I tried to point out in the presentation, the above conditions are commonly present in infants delivered prematurely. Although the mother's zinc stores may be adequate, premature delivery would prevent normal zinc accretion during the third trimester. If total parenteral nutrition is required and zinc is not added then zinc depletion is imminent. It is this group of infants that are at greatest risk to develop clinical and biochemical signs of zinc deficiency within the first few months.

J.C.L. Shaw: There has been an attempt to accociate zinc deficiency in the mother with events in the child (JAMESON, S. (1976) Acta Med. Scand. (suppl.) 593:4). He attempted, by measuring plasma zinc levels in the mothers, to relate these plasma zinc levels to events around delivery and effects on the fetus.

H.L. Greene: In children of patients who have acrodermatitis enteropathica with a very low plasma zinc concentration, there appears to be a very high incidence of congenital malformations. Such observations are in agreement with the findings in animals which indicate a high degree of fetal wastage and congenital malformation in pups of zinc depleted animals. Thus it appears that zinc is important for normal fetal development. It has been suggested that a number of congenital malformations might in fact be due to zinc depletion in the mother during a critical phase of development. I think this is yet to be shown.

G.E. Gaull: Ganschow and Piletz (PILETZ, J.E. and R.E. GANSCHOW. (1978) Science 199:181.) recently reported a mouse mutant with a failure to have a zinc-binding protein in the milk.

J.C.L. Shaw: This is the lethal milk mutant in mice. I don't know if it's due to a failure of the zinc-binding ligand, but there is certainly an inadequate amount of zinc in the milk of the mice. If you take pups from normal mothers and suckle them on the zinc–deficient milk mice, they all die. If you take the pups from the zinc-deficient mothers and suckle them on normal dams, they grow normally. So that they're not zinc-deficient in utero, they're only zinc-deficient post-natally and it appears to be a specific deficiency of zinc in the milk of the mother. We hear frequently today that mother's milk is best—and it is just possible that there may be mother's milk among the human population that in fact is deficient in a similar way. There's been another mutant mouse strain described that secretes toxic amounts of tin in its milk and kills its offspring (RAUCH, H. (1977) Mouse News Letter 56:48). I think we ought to bear in mind that, if we find a baby on the breast who is not thriving, there is a possiblility that the milk may be toxic in some way, either through some toxic substance secreted in excess or some deficiency.

G.E. Gaull: That is sort of what I had in mind a propos of the remarks about zinc deficiency in development, because a newborn mouse is roughly equivalent to a second-trimester human fetus.

GENERAL DISCUSSION

A. Ballabriga: Regarding parenteral alimentation with fat, I would like to call attention to two points. The first with relation to fat stores in the pulmonary vessels in some cases observed during post-mortem examinations of low birthweight newborns. In an autopsy series of 22 infants from 7 to 123 days of life who had been submitted to parenteral lipid nutrition from 4 to 27 days, lipid droplets in alveolar capillaries were found in 8 cases (36.4%), lipoid alveolitis in 3 (13.6%) and severe changes associated with fat deposition in intrapulmonary arteries from 0.1 to 0.6 mm in diameter in 17 (77.3%). According to the prevalent type of arterial lesions the cases were classified in stages I to IV (early lesions, acute florid stage, lipophagic florid stage and regressive stage) which showed a good correlation with the length of lipid treatment or the lapse of time between beginning of treatment and death of the infant. Segmentary changes in the intrapulmonary branches of the pulmonary artery without involvement of the more proximal ramifications were characterized by an early phase of subendothelial lipid deposition, evolving apparently to massive fat penetration within the intimal layer, with a singular mechanism of transportation of lipids through the vessel wall towards its periphery, mediated in part by lipophagic cells. The deposition of lipids subsided with the progression of the treatment and the changes evolved to a fibrotic thickening of the intima with progressive disappearance of lipophagic cells. The reduced lumen of the vessels persisted. The penetration of lipidic material in the intima elicits in a number of cases the engulfing of lipid droplets by macrophages that predominate in the lipophagic florid lesions. All the early cases and 87.5% of florid acute cases were found in infants treated up to 8 days. A main factor in pathogenesis of the lesions is ascribed to the existence of previous injury of the arterial wall mediated by hypoxia or acidosis. It is assumed that the degree of lipidization does not depend primarily on the length of lipid treatment. It is unknown if a persistent narrowing of pulmonary vessels could lead to pulmonary hypertension in later life.

The second point concerns changes in the chemical composition of organs during parenteral nutrition with fat. Under the influence of parenteral alimentation with fat preparations a great increase of linoleic acid was found in both liver phosphoglycerides and in brain choline phosphoglycerides (CPG). No accompanying increase of arachidonic acid was found, as if some protective mechanism prevented the increase of 20:4 (n–6) above the normal limits. In liver the 22:6 (n–3) decreased to half the normal value at this age. The resulting n–3/n–6 index showed then a regression to the values found in very immature infants. After parenteral nutrition with high amounts of 18:2 (n–6), some changes in the aorta phosphoglyceride fatty acids, parallel to those occurring spontaneously with maturation, took place, like the decrease of 18:0 and 18:1 (n–9) in ethanolamine phosphoglycerides (EPG) and the increase of 18:2 (n–6) in CPG. In these children, however, the increase of the n–6 fatty acids was due exclusively to the contribution of linoleic acid (which in this case increased also in EPG), whereas its product, arachidonate, did not increase – and it even decreased – in CPG. On the other hand, the decrease in the aorta of the n–3 fatty acids in CPG, although very slight, was opposite to the findings with maturation and is consistent with the competition between linoleate and linoleate families. In the total fatty acids of the subcutaneous fat, the percentage of linoleic acid and the 18:2 (n–6)/18:1 (n–9) index increased. There are also some modifications in the value of the C18:2, elongation of C20:4 (n–6) and in the triene/ tetraene index in the red cell lipid stroma during administration of fat by intravenous route.

J. Senterre: What was the lipid concentration in the blood of these infants? It was very high, I suppose.

A. Ballabriga: No. It's not a problem of the clearance of the lipids, it's not a problem of the turnover of triglycerides into free fatty acids; we have given 3 grams per kilogram during 24 hours around the clock, with pump and slow perfusion. The problem is the existing lesion in the arterial tree. That means that when you give the infusion at the same rate to a normal infant, you will observe nothing. If this infant got previously these lesions connected with anoxia or acidosis especially, then you can produce these deposits of fat in the lung.

D. Hull: I was very interested in these findings. Have you made similar studies of babies who have not been given intralipid, because I am reminded of the study a long time ago by Aherne in which he reported that in babies who were 5, 6, 7 days old on normal nutrition, there was a lot of lipid, I remember, in the mucosal cells of the lung. But I have no recall whether he actually looked at the intima. I wonder if similar findings to a lesser degree are seen in babies who are not actually given intralipid.

A. Ballabriga: In my opinion, this phenomenon is quite different. In infants who have not received any kind of fat intravenously, but have been fed with normal milk, you can find in post-mortem examinations some fat droplets in the lung vessels but none ever included in the intima.

R.D.G. Milner: I want to ask a question–addressed really to all the speakers and the audience–because the theme this morning has been that of parenteral versus enteral nutrition. It's been accepted and particularly by Dr. Heird who was explicit in the introduction to his paper, that there are, presumably, an important group of preterm infants who cannot be fed enterally and therefore–and this is a deduction–there is a clinical need to develop parenteral nutrition in neonatal medicine. Now, I accept, as a clinician, that there is a need for total parenteral nutrition in a group of surgical neonates. I remain unconvinced, today, that there is an a priori case for developing total parenteral nutrition for preterm medical neonates. Could we have this discussed, please?

J.C.L. Shaw: I'm not going to give you an answer. I think there is no evidence anywhere that any infant has been saved by parenteral nutrition in so far as there's been no control trial. Nobody is going to let babies die of starvation, so what is your end point in a control trial? But there is no doubt that weight gain in parenterally fed babies is better than babies maintained on a glucose drip (SHAW, J.C.L. (1973) Ped. Clin. N. Am. 20:333.) So that, to this extent, there is some purpose in it. You talk about total parenteral nutrition, I don't think it has to be total. I think that you can give parenteral feeding while the gastrointestinal feeding is being built up. There is abundant evidence that the intestinal function of newborn babies–particularly premature babies–is not fully developed. Many babies are in negative zinc or copper balance, they may be in negative magnesium balance, there are certainly many in negative calcium balance; they find it difficult to tolerate large volumes of feed and we start them off with something like well under one-half their actual nutritional requirements. Added to that is the excellent calculation made by Bill Heird and his colleagues (J. Pediat. 80:351, 1972) on survival time in starvation. I don't think they claim any great precision in these figures, but, roughly, the survival time in starvation for any one of us is about 100 days. For a premature baby, it's about 4 days.

I think it puts the whole question of parenteral nutrition into a completely different perspective. I think there is quite a lot of evidence to suggest that it's a good thing.

R.A. McCance: I have no excuse for coming in on this at all, except that I think a general principle is involved here. I entirely agree with Professor Milner, I would like to see the necessity for any parenteral nutrition justified. On the other hand, I agree with what Dr. Shaw has said. I think its use is much more likely to be practised first in surgical cases. In the interest of progress, one would like to see all our procedures justified. It's not quite time yet for us to come to a final decision.

In medicine it's very unwise to suggest that a generalization should be applied to every case; one can only generalize. Each individual dealing with his own particular case must make his own decisions. All we can do is to offer guidelines after the matter has been studied from all angles by the experts.

B.S. Lindblad: In my paper I referred to 20 cases of surgical newborns and infants with intractable diarrhea, the two major indications for parenteral nutrition during early infancy. We made rather careful estimations and found that three of those 20 cases had survived because of the treatment and two were greatly helped by the treatment. Since that time, our definite clinical impression is that the omphaloceles in particular are greatly helped and survive because of this treatment.

C.A. Canosa: At the end of the meeting–mainly after Dr. Gaull's and Dr. Senterre's presentations about protein requirements for low birth weight infants, we still do not know. The figures given by these two authors vary between 1.8 and 4.0 g/kg/day. Also, it still remains to be decided whether breast milk is the ideal food for very low birth weight infants. These two important questions will undoubtedly stimulate further research in these relevant issues of early infant nutrition.

J.H.P. Jonxis: Whatever the subject, when you ask a number of experts, they will never give you one answer. Experts always differ in their opinions and, in this rapidly changing field of nutrition, I believe it is impossible to give a definite answer. On the other hand, I believe that by talking together and by comparing different approaches we learn much. When you look back a few years, you can see how much our knowledge has increased and I believe it has been–as you have heard now–for the benefit of newborn infants.

Before handing over the chair to Professor Visser, I would like to thank him on behalf of the whole group for organizing this symposium. I would also like to thank all the speakers and those who participated in the discussions for the very nice days we had together. We all would like to thank Nutricia for making this symposium possible. I believe cooperation between industry and science is very important. We need each other. Without industry, we miss possibilities in medicine. On the other hand, industry needs us for ideas and criticism. For these reasons, a symposium such as this one is very important.

When I look back on the five Nutricia Symposia, I think they have been quite a success. And I have asked myself: why? Every time we concentrated on the same subject, with different audiences and different speakers, but still with a certain continuity as several of the speakers and guests have attended more than one symposium. Another important factor is that the group is small. When you bring scientists together, you have to have a small group – it is the only way to have good communication and a good exchange of thoughts. I believe we succeeded in this. I hope this will not be the last time that Nutricia will make it possible to organize a symposium along those lines.

CLOSURE OF THE SYMPOSIUM BY PROFESSOR VISSER

Thank you, Professor Jonxis. Ladies and gentlemen, before closing this symposium, I would also like to express my thanks. First of all to the Nutricia Company for making it possible to organize this symposium. All speakers and guests: thank you for coming, thank you very much for your contributions–in particular during the lively discussions. I would like to thank the chairmen for their help. My special thanks go to my friends from the audiovisual department of this hospital, Mr. Kempers and his co-workers who did so much, quietly, behind the scenes, the projectionists and the two students who were so helpful during the discussions. I would like to thank the managing board of this hospital for providing the facilities. In particular, I am thankful to the domestic service of the hospital, Mr. Steketee and his co-workers who served us lunch, coffee and tea. Very special thanks to both secretaries, Mrs. Hermans-Zandbergen, Mr. Weber's secretary, and Mrs. Hellingman-van Holten, my secretary for their invaluable help during the last year and particularly during these days.

I think this has been a good meeting. It has been a reunion of old friends, but we also have made many new friends. When I gave a summing-up at the end of the second symposium – the Nutricia Symposium in 1968 – I said 'progress has been defined as the activity of today and the assurance of tomorrow. The art of progress is to preserve order amidst change and to preserve change amidst order.' I think that this symposium has been a stimulus for future work. We have put some things in order, but at the same time we have learned that almost everything is changing. This means that we will be ready for another symposium within some years.

I wish you all a good journey home. Thank you all and goodbye.

INDEX OF SUBJECTS

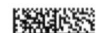